LEIGHTON E. CLUFF, M.D.
Professor and Chairman
Department of Medicine
University of Florida College of Medicine
Gainesville

GEORGE J. CARANASOS, M.D.
Associate Professor of Medicine
University of Florida College of Medicine
Gainesville

RONALD B. STEWART, M.S.
Assistant Professor of Pharmacy
University of Florida College of Pharmacy
Gainesville

CLINICAL PROBLEMS WITH DRUGS

VOLUME
V
IN THE SERIES
MAJOR PROBLEMS IN INTERNAL MEDICINE
Lloyd H. Smith, Jr., M.D., *Editor*

W. B. SAUNDERS COMPANY • PHILADELPHIA • LONDON • TORONTO • 1975

W. B. Saunders Company: West Washington Square
Philadelphia, PA 19105

12 Dyott Street
London, WC1A 1DB

833 Oxford Street
Toronto, Ontario M8Z 5T9, Canada

Library of Congress Cataloging in Publication Data

Cluff, Leighton E

Clinical problems with drugs.

(Major problems in internal medicine; v. 5)

Includes index.

1. Chemotherapy. 2. Drugs—Side effects. 3. Iatrogenic diseases. I. Caranasos, George J., joint author. II. Stewart, Ronald B., joint author. III. Title. [DNLM: 1. Drug therapy—Adverse effects. W1 MA492T v. 5 / QZ42 C649c]

RM262.C56   615'.7'04   74-24512

ISBN 0-7216-2613-0

Clinical Problems with Drugs   ISBN 0-7216-2613-0

© 1975 by the W. B. Saunders Company. Copyright under the International Copyright Union. All rights reserved. This book is protected by copyright. No part of it may be reproduced, stored in a retrieval system, or transmitted in any form or by any means, electronic, mechanical, photocopying, recording or otherwise, without written permission from the publisher. Made in the United States of America. Press of W. B. Saunders Company. Library of Congress catalogue card number 74-24512.

Last digit is the print number: 9   8   7   6   5   4   3   2   1

MAJOR PROBLEMS IN INTERNAL MEDICINE

Shearn: Sjögren's Syndrome
Cogan: Ophthalmic Manifestations of Systemic Vascular Disease
Williams: Rheumatoid Arthritis as a Systemic Disease
Cluff, Caranasos and Stewart: Clinical Problems with Drugs

In Preparation

Gorlin: Coronary Artery Disease
Ingbar: Pathophysiology and Diagnosis of Disorders of the Thyroid
Kass: Pernicious Anemia
Krugman and Ward: Viral Hepatitis
Potts: Disorders of Calcium Metabolism
Felig: Diabetes Mellitus
Ranny and Bunn: Normal and Abnormal Hemoglobins
Sleisenger: Malabsorption
Havel and Kane: Diagnosis and Treatment of Hyperlipidemias
Siltzbach: Sarcoidosis
Scheinberg and Sternlieb: Wilson's Disease and Copper Metabolism
Braude: Principles of Antibiotic Usage
Fries and Holman: Systemic Lupus Erythematosus
Atkins and Bodel: Fever
Lieber and De Carli: Medical Aspects of Alcoholism
Merrill: Glomerulonephritis
Bray: The Obese Patient
Goldberg: The Scientific Basis and Practical Use of Diuretics
Laragh: Reversible Hypertension
Kilbourne: Influenza
Deykin: Diseases of the Platelets
Schwartz and Lergier: Immunosuppressive Therapy
Cohen: Amyloidosis
Seegmiller: Gout
Weinstein: Infective Endocarditis
Sasahara: Pulmonary Embolism
Zieve and Levin: Disorders of Hemostasis

FOREWORD

Voltaire said, "Doctors pour medicines about which they know little, for diseases about which they know less, into human beings about whom they know nothing." Strong words with perhaps some Gallic garnishing, but with enough satirical truth to haunt us for the past two centuries. It is impossible now to imagine the practice of medicine without the vast array of chemical agents with which we attempt to distort or restore the body's internal environment, or to create a selective disadvantage for bacteria, viruses, neoplastic cells, and other alien agents that threaten man's well-being. There has been immense progress in the creation of new therapeutic drugs. Some of this progress has been empirical, but increasingly it is based on scientific analyses of mechanisms of drug action. By and large, the new insights in molecular pharmacology are derived from the general progress in biochemistry, molecular biology, virology, immunology, and the other disciplines which collectively have shared in the extraordinary advances in biomedical research in the past 30 years.

Through the ingenuity and resourcefulness of scientists, stimulated in considerable measure by the competitive pressures of a multibillion-dollar pharmaceutical industry, we have large numbers of new and potent compounds. Some are available directly to the patient, although most of them must be prescribed by a physician. Beyond defined "drugs," many other strange molecules assail us almost inadvertently in food preservatives, hair sprays, insecticides, plastics, and other miracles of chemistry thought necessary for human progress. Thus with each year that passes we are exposed by chance or by therapy to new classes and varieties of carbon compounds of increasing number and complexity. Even if we would, therefore, we cannot adhere to the paraphrase of Shakespeare quoted by Goodman and Gilman:

> Those drugs thou hast, and their adoption tried
> Grapple them to thy soul with hoops of steel;
> But do not dull thy palm with entertainment
> Of each new-hatch'd, unfledged remedy.

It is not surprising, therefore, that a heavy price is being paid in adverse drug reactions. Such adverse reactions either trigger or complicate large numbers of hospital admissions, and are important causes of disability and of death. It is not unusual for a hospitalized patient to receive 10 to 15 drugs simultaneously. Beyond their individual toxicities, these drugs may interact in subtle and occult ways, the anticipation or recognition of which may tax the acumen of the physician. The new specialty of Clinical Pharmacology has arisen in response to the widespread effects of drug toxicity, as well as in response to the desire to improve drug efficacy. An analysis of past and present drug therapy is now central to the study of every patient. Many of the disturbances that we note and measure in the individual patient are more related to our therapeutic efforts than to the original or underlying illness.

In this monograph, *Clinical Problems with Drugs*, the authors have presented a systematic analysis of adverse drug reactions. The physician who reads this book will have an improved ability to anticipate and therefore to prevent drug toxicity. When drug toxicity does appear—and inevitably it will in some patients, despite the most skillful therapeutic interventions—he will be able to recognize and to understand more readily what has occurred and to plan treatment more rationally. The book is likely, therefore, to become a standard reference which will be consulted frequently in the office, clinic, and hospital.

LLOYD H. SMITH, JR., M.D.

PREFACE

Chapters or sections on drug-induced diseases have been included in many medical textbooks in recent years, in recognition of the increasing frequency and importance of these clinical problems. Initially, primarily allergic reactions to drugs were discussed, and these chapters were included in sections on immunologic diseases. Most drug-induced diseases, however, are attributable to pharmacologic rather than immunologic mechanisms. This fact, added to the growth of the field of clinical pharmacology, has been associated with the development of sections on clinical pharmacology in some medical textbooks, including discussions of drug-induced diseases. Discussion of adverse reactions to drugs, however, is being included more and more in chapters on diseases affecting different systems or organs, either because such diseases may be induced by drugs, or because drug therapy for these system or organ diseases often results in adverse drug effects. Most medical textbooks, however, can not and do not provide a full account of the importance of the mechanisms and manifestations, and the diagnostic, therapeutic, and preventive aspects of clinical problems with drugs.

Drugs are the cornerstone of patient management for surgical, medical, pediatric, psychiatric, obstetric, and other physicians. Radiologists, anesthesiologists, and others involved in diagnostic or therapeutic procedures also use drugs that may cause adverse effects, either during or after their involvement with patients. Nurses responsible for drug administration also must be aware of the effects of the medication they give to patients in order to be able to detect adverse reactions. Pharmacists dispensing drugs or providing drug information to physicians, nurses, and patients should be familiar with their possible adverse consequences. Health professional students or trainees should have an understanding of drug problems in order to condition their expectations of drug use, and to assist them in more rational practices of drug prescribing and administration. Finally, patients should be more aware of the wide array of illnesses that drugs may cause, as they are the ones who either may become ill or may experience the benefits of drug therapy.

Clinical problems with drugs, therefore, are pertinent for all health professionals participating in the care of patients, and this book is intended to assemble information that will assist them in their understanding, recognition, management, and prevention of drug-induced diseases.

In many ways, a book on clinical problems with drugs resembles a medical textbook in that there are very few manifestations of illness, organ or system diseases, pathologic lesions, or physiologic and biochemical abnormalities that may not be caused by drugs. Today, a thorough knowledge of medicine requires familiarity with the clinical problems of drugs.

It seems certain that as new drugs are introduced and drugs are used with greater frequency, particularly as our population becomes proportionately older, and as we become more astute in recognizing diseases caused by drugs, the study of clinical problems with drugs will become more and more important. This book, hopefully, will provide a means of viewing these problems collectively and within an overall perspective.

This book is dedicated to Dr. A. M. Harvey, Emeritus Professor of Medicine, the Johns Hopkins University School of Medicine, who encouraged the beginning of studies on adverse drug reactions by one of us (L.E.C.). In addition, we deeply appreciate the long and productive assistance and support of the professional staff of the Food and Drug Administration in helping us develop our understanding and knowledge of drug-induced disease.

LEIGHTON E. CLUFF
GEORGE CARANASOS
RONALD STEWART

CONTENTS

Chapter 1
PERSPECTIVES.. 1

Chapter 2
PHARMACOLOGIC MECHANISMS... 21

Chapter 3
IMMUNOLOGIC MECHANISMS... 60

Chapter 4
CLINICAL MANIFESTATIONS.. 80
    1. Dermatologic Manifestations... 80
    2. Hematopoietic Manifestations 97
    3. Cardiovascular Manifestations 115
    4. Gastrointestinal Manifestations 126
    5. Liver Manifestations 131
    6. Respiratory Manifestations 142
    7. Endocrine Manifestations.. 150
    8. Urinary Tract Manifestations 158
    9. Gynecologic Abnormalities.. 164
   10. Fetal and Neonatal Manifestations................................. 166
   11. Metabolic Manifestations.. 171
   12. Musculoskeletal Manifestations.................................... 181
   13. Neurologic Manifestations 184
   14. Behavioral Manifestations... 194
   15. Multisystem Manifestations 197
   16. Infections.. 204
   17. Ocular Manifestations.. 207
   18. Ear Manifestations.. 213

Chapter 5
INDIVIDUAL DRUGS AND THEIR ADVERSE EFFECTS 228

Chapter 6
DRUG INTERACTIONS 261

Chapter 7
CONTROL AND PREVENTION 272

INDEX 279

CHAPTER 1

PERSPECTIVES

HISTORICAL PERSPECTIVES

Major advances have been made in the research, development, and regulation of drugs, in standardizing their chemical constituents, and in improving their uniformity, claims of effectiveness, distribution, and availability. The physician may prescribe a vast array of agents capable of affecting almost every bodily function, and of altering the manifestations, if not the outcome, of many diseases. Most of the drugs now available, however, have been introduced since many physicians completed their formal medical training, and physicians frequently have insufficient familiarity with many drugs to use them well.

Extensive displays of over-the-counter (OTC) drugs in pharmacies and in shops not specifically devoted to selling drugs, such as supermarkets, are often confusing and incomprehensible even to the well-informed buyer. The public usually has little, if any, understanding of pharmacology and is faced with bewildering problems in selecting drugs for personal or family use.

Today, no one except experts in the drug field can claim to be qualified to know how to use more than a few drugs. It is no surprise, therefore, that many OTC drugs are used unwisely by the public, and that restricted drugs are often prescribed incorrectly by physicians. Most, if not all, prescription drugs may cause serious harm, even when used appropriately; but when they are used improperly, this risk is certainly increased. Many nonprescription drugs are used irrationally and also may cause harm, whether they are taken appropriately or inappropriately. No drug is completely safe, and all drugs should be used only with full understanding of their proper administration and their potential adverse effects.

In a sense, the medical profession and the manufacturers and distributors of drugs have promulgated a concept of the effectiveness of drugs which is unwarranted. In accordance with this concept, the public has demonstrated attitudes indicating its belief that any misery, discomfort, or distress should be resolved by taking a medicine or a drug. Too little attention has been given to the need for rational discrimination among types of drugs; to the need for avoidance of drugs at times; and to the often limited usefulness of drugs.

The cost to the patient and the public for OTC and prescription drugs accounts for about 10 per cent of the total health budget, or about 8 to 10 billion dollars per year. Although the price of individual drugs may decrease, the total cost of drugs will probably increase, since there is no indication that overall consumption will level off or decline. Unfortunately, those groups who are often economically deprived, such as the elderly, use a large amount of drugs. Emergence of national systems to reimburse for the costs of drugs and medical care may increase the use of drugs even further, unless more stringent methods of regulation are developed. The prescribing of drugs by their generic rather than their trade names may reduce their cost, but it will not influence their excessive or inappropriate use.

Consumption of drugs represents an important form of environmental chemical exposure and pollution. It is probably a more important cause of environmentally-induced disease than other forms of environmental exposure which receive greater attention and precipitate more concern. It seems absurd to clean up the air, the water, and the food we eat to improve our health, while simultaneously promulgating drug use which increases the frequency and severity of drug-induced disease. Unfortunately, we are developing better methods for monitoring air pollution than for monitoring drug utilization.

Excessive consumption of drugs is of concern because of (1) its cost, (2) the diseases it may induce, and (3) its irrationality. Irrational behavior should be corrected by education, but may require control measures if it results in harm to the public or in unacceptable increases in public cost. Irrational use of drugs may be modified by education and the provision of more accurate and appropriate information by government agencies, drug manufacturers, and physicians, rather than coercive or biased information by advertising and promotion. Formulation of the educational requirements and information needed, however, depends upon an appreciation of the areas of deficiency. If the public and physicians use drug A well and drug B badly, there is little to be accomplished by emphasizing and providing further information about drug A. If advertising or promotion of drugs is not in the public interest, or is biased and misleading, it must be controlled. If the drugs available are ineffective, unsafe, or unnecessary, they should be eliminated. Actions and decisions in these directions must be based upon familiarity with areas requiring attention and causing concern. To obtain such knowledge, monitoring of patterns of drug utilization and of adverse drug reactions is necessary. Groups of individuals differ in geographic location, sex, age, race, social and economic characteristics, and they also vary in their use of drugs, their needs, and their powers of discrimination and susceptibility to promotional efforts. Familiarity with these differences is essential in order to institute measures for improving drug utilization. It is important to identify how drugs are used by different groups of the population and by different groups of physicians, so that we may increase the probability of directing efforts to improve drug utilization toward those most in need and those who will be most benefited. It must be remembered, as Alfred Stillé stated, "The virtues of a medicine depend less upon its intrinsic properties and powers than on the capacity of the physician who administers it—or the person who uses it—just as the efficiency of firearms depends less on the explosives and missiles they contain than on the judgment and accuracy of aim of the man who discharges them."

Diseases caused by drugs have become a major public health problem, sometimes reaching epidemic proportions. Several studies indicate that hundreds of thousands of persons are hospitalized in the United States each year because of diseases caused by OTC and prescription drugs. When this incidence is added to the rate of frequency of adverse drug effects occurring in hospitalized patients and in nonhospitalized persons, the magnitude of the problem becomes astounding. Furthermore, if the cost of caring for these patients were determined or estimated, it would become apparent that hundreds or thousands of millions of dollars are involved. Whether or not the overall benefits provided by some drugs counterbalance their hazardous effects is not known. Even if the benefits provided by drug administration are as important to our health as their frequent use implies, we still might question whether or not we would be better off without so many drugs. Decreased drug use would lead to a reduction in the prevalence of drug-induced illness. Very few have questioned the value of a drug which is important in the treatment of a specific problem in a specific patient, used to accomplish a particular beneficial purpose. However, in many instances the statistical probability of harm to the patient may not be much less than the statistical probability of benefit.

Everyone, including the public, the medical profession, the drug manufacturers, and the government is or should be alarmed by the present patterns of drug utilization and high incidence of drug-induced disease: the public because of the impact upon its health and economy; the patient because of his or her susceptibility of drug-induced disease; the physician, pharmacist, and other health professionals because of their involvement in prescribing, dispensing and administering drugs which cause illness; and the government, because of its responsibility to protect the public interest and control costs, and its educational obligations. Without substantial understanding of the problem, the responses of these groups, at best, will be erratic, often irrational, unenlightened, and inadequately informed.

THE DEVELOPMENT OF DRUGS

Before the mid-19th century, few effective drugs were available. Most of these were derived from natural materials, particularly plants, and often proved ineffective, noxious, or hazardous. This led to a tendency toward therapeutic nihilism regarding drugs and the belief, as expressed by Oliver Wendell Holmes, that "if the whole materia medica, as now used, could be sunk to the bottom of the sea, it would be all the better for mankind and all the worse for the fishes." Then, development and recognition of ether, chloroform, and nitrous oxide as anesthetic agents, together with the isolation of plant alkaloids for use in drugs, including morphine, codeine and heroin, and the synthesis of salicylic acid in drug preparations about 1850 to 1860, heralded the beginning of synthetic pharmaceutical chemistry. During the next few decades these events coincided with the development of nosology and the identification of microbial causes of diseases. Application of new chemical agents to treat illness was a natural consequence of the merger of these two occurrences.

In the *Pharmacopeia of the United States* (USP) published in 1916, only 11 per cent of all drugs listed were synthetic; others were often worthless, but included some effective medicinals derived from natural sources such as plants, and a few derived from animal sources, such as thyroid gland derivatives and cod liver oil. Following World War I, and particularly during and after World War II, the chemical synthesis and development of new drugs entered a period of expanding growth, and the USP published in 1965 contained 179 synthetic chemicals, accounting for 63 per cent of all drugs listed. Only 19 per cent of the drugs were of plant origin. Today, the total number of different drug products available in the United States is not known, but it exceeds 20,000, and most are synthetic chemicals. Within this century, therefore, the development and availability of chemically synthesized drugs have been remarkable in their volume and confusing in their array. These extraordinary expansions of pharmaceutical chemistry have provided medical practitioners with a vast number of agents capable of influencing human beings and human illness. Few drugs, even today, however, are curative; most are palliative. This does not diminish the importance of those drugs capable of relieving the discomfort and manifestations of disease, but it does illustrate the still largely primitive state of therapeutics in eliminating, preventing, or curing disease. Curtailment or restriction of further drug development would ignore these inadequacies, and decrease the possibility of evolving a rational therapeutic supply. A rational basis for drug design is essential but not now generally possible because of the limitations of our knowledge in this area.

The immense number of drugs available for OTC or prescription purposes points to an ever-growing possibility of the rise of drug-induced illnesses, because no drug is completely innocent or incapable of causing harm. Drug-induced disease, however, is not a problem of recent origin. More than 2500 years ago, Hippocrates cited physicians as a cause of injury to patients and cautioned them to treat with compassion and not to cause harm. George Washington died on December 14, 1799, possibly as a result of the application of cantharides to his pharynx to treat a sore throat. One of the first attempts to scientifically evaluate the adverse effects and efficacy of a therapeutic measure was conducted by P. C. A. Louis in 1828, at the Charité Hospital in Paris. His studies on the effectiveness of treating patients who had pneumonia by bleeding them indicated that the outcome might be improved if bleeding were not done at all. Conceivably, similar studies on therapeutic procedures used today might have similar findings. The introduction of chloroform and ether in the mid-19th century resulted in the death of occasional patients after induction of chloroform anesthesia. One of the first collaborative studies of an adverse drug effect was conducted by the British Medical Association in 1877 as a result of this problem, but 13 years of effort were required before it was settled that chloroform sensitized the myocardium and predisposed the heart to major cardiac arrhythmias which can cause death.

After World War I, the possible implications of salvarsan and its substitutes as causes of acute yellow atrophy of the liver were investigated. These studies illustrated the great difficulty involved in distinguishing a possible drug-induced disease from a disease attributable to other causes. It seems probable now that many of the instances of jaundice suspected of being related to the use of neoarsphenamine were attributable to the transmission of viral hepatitis through contaminated equipment and solutions.

The delay in identifying the relationship between a disease and the administration of a drug is well-illustrated by the lapse of almost 45 years, between 1889 and 1933, before amidopyrine was associated with the occurrence of agranulocytosis. Once the association was suggested, a large number of patients with amidopyrine-induced agranulocytosis were identified within the next year and the drug was prohibited for OTC use in 1936 in the United Kingdom and in 1938 in the United States.

The development and use of the sulfonamides in the 1930's increased the familiarity of physicians with the problems of adverse drug reactions. Sulfonamide drugs had real curative powers, and were among the very first synthetic compounds with such an action, leading to their widespread use in treatment of many common pyogenic infections. Crystalluria, renal failure, hemolysis, and allergic reactions were soon recognized as deleterious consequences of the administration of sulfonamides, but the powerful effectiveness of these drugs overshadowed concern about their untoward side effects. Chemical modification of sulfonamides directed at avoiding some of their adverse effects increased their solubility and reduced the probability of crystalluria and renal failure. These efforts, however, led to the development of the long-acting sulfonamides, which became responsible for an increased occurrence of Stevens-Johnson syndrome, a different but equally serious drug-induced disease.

Allergic reactions to penicillin and adverse effects of other antibiotics introduced after World War II appeared insignificant in comparison with the impressive therapeutic powers of these drugs in the treatment of infectious diseases which were a major cause of morbidity and death. This sublimated the alarm which might have been voiced if similar reactions had been caused by less effective agents.

THE REGULATION OF DRUG USE

The most recent dramatic instance of drug induced-disease which led to worldwide alarm and fear occurred just over ten years ago, and focused attention more forcefully than ever before upon the rising problem and catastrophic possibilities of deleterious drug reactions. In 1961, thalidomide was suspected as a cause of phocomelia or hypoplastic and aplastic limb deformities in newborn infants. The drug had first been marketed in Germany in 1956. The disastrous implications of this problem, and the demonstration of clear proof of birth defects in many of the infants born to women who had been administered this drug while pregnant, were followed by removal of thalidomide from the market. It was found that thalidomide had been distributed to 1125 physicians in the United States for clinical trials; but when the drug was withdrawn from the market, it proved impossible to locate all of the drugs which had been distributed, or to identify those patients to whom it had been given. Relatively few congenital abnormalities in infants caused by the use of thalidomide were recognized in the United States, but the alarming effects of the drug were widely published, and precipitated action by the United States Congress to strengthen the regulations of the Food and Drug Administration concerning drug investigation and marketing. Other governments also established control mechanisms to ensure adequate and appropriate testing of toxicity before new drugs were used to treat human beings. These events augmented growing public and governmental concern about drug-induced disease, drug investigation, drug safety, and drug efficacy. A Committee on Safety of Drugs was established in the United Kingdom in 1964, and further requirements for drug control and regulation were incorporated in the legislation on medicines enacted by the British Parliament in 1968.

In 1906, the first Pure Food and Drug Act was passed by the United States Congress, following the death of ten children because of contaminated tetanus antitoxin in 1901, and as a result of growing concern about unsanitary and fraudulently represented foods. Objections to such legislation by the respective industries were loud, but the anger of President Theodore Roosevelt over the abysmal quality and conditions of food production in this country was stronger, and resulted in its enactment. The early legislation provided means for improving the production of foods and drugs, but continued baseless and dishonest claims of efficacy by the drug manufacturers led to passage of the Shirley Amendment in 1912, which classified a product as misbranded if claims in labeling of therapeutic or curative effects of drugs were false or fraudulent. However, the government was required to prove a deliberate intention to defraud on the part of a manufacturer before regulatory action could be taken.

In 1927, the Food and Drug Administration (FDA) became an independent regulatory agency. Between 1906 and 1927, the main emphasis of control legislation had been on foods, in part because little was known about the dangers of drugs and very few effective drugs were available. Dangerous drugs continued to be sold legally up until 1927 because testing for safety before marketing was not required. Flagrant violations by manufacturers were identified, but the government was not empowered to take any action. Manufacturers objected to regulation of drug advertising, and monitoring such advertising was the responsibility of the Federal Trade Commission. Establishment of the FDA as an independent agency represented an attempt to control deficiencies regarding testing and marketing in the Commission's regulatory activity.

The use of sulfonamides dissolved in diethylene glycol, which were not tested for toxicity prior to distribution for human use, produced extensive lethal effects in the early 1930's. At least 100 persons, mostly children, died from use of the drug. An FDA agent reported, "The most amazing thing about the company (manufacturing Elixir of Sulfonilamide) was the total lack of testing facilities. Apparently they just throw drugs together and if they don't explode, they are placed on sale." Defects in the regulatory law, however, prevented legal action from being taken. A new law was enacted by Congress in 1939, broadening the previously narrow definition of a drug to include cosmetics and therapeutic devices, and requiring demonstration of proof of safety before marketing. The individual ingredients of a drug product had to be listed on the label, as well as directions for its use. Subsequently the spirit and letter of the law were quietly implemented, in many cases with voluntary compliance by manufacturers. When necessary, however, regulatory authority was exercised to enforce the law as it was interpreted. In the course of the next 25 years, 14,000 applications for new drugs were received by the FDA. Certification of batches of some drugs as to strength, quality and purity, as set by the USP was inaugurated, and the FDA developed testing laboratories to evaluate the safety and quality of some drug products. There was little need felt or effort made to enlarge the FDA's function until about 1960, when concern with the prices of drugs prompted further congressional investigation by the Antitrust and Monopoly Subcommittee of the Senate Judiciary Committee, chaired by Senator Estes Kefauver. This committee revealed the exorbitant gross profits realized by drug manufacturers from the sale of many drugs, the pressures brought to bear upon physicians from advertising and detail men representing individual drug companies, and brought attention again to the widespread lack of knowledge about the actions or adverse effects of drugs. The public became aroused and the drug industry was horrified. In the midst of considerable harangue, polarization of the views of both sides, and confusion, the thalidomide disaster occurred, and this resulted in the emergence of strengthened legislation, and of the Drug Amendments of 1962. This new legislation required the registration of drug manufacturers, and their subjection to periodic inspection of factories, records, and testing procedures. Drugs had to be approved by the FDA as effective as well as safe before they could be marketed. Approval of older drugs could be withdrawn if new information was uncovered which seriously questioned their safety and efficacy. Testing of new drugs in human beings required "informed consent," and investigators of new drugs had to be registered by the manufacturer and the FDA. Official names of drugs had to be approved by government authority, and labeling of drugs and information provided to physicians had to include valid and proven statements of efficacy, safety, and contraindication.

During the past decade implementation of these new laws has been progressive. At times it has resulted in controversy, required making decisions with limited available information, and occasionally been stumbling and ineffective; it has also probably reduced the efforts of manufacturers in the area of new drug development. But overall, it has improved the quality of drugs available to the American public and for prescription by physicians. It seems unlikely that the existing legislation will remain unchanged. New problems will emerge; methods for detecting previously unknown adverse drug effects in man are still poorly developed, means for monitoring drug utilization are limited in scope, and monitoring of adverse drug reactions to evaluate them as public health problems is minute and incomplete. Many of these remaining problems may be resolved by modifications within the existing legislation. The broad responsibilities of the FDA, however, are difficult to reconcile with its predominantly regulatory function. Resolution of this difficulty remains for the future.

It is important to emphasize that both private and public groups also have been instrumental in improving and regulating drugs. Through the efforts of physicians and pharmacists, over 150 years ago both the United Kingdom and the United States established pharmacopeias setting standards for drugs. Pharmacopeias had also been published in Germany and elsewhere before that time. The USP, however, is primarily a book of standards containing descriptions, chemical tests, and formulas, which largely serves the needs of pharmacists. The USP, therefore, is not a therapeutic guide. The American Medical Association (AMA) has attempted to remedy this failure by preparing a book, *AMA Drug Evaluation* (1971), to serve the needs of physicians, but the impact of this book still remains to be seen. In 1888, the American Pharmaceutical Association began publication of *The National Formulary* (NF), to list standards for drugs prescribed by physicians but not listed in the USP, including drug mixtures and combinations. The role of both the NF and USP, however, is now questionable, since the FDA now has the responsibility to evaluate and set standards for drugs.

Since the end of the 19th century, the AMA has contributed greatly to improving the safety and efficacy of drugs, and has considered means to restrict advertising in its publications in order to eliminate quackery and false claims. An AMA Council on Pharmacy and Chemistry was developed in 1905, becoming the Council on Drugs in 1956. Several publications on drug information were begun, and have proved useful. Concern about the incidence of aplastic anemia attributed to chloramphenicol resulted in the establishment of a Committee on Blood Dyscrasias in 1953, which broadened into a Registry on Adverse Reactions in 1960. The AMA then developed a nationwide system for physicians to report adverse drug effects, in the hope that this would better define the problem and facilitate earlier reporting and recognition of serious drug-induced disease. The program attracted much attention, but it had serious defects. Issues of malpractice involving reporting physicians emerged, and the system did not appear to serve its main function, i.e., circulating early warnings of serious drug effects. Much valuable information was obtained, but when the FDA assumed responsibility for developing methods for monitoring adverse drug reactions in 1960, the AMA program ceased to function. If this task were reassessed, the AMA could continue to develop valuable methods for the distribution of drug information to physicians, and provide a ready means for collecting and soliciting material on suspected new adverse effects of drugs through its membership.

In the past decade, many countries have developed national centers for monitoring adverse drug reactions. Some of these have been effective, but many have had only limited value. The United Kingdom has perhaps been most successful in this effort, even though the United States (FDA) has spent far larger sums of money in its somewhat erratic efforts to keep track of adverse drug reactions. Along with these efforts to establish national centers, about eight years ago the World Health Organization (WHO) initiated a pilot project (1) to develop computerized systems for international monitoring of adverse drug reactions by integrating data obtained from several national centers, and (2) to assist in the establishment of new national centers and to facilitate the development of methods for intensive drug monitoring in order to provide epidemiologic information on drug utilization and rates of adverse drug reactions. The success of this pilot project resulted in establishment of a permanent Drug Monitoring Program under WHO. This development is essential to the advancement of the proper use of drugs because of the worldwide problem of adverse drug reactions and the need for international collaboration to aid in early recognition of drug-induced disease.

Modern medicine is a reflection of the Western European Judeo-Christian ideals of individuality, extended to concern for the people of an entire nation and of the world. Extrapolation of the physician's concern for an individual patient to the concern he and others must have for all individuals in a population involves important and complex organizational, financial, and philosophical considerations. Drug-utilization patterns and adverse drug reactions are part of these considerations, and monitoring them is important. Without the understanding which may be derived from drug monitoring, studies of adverse drug reactions, and clinical pharmacology, irrational regulations may be established. Restrictions on drug use are inevitable. However, additional catastrophic drug-induced diseases may affect excessively large numbers of persons before they are recognized, and essential information is needed to meet educational objectives. Vision and patience, perseverance, public and medical support, and industrial and governmental assistance will be required. The problem is urgent and the time to progress is now, so that a future of more rational care may evolve.

EPIDEMIOLOGIC PERSPECTIVES

Intensive epidemiologic surveillance of hospitalized patients in the United States and abroad has shown that 2 to 5 per cent of patient admissions to the medical and pediatric services of general hospitals are attributable to drug-induced diseases. Five to 30 per cent of patients experience adverse reactions to drugs during hospitalization. An unknown proportion of fetal abnormalities may be attributable to drugs taken by the mother during pregnancy or administered during parturition. An undetermined number of illnesses caused by drugs are responsible for visits of patients to physicians' offices. Conceivably, some diseases for which causes have not been demonstrated or which are widespread may have been induced by drugs.

Unquestionably, adverse drug reactions occur commonly and will become an even more serious problem as the arsenal of medicines available OTC and prescribed by physicians becomes larger. All drugs may cause harm with varying frequency and severity. Even when used with the most scrupulous care, drugs will cause illness in some patients. To reduce this risk to a minimum, however, drug usage must be based upon an understanding and appreciation of its value, limitations, and the probability and severity of illnesses for which a drug may be responsible. This requires epidemiologic and statistical information about the risks and benefits of drug administration.

The diseases induced by drugs are protean and may mimic other diseases. They may be acute or chronic, and may occur during brief or prolonged use of a drug. Most patients take several drugs at one time, and identification of the one specifically causing an adverse reaction is often difficult. Increasingly, it has also been recognized that interaction of two or more drugs is responsible for untoward effects which neither drug alone will produce. Very few diagnostic studies are available which confirm the causal relationships between a drug and a disease, or which predict an individual's predisposition to an unfavorable drug effect. Very few individuals receiving a particular drug may experience adverse effects, and circumstantial evidence alone does not establish, even though it may suggest, a relationship between the drug and a disease. The use of statistical evidence to determine an epidemiologic relationship between a drug and a disease, however, has proved to be a reliable and effective method in identifying and defining adverse drug reactions and characterizing drug utilization. Epidemiological associations, nevertheless, may be misused in evaluating individual patients with suspected drug-induced disease. For example, although thromboembolic disease occurs in women who do not take oral contraceptives, appearance of this problem in a woman receiving these drugs today will often be interpreted as having been caused by the drug, although there is no substantiating evidence. Without epidemiologic study, however, such an association may not have been recognized at all.

Adverse reactions to drugs when their pharmacologic effects are known (e.g., hypoglycemia following administration of insulin) usually are readily identified and related to the drug, but those reactions not known to be caused by a drug's pharmacologic action, or attributable to allergies or other mechanisms, often are not as easily related to a specific drug. Familiarity with the diseases caused by drugs, analysis of the drugs a patient is taking, and evaluation of the drugs a particular patient has been taking prior to or at the onset of illness are important in recognizing drug-induced disease.

Adverse reactions to drugs range from the very minor to the very serious: they may be insignificant and of little consequence; may require extensive medical care, or may result in death. Minor reactions may be very important or disquieting to the patient, seem to be a nuisance to the physician, and are often subjective. "Minor" manifestations of adverse drug reactions such as nausea, vomiting, and dizziness are common, but incrimination of a specific drug as responsible for them is most difficult, because they are common symptoms of many illnesses which are not drug-related. Seemingly insignificant adverse drug reactions, however, may be premonitory signs of more serious disease and should not be overlooked. For example, the occurrence of pruritus may seem unimportant, but it may precede the development of exfoliative dermatitis. Nausea and vomiting may indicate drug-induced gastritis preceding gastric hemorrhage.

THE UTILIZATION OF DRUGS

With exceptions, many physicians have limited perception of how drugs are used in medical practice, and little effort has been spent in evaluating physicians' prescribing practices as a means of improving the use of drugs. Individual physicians, however, prescribe a limited number of different drugs which seem to suit the needs of their patients, and of which they have some understanding. It is likely that most physicians use no more than 50 drug products in their practice.

The drug needs of patients differ depending upon their illnesses, preferences, and idiosyncrasies. In the hospital, the community, the region, and throughout the nation, many different drugs are administered to patients by many different physicians, and drug-utilization patterns frequently seem complex and irrational.

Patients are not usually given only one drug by their physician. They often are cared for by more than one physician, each of whom may prescribe different, or the same, drugs for the same or different clinical problems. Moreover, they frequently use OTC drugs sporadically or regularly on their own.

The many different drugs which exist and are prescribed by physicians with varying skills and drug preferences, administered to individuals with unpredictable susceptibility to drug action, and purchased OTC by patients with little understanding of the drugs they use, illustrate the complexities of drug utilization. It is in this setting, however, that adverse reactions to drugs occur. Understanding drug utilization, therefore, is essential to understanding drug-induced disease.

Persons who should be knowledgeable about drugs a patient consumes include the patient himself, the physician caring for the patient, and the pharmacist dispensing the drugs. Unfortunately, the degree of familiarity of each of these individuals with drug utilization is poor. Hospitalized patients are frequently not advised of the medications they receive until their discharge, when they may be informed about the prescriptions they are to have filled to continue taking the medication at home. Only one-third of the medications consumed may be known to ambulatory patients by name, and some medications may be incorrectly identified. In addition, some (5 to 10 per cent) of patients may be incorrectly informed as to the purpose of a drug they are taking, and may correspondingly misuse it. Twenty-five to 50 per cent of patients may make errors in self-administration of prescribed medications, and in many instances (4 to 35 per cent) the erroneous method of drug administration may prove a serious threat to the patient's health. The older the patient, the more likely is he or she to commit such errors. Patients also may fail to take their prescribed medications. In one study, 31 per cent of "reliable" patients took less than 70 per cent of their medications. Lower socio-economic background and particular psychological features of patients are among the factors which determine patients' degrees of compliance in taking prescribed medications. Physicians must appreciate that once they prescribe a drug, their instructions are not automatically or regularly followed by the patient obtaining or taking the drug.

The ambulatory patient is usually the only one who knows the prescription and nonprescription drugs he or she has obtained, has taken in the past, or is now using. Therefore a drug history given by the patient, and confirmed when possible by the patient's family, dispensing pharmacist, and prescribing physician, is a critical part of the clinical evaluation of every person. This history is a key to avoiding administering drugs hazardous to the patient, preventing potential adverse drug interactions, and advising the patient as to the appropriateness or inappropriateness of his drug practices. Several studies have been done to develop interview techniques for obtaining a patient's drug history. A method we have developed has proved most successful. It is now being used regularly in our general medical clinic, and is included in the educational program for medical students that instructs them in interview and history-taking techniques. As part of this procedure, prior to his first appointment each patient is instructed to bring any medications he or she has used during the preceding 30 days to the office or clinic on the appointment day. These drugs are then examined and the patient is questioned in order to obtain a detailed history of his or her medications, and any adverse reactions to them. Thus information about drug use and reactions becomes an integral part of the record, and reinforces for the patient and the physician the importance of preventing drug-induced illness. A structured interview form is used, including a checklist of types of therapeutic drugs that might have been used. Patients initially indicating they have taken no medication or have had no "bad reaction" to a drug, often identify drugs taken or remember adverse drug reactions experienced previously while they are reviewing the checklist. The interviewer then identifies a therapeutic drug category, such as cold medicine or constipation remedies, and suggests several brand names of medications in these categories. Frequently, patients may state that they could not take a particular drug product named because it caused vomiting, dizziness, or a rash; this facilitates identification of drug idiosyncrasies or allergies. The checklist also serves to identify drugs the patient has taken which had been prescribed for someone else. Such drug misuse is, otherwise, often overlooked by the patient. The information obtained can have profound importance in diagnosing a possible drug-induced illness and in some cases, in safely treating the patient.

Failure of the physician to obtain an adequate drug history from his patient is as culpable as failure to inquire about an obese patient's dietary habits. Lack of success in recognizing and treating a drug-induced disease appropriately is directly related to failure to obtain a drug history. Most physicians do not obtain adequate drug histories. They routinely identify fewer than one-half of the medications taken by their patients, and only one-third of their adverse drug reactions.

Unfamiliarity of the physician with his patients' drug utilization undoubtedly contributes to the occurrence of drug-induced disease. Potentially deleterious interactions between drugs being taken can be identified in over one-half of ambulatory patients studied. Later on, continued administration to patients of pharmacologic classes of drugs similar to those which have already produced an adverse reaction can result in serious consequences. Such consequences are often characterized by exaggerated therapeutic responses, such as personality change, and by somnolence in patients taking more than one psychoactive agent, even including alcohol. Some drug interactions may decrease the therapeutic efficacy of a medication, as exemplified by decreased absorption of some antibiotics taken with antacids. Other drug interactions may result in disease which would not occur if either drug were given alone, as illustrated by gastric hemorrhage in patients taking an anticoagulant and aspirin, or hypertensive crisis in patients taking an amphetamine and a monoamine oxidase inhibitor.

Almost half of all patients take medication prescribed by more than one physician, and there is a relationship between the number of physicians prescribing for a single patient and the potential for adverse drug interaction. About one-third of single prescribers, however, may administer drugs to patients that may interact adversely. Nevertheless, the possibility of an adverse drug interaction increases to two-thirds or more in patients being cared for by multiple prescribers. In addition, as might be expected, the average number of prescription drugs taken by patients is directly related to the number of physician prescribers, varying from 2.6 in patients with one prescriber to 8.8 in patients with three or more prescribers. These findings emphasize that physicians are not familiar with the drug-utilization experience of their patients, and are often unaware of potentially deleterious drug interactions.

The pharmacist is a focal point in the use of prescription and nonprescription drugs. He is often the only health professional with access to information concerning almost all drugs used by patients. Unfortunately, however, he often does not use this information to examine drug-utilization patterns of patients, or to evaluate drug-prescribing practices of physicians. Appropriate utilization of the information obtained or obtainable by community pharmacists could help in avoiding patient use of drugs that may adversely interact, and could serve as both a resource for physicians in obtaining drug histories of patients and a tool for improving drug utilization.

Community pharmacies in 1970 dispensed over 1.2 billion prescriptions at a cost of nearly $5 billion. The sheer magnitude of this is further increased by similar data on the dispensing and cost of nonprescription drugs. The pharmacist maintains an inventory; he is often required by law to keep records of prescription drugs dispensed, but this information has usually not been used to improve drug utilization. Fortunately, studies reveal that most patients have their prescriptions filled at a single pharmacy. The volume of data in a single pharmacy, however, is too extensive and complex to serve the needs of drug-utilization review without first being subject to automatic data processing. In addition, the collation of drug purchases made by patients in different pharmacies requires standard systems for data collection. Systematizing methods used to gather data would enable the integration of data on a single patient using different dispensers. At some time in the future a system for handling such data must be developed and constructed, at least on a regional basis, and methods must be evolved to apply such data to improve drug use.

A need has rapidly arisen for peer evaluation of medical practice, which could be used in part for monitoring the prescribing practices of physicians in hospitals and in communities. If appropriately developed to provide better and more accurate information for physicians and patients, rather than for punitive or regulatory functions, such monitoring of drug utilization could go far in reducing the misuse of drugs and the occurrence of drug-induced disease.

The risk associated with the administration of a drug to a patient is determined by the rate of occurrence of an adverse reaction, the physician's awareness of factors influencing an individual's susceptibility to adverse drug reactions, and the physician's familiarity with the severity of the illness which may be drug-induced. The rate of occurrence of an adverse reaction to a particular drug can be determined accurately only by knowing the proportion of patients receiving the drug who develop the reaction. Calculation of the population at risk, i.e., those receiving the drug, and detection in this population of adverse reactions to the drug are essential to determine the rate of adverse drug reaction. Characterization of the population at risk is necessary to detect factors responsible for individual idiosyncrasies to drugs. Familiarity with a drug's metabolic effects and its pharmacologic action may indicate factors probably important in predisposing some patients to adverse reactions. Knowing about drug utilization and the pharmacologic properties of drugs is an integral part of understanding, detecting, and preventing drug-induced disease.

Adverse Drug Reactions

Adverse reactions to drugs occur with varying frequency and severity. The factors determining why some, but not all, patients receiving a drug develop an adverse reaction are largely unknown. Only after 1960 were concerted efforts made to investigate the frequency, characteristics, and predisposing factors responsible for adverse drug reactions in ordinary clinical settings, and in sick patients under the care of many different physicians, using a large variety of prescribed and OTC drugs and drug products.

Some epidemiologic studies of adverse drug reactions have identified factors important in preventing their occurrence. There is a direct relationship between the rate of occurrence of adverse drug reactions in hospitalized patients and the number of different drugs they are given. In one study, it was found that less than 5 per cent of patients receiving fewer than six drugs during hospitalization developed an adverse reaction. If the number of different drugs administered exceeds 16, the probability of a reaction occurring during hospitalization increases to over 40 per cent. This observation should be used to caution every physician to exercise care in prescribing multiple drugs for his patients, and to warn the public to be as discriminating as possible in its use of OTC drugs. Patients receiving many different drugs usually are sicker than those receiving fewer drugs, at least as defined by mortality, duration of hospitalization, and presence or absence of renal failure. The combination of multiple drug treatment, renal failure, disturbed cerebrovascular activity, and disturbed hepatic function which are often associated with severe illness compounds the problem of adverse drug reactions, not only because of possible adverse drug interactions, but also because multiple drug administration may contribute to further impairment of the metabolizing, excretion, and distribution of drugs. Although very sick patients may require many drugs, it is important to recognize the predisposition of these patients to adverse drug effects, and to avoid administering all but the most essential drugs.

Patients who experience or who have experienced an adverse drug reaction are predisposed to developing others. For example, patients who give a genuine history of a reaction to a drug, who have a reaction when hospitalized, or who develop one during hospitalization, are two to three times more likely to develop another adverse drug reaction than patients without such drug experiences. The subsequent adverse drug reactions are not necessarily attributable to the same or a similar drug, and may differ in manifestation. An adverse reaction to any medication, therefore, should be considered as evidence of predisposition to adverse reactions to other and all drugs. At least until more information is available, administration of drugs to such patients, therefore, requires greater care and more critical observation for adverse drug effects.

Factors known to be predisposing to adverse drug reactions are sex (female), age (older persons), certain racial characteristics, the presence of renal or hepatic disease, diseases of the intestinal tract, possibly a history of atopic disease, and some heritable or acquired diseases. Familiarity with such conditions in the patient, therefore, is necessary to avoid inadvertent induction of a drug-induced disease.

When treating children it is a standard practice to administer medication in doses regulated by the patient's weight, body surface, or age. In contrast, adults are usually given drugs without significant consideration of weight, size, or age. Although it seems logical to suppose that this practice would result in a reduced frequency of adverse drug reactions in pediatric patients, the frequency of such reactions in children is no lower than that in adults. This observation strongly indicates the inadequacy of present systems used for determining the dosage of a medication. The known variability in blood levels or bioavailability of drugs following administration of a standard dose to a reasonably uniform group of patients suggests that methods for determining bioavailability of an administered drug in patients may be necessary, particularly with some drugs, to determine the dose necessary to achieve a desired therapeutic effect while avoiding an adverse reaction. With rare exceptions, however, studies of bioavailability are not generally available. Illustrative of the possible usefulness of such methods of measurement is the use of sulfonamide blood levels to avoid crystalluria and to achieve the desired therapeutic benefits in treatment of infection.

The Promotion of Drugs

Physicians often show considerable interest in a newly marketed drug, and their use of these drugs shortly after they become available is frequently excessive, often inappropriate, and may have serious adverse consequences. For example, after the marketing of ethacrynic acid and furosemide as diuretics, a large number of patients who had been administered these drugs by their physicians were admitted to hospitals with severe dehydration and electrolyte depletion. After a time, this problem was no longer observed as frequently, probably owing to decreased and more appropriate use of these drugs by physicians. It is essential for physicians planning to use a new drug to familiarize themselves with its pharmacology, use, and hazards prior to prescribing it. Unfortunately, however, many physicians will use a new drug when they have only been exposed to advertising information or material provided by pharmaceutical detail men, or hearsay, and such information is too often biased, poorly presented, and inadequate. Physicians must not depend solely upon these sources of information in deciding to use a drug; otherwise, it is certain the drug will be misused.

Promotional activities of manufacturers and distributors of drugs have been found to be more important than other sources of information in influencing both the purchasing of OTC drugs by the public and the prescribing of drugs by physicians. Scientific journals, carefully developed expert opinions, books, lectures, seminars, compendia, reviews, and many other means to inform the medical profession about drugs are now available, and others are being developed with considerable speed. Such sources of information are often of great value, but investigation of factors influencing physicians' practices of prescribing drugs has shown them to be less influential than promotional efforts. Similarly, drug advertising more often determines OTC drug purchases than advice or counsel of physicians or pharmacists. The promotional intent of materials released by manufacturers and distributors invariably emphasizes the claims of effectiveness, and usually encourages use of a drug by subtle and not so subtle suggestion and inference. Anyone watching television, reading advertisements in magazines, or examining displays in stores selling drug products can easily recognize the biased and coercive nature of promotional literature. It is no wonder that drugs are overused, misused, and abused. Countermeasures have been developed and used to provide a more balanced understanding of drugs and drug use, but these would be unnecessary if the promotion of drugs was conducted rationally, responsibly, and with the objective of meeting public interests and needs. It is not justifiable to promote drugs as the means to complete social, physical, and emotional well-being.

Some medical institutions providing medical care have adopted restrictive drug formularies in order to limit the prescribing of drugs to those accepted as most important, useful, and economical by informed physicians and pharmacists; to provide for purchasing of particular drug products shown by scientific study to be reliable, effective, and safe; and to enable prescribing of a drug by its generic rather than its trade name. Such formulary systems can have important influences upon drug utilization in medical institutions. Development of restrictive formularies in many medical institutions and in noninstitutionalized medical settings, however, has been very controversial and often has been prohibited by the physicians involved, largely because of concern about the limitations the formulary is thought by some to impose upon the freedom of physicians to practice medicine, and upon the merchandising interests of pharmacists. A restrictive formulary probably is essential in every medical-care setting to improve patient care, to reduce the problems of adverse drug reactions, to provide the understanding physicians require to prescribe drugs well, and to control costs to patients and to dispensers of drugs who are otherwise required to carry excessively large and diverse inventories.

Sale of OTC drugs is now a multibillion dollar business and is no longer confined to pharmacies. The public deserves and should demand better guidance and advice about the use of OTC drugs than is now available in promotional materials or is provided by uninformed clerks, salespersons, and displays. It is questionable whether or not we, as a public and a nation, can justify the large number of different OTC drug products now being manufactured, distributed, and sold in establishments where inadequate, inappropriate, and usually misleading advice and counsel are available.

Increasing attention to factors influencing drug utilization and prescription, and to the types and numbers of different drug products available, is probably most likely to improve drug utilization practices and to diminish the problems of drug-induced disease.

REFERENCES

Historical Perspectives

Barber, B.: Drugs and Society. New York, Russell Sage Foundations, 1967.
Burack, R.: The Handbook of Prescription Drugs. New York, Pantheon Books, Random House, 1973.
de Haen, P.: Drugs and drug use. Med. Sci., *18*: 1967.
Dowling, H. F.: Medicines for Man. New York, Alfred A. Knopf, Inc., 1971.
International Drug Monitoring: The Role of National Centers: WHO Tech. Rep. Ser., no. 498: 1972.
Lasagna, L., ed.: Clinical pharmacology. *In* International Encyclopedia of Pharmacology and Therapeutics, vol. 1, Oxford, Pergamon Press, 1966.
Lennard, H. L., Epstein, L. J., Bernstein, A., and Ransom, D. C.: Mystification and Drug Misuse: Hazards in Using Psychoactive Drugs. San Francisco, Jossey-Bass, Inc., 1971.

Royall, B. W.: International aspects of the study of adverse reactions to drugs. Biometrics, 27:689, 1971.
Royall, B. W.: The use of computers in international drug monitoring. WHO Chron., 27:469, 1973.
Stillé, A.: Of therapeutics. In Brian, W. R., ed., The Quiet Art, A Doctor's Anthology, Edinburgh, E.&S. Livingston, 1952.
Talalay, P., ed.: Drugs in Our Society. Baltimore, The Johns Hopkins University Press, 1964.
Wade, O. L.: Adverse Reactions to Drugs. London, Heinemann, 1970.

Epidemiologic Perspectives

Borda, I. T., Slone, D., and Jick, H.: Assessment of adverse reactions with a drug surveillance program. JAMA, 205:645, 1968.
Boston Collaborative Drug Surveillance Program: Drug surveillance: problems and challenge. Pediatr. Clin. North Am., 10:117, 1972.
Brodie, D. C.: Drug Utilization and Drug Utilization Review and Control. National Center for Health Services, Research and Development, U.S. Dept. of Health, Education, and Welfare, Washington, D.C., U.S. Government Printing Office, 1971.
Cluff, L. E.: Adverse reactions to drugs: Methods of study. In: Lasagna, Leo, ed., International Encyclopedia of Pharmacology and Therapeutics, vol. 2, Oxford, Pergamon Press, 1966.
Cluff, L. E.: Prescribing habits of physicians. Hosp. Prac., 2:100, 1967.
Cluff, L. E., and Stewart, R. B.: Studies on the epidemiology of adverse drug reactions, VI, Utilization and interactions of prescription and non-prescription drugs. Johns Hopkins Med. J., 129:319, 1971.
Crooks, J., Weir, R. D., Coull, D. C., et al.: Evaluation of a method of prescribing drugs in a hospital, and a new method of recording their administration. Lancet, 1:668, 1967.
Finney, D. J.: The design and logic of a monitor of drug use. J. Chronic Dis., 18:77, 1965.
Gardner, P., and Cluff, L. E.: The epidemiology of adverse reactions: A review and perspective. Johns Hopkins Med. J., 126:77, 1970.
Hurwitz, N., and Wade, O. L.: Intensive hospital monitoring of adverse reactions to drugs. Br. Med. J., 1:531, 1969.
Jick, H., Miettinen, O. S., Shapiro, S., et al.: Comprehensive drug surveillance. JAMA, 213:1455, 1970.
Maronde, R. F., Lee, P. V., McCarron, M. M., et al.: Physician prescribing practices – A computer based study. Am. J. Hosp. Pharm., 26:566, 1971.
Reidenberg, M. M., and Lowenthal, D. T.: Adverse non-drug reactions. Engl. J. Med., 279:678, 1968.
Schimmel, E. M.: The hazards of hospitalization. Ann. Intern. Med., 60:100, 1964.
Smith, J. W., Seidl, L. G., and Cluff, L. E.: Studies on the epidemiology of adverse drug reactions, V, Clinical factors affecting susceptibility. Ann. Intern. Med., 65:629, 1966.
Stewart, R. B., and Cluff, L. E.: A review of medication errors and compliance in ambulant patients. Clin. Pharmacol. Ther., 13:463, 1972.
Stollacy, P. D., and Lasagna, L.: Prescribing patterns of physicians. J. Chronic Dis., 22:395, 1969.
Task Force on Prescription Drugs. U.S. Dept. of Health, Education, and Welfare, Office of the Secretary, Washington, D.C., U.S. Government Printing Office, 1969.

CHAPTER 2

PHARMACOLOGIC MECHANISMS

The pharmacologic actions of drugs used for ordinary diagnostic, therapeutic, or prophylactic purposes may produce desirable or undesirable, expected or unexpected, intended or unintended, minor or serious effects. Although drugs may also produce adverse effects when they function as antigenic haptens resulting in allergic reactions, epidemiologic studies have demonstrated that over one-half of observed adverse drug reactions are attributable to pharmacologic rather than immunologic mechanisms.[17,58]

Most drugs have several pharmacologic actions, some of which may be responsible for both desired therapeutic effects and adverse effects. Irrespective of whether the effect produced is therapeutically desired or undesired, the responsible pharmacologic mechanisms may be the same. It is generally held that the pharmacologic action of drugs is evoked by interaction of the drug with receptor sites of responsive cells located in the plasmic membrane, and the intensity or magnitude of the response is a function of the quantity or amount of the drug administered, and of the availability and affinity of the receptor site for the drug.

There is wide variation in the quantity of a drug required to produce a given response (either therapeutic or toxic) in different individuals, and this corresponds to a normal frequency distribution curve. This curve has been graphically represented as the quantal dose response curve (Fig. 2–1). The curve is developed by relating the dose of the drug to the cumulative percentage of subjects exhibiting a response. Any point along the curve gives the percentage of patients responding to a corresponding dose of the drug.

A certain concentration (dose) of a drug is required to produce a therapeutic response. Increasing the dose above this threshold will result in an increase in the response, until a maximal response is

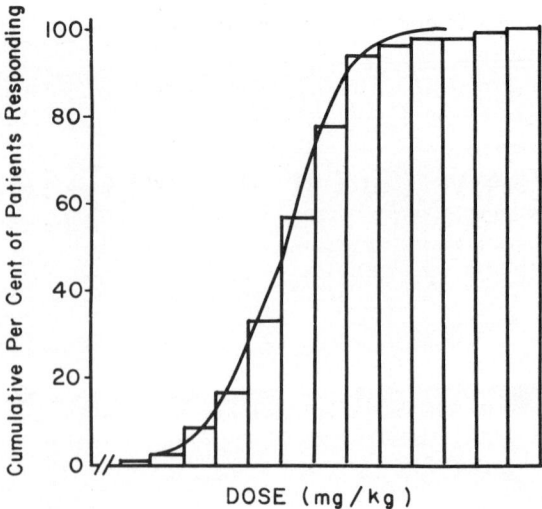

Figure 2-1. Quantal dose response curve. Variation of drug dose required to produce a given response in a group of patients.

attained which may remain unaltered even with further increases in the dose, although pharmacologic effects unrelated to the therapeutic response may occur and cause unfavorable reactions.

The response curve of a single dose cannot adequately characterize the action of a drug in a complex biological system. For example, the concentration of digoxin required to exert a desirable therapeutic effect upon the cardiovascular system also may produce a toxic effect upon the gastrointestinal system. Ideally, a drug should produce its desired effect without inducing adverse effects. For every drug, there is some dose that will cause a toxic effect, and often the toxic dose may fall well within the range of the therapeutic dose.

Types of Adverse Effects

The adverse effects of a drug may consist of exaggerated extensions of the therapeutic purposes for which the drug is given, or may be attributable to pharmacologic actions which are not directly related to the desired therapeutic effect. The first process is illustrated in the following examples:

ANTICOAGULANTS. Anticoagulants are therapeutically useful because they inhibit blood-clotting mechanisms. Bleeding, however, is a logical extension of their main action.

ANTIHYPERTENSIVE ACTION. Guanethidine exerts antihypertensive action by creating an adrenergic blockade. This in turn may produce severe adverse effects, including orthostatic hypotension,[132] which also may result from administration of other antihypertensives, including methyldopa and ganglioplegic agents.[90,96]

ANTINEOPLASTIC THERAPY. Most agents used to treat malignant disease interrupt DNA synthesis or alter DNA macromolecules.[31] Through this action proliferation of malignant cells is curtailed, but normal cells having a high rate of cellular proliferation also will be affected. These include cells in bone marrow, in the gastrointestinal tract, and in the hair follicles. Therefore, anemia, diarrhea, and alopecia are common side effects of antineoplastic therapy.

Since these adverse effects are closely associated with the therapeutic action of a particular drug or drugs, they are often not unexpected and, in fact, are usually anticipated. For these reasons they may not be classed as toxic by prescribing physicians.

Many adverse reactions are not extensions of the therapeutic effect of a drug but are attributable to other pharmacologic actions. These types of reactions are often obscure, and a cause and effect relationship is difficult to establish. For example, 80 years of clinical experience transpired before gastric bleeding was related to the administration of aspirin.[124] Several examples that follow illustrate adverse effects not normally related to the therapeutic purpose for which a drug is given.

CARCINOGENIC EFFECTS. Adverse effects of drugs are more readily identified when they occur shortly after administration of a drug. Unfortunately, drug-induced carcinomas may take years to develop, and identification of the relationship of such carcinomas to the administration of a particular drug may take even longer. For example, the association of adenocarcinoma of the vagina with maternal stilbestrol therapy was not recognized for two decades.[76]

BONE MARROW DEPRESSION. Aplastic anemia has been associated with the use of many drugs, including chloramphenicol, propylthiouracil, and indomethacin.[26,116,117] The mechanisms by which these agents induce this disease are not clearly established.

METABOLIC EFFECTS. Thiazide diuretics had been used in clinical practice for only a few months when reports appeared suggesting that they could induce a diabetic state.[45] Barbiturates have long been known for their capacity to alter metabolism of liver porphyrin in man. Many agents have now been identified which can induce liver microsomal enzymes and alter metabolism of drugs.

NEPHROTOXICITY. Many compounds have been demonstrated to be toxic to the kidney. Notable drugs in this category include those containing heavy metals, aminoglycoside antibiotics, and some analgesics.[114] Again, these toxic effects are not related to the drug's therapeutic purposes and are clearly undesirable and unintended.

HYPERPLASIA. Quite apart from their therapeutic effects, the hydantoin anticonvulsants will induce gingival hyperplasia in nearly

40 per cent of the patients using the drug.[110] This effect does not appear to be related to the dose administered, and in most cases the gums will return to normal within a year after use of the drug is discontinued.[18]

PSYCHOGENIC EFFECTS. Emotional change can be an adverse effect which is dissociated from the therapeutic purposes for which some drugs are given. This is seen in the behavioral and emotional side effects produced by drugs used for nonpsychotherapeutic purposes.[88] Prednisone and isoniazid produce emotional or behavioral disturbances in 2.6 and 1.9 per cent, respectively, of all patients receiving these drugs.

TERATOGENIC EFFECTS. Drugs which reach the embryo during the first trimester of pregnancy can have a significant impact on the future development of the fetus. The teratogenic effect of these drugs may be unrelated to the therapeutic action of the drug, as illustrated by thalidomide, which was used as a sedative.

ARGYRIA. Skin discoloration occurring in patients using silver salts over a prolonged period is a classical illustration of tissue distribution of a drug leading to an adverse effect. The silver granules deposited throughout the dermis cause a bluish-grey color. Another example of reactions caused by physical deposits occurs in the administration of tetracycline, which, when used in children, may deposit in teeth and cause permanent staining.[120]

Adverse reactions to drugs can mimic almost any disease, and are often difficult to diagnose. These drug-induced diseases, like other diseases, may be characterized predominantly by physiologic or biochemical abnormalities, or may be associated with anatomic or pathologic changes. Examples of these adverse effects are given below.

PHYSIOLOGIC OR BIOCHEMICAL ABNORMALITIES. Drugs often alter gastrointestinal function and produce digestive disorders[164] most often characterized by nausea, vomiting, diarrhea, or constipation. These manifestations of adverse drug effects are not ordinarily associated with anatomic or pathologic change, and may occur following either oral or parenteral drug administration.

Acute dystonic reactions, such as oculogyric crises or torticollis, which are caused by some drugs, may be mistaken for tetany or hysteria.[122] Severe coma, depression, paranoia, hallucinations, vivid dreams, and other psychophysiologic, behavioral, or neurophysiologic abnormalities may be induced by drugs and are not known to be associated with histopathologic changes.[23,64,187]

Levels of serum enzymes, as illustrated by glutamic-oxaloacetic transaminase, may rise following administration of drugs such as methyldopa, phenothiazines, and sex hormones. Hyperuricemia has been caused by the use of thiazide diuretics. These biochemical aberrations caused by drugs may not be accompanied by demonstrable pathologic lesions, although such lesions may become evident, as when gout occurs in association with thiazide-induced hyperuricemia.

ANATOMIC-PATHOLOGIC ABNORMALITIES. Many adverse drug reactions are characterized by gross or histopathologic changes. The irritant effects of drugs applied to the skin and causing dermatopathologic abnormalities are probably the most common of these. A striking example of an anatomic lesion caused by a drug is the retroperitoneal fibrosis observed in patients given methysergide in treatment of migraine headache.[68] Fibrotic changes have also been caused by other drugs and affect the lung parenchyma, the heart, and other organs.

The multiplicity and variety of biochemical, physiologic, and pathologic effects of drugs resulting in adverse consequences and disease will become increasingly evident in this book. Recognition that drugs may produce both functional and anatomic abnormalities because of their pharmacologic action is important in fully appreciating the ramifications of drug-induced disease.

BIOLOGIC DETERMINANTS OF ADVERSE DRUG REACTIONS IN "NORMAL" PERSONS

The organism's biologic responses to a drug's pharmacologic action, leading to desired or undesired effects, are related to dose, as mentioned before, but also are influenced by variations among individuals, administration of other drugs, environmental conditions, and many other factors. Individual differences affecting drug action include the rate of drug absorption, age, sex, weight, and hepatic and renal functions of the patient, heritable traits, and whether or not the patient is pregnant.

Generally, adverse effects of drugs which are attributable to their pharmacologic action occur most frequently in the very young and the very old. Incomplete organ and physiologic development in the newborn and in infants may influence their absorption, distribution, metabolism, and elimination of drugs. Illustrative of the influence of the stage of physiologic development upon drugs is the lower rate of elimination of sulfobromophthalein in newborn infants, and the increasing rate of elimination of this drug as children mature. In addition, the half-life of chloramphenicol in infants is longer than in children or adults, resulting in high blood levels for a longer period of time, and this may lead to the "gray syndrome" and death.[112] This effect of chloramphenicol in infants is attributable to an incompletely developed system for metabolizing the drug. Aged patients, on the other hand, also have less ability to metabolize and excrete drugs, probably as a result of degenerative processes which reduce rates of excretion and metabolism of drugs. For example, elderly patients with no urinary symptoms and normal serum creatinine levels may have reduced renal clearance of endogenous creatinine, and the half-life or blood levels of drugs excreted by the kidney may be increased, including penicillin, aminoglycoside antibiotics, and digoxin.[49,71] The hazard of adverse pharmacologic action of these drugs, therefore, may be significantly increased in the aged individual. Comparative studies of blood levels in young adult men and octogenarians given a standard dose of sulfamethoxypyridazine demonstrated that peak blood levels in the elderly men were three times higher than in the younger men.[21] These variations in response to drugs in old and very young patients often have led to the practice of reducing the dose of a drug given to these individuals.[35]

Sex differences probably are not of great importance as a determinant of the pharmacologic response to drugs, except when these differences affect the type and number of drugs taken. Women, however, do experience adverse drug reactions affecting the gastrointestinal system more frequently than men.[164] In addition, women over 60 years of age receiving heparin therapy appear to develop bleeding complications more often than men.[86]

Weight has long been considered an important factor in calculating the approximate drug dosage. A 2-year-old child weighing 30 pounds should not receive the same dose of medication as an 8-year-old weighing 60 pounds. The drug dose to be administered often is measured on a mg/kg basis, in an attempt to adjust for the effect of weight upon the pharmacologic action of the drug.

In many instances the weight of the individual has not been considered as important a factor in determining drug dosage for adults as it is for children. The ratio between the amount of the drug administered and body weight generally determines the concentration of the drug at the site of action. It is reasonable, then, to adjust dosages according to the patient's weight. Dosages usually recommended for an adult in several drug compilations or compendia are for a patient weighing from 132 to 154 pounds.[145] These doses, however, might not be appropriate for a 250-pound man or a 100-pound woman. It has also been shown that the dosage for obese patients may be different than that required for a patient with a lean build, since many drugs are distributed principally in the water and lean mass of the body and not in the fat. The importance of weight as a determinant of peak blood levels of drugs (Fig. 2–2) has been demonstrated in a study of bromides. The blood level resulting from daily doses of bromides can be directly correlated to the weight and distribution of water, lean mass, and fat in the patient.[171]

Renal function has a profound influence upon blood levels of many drugs, and upon their adverse effects. When administered to a patient with decreased renal clearance, a drug excreted primarily by the kidney will result in blood levels of that drug higher and more prolonged than in normal individuals. The relationship of creatinine

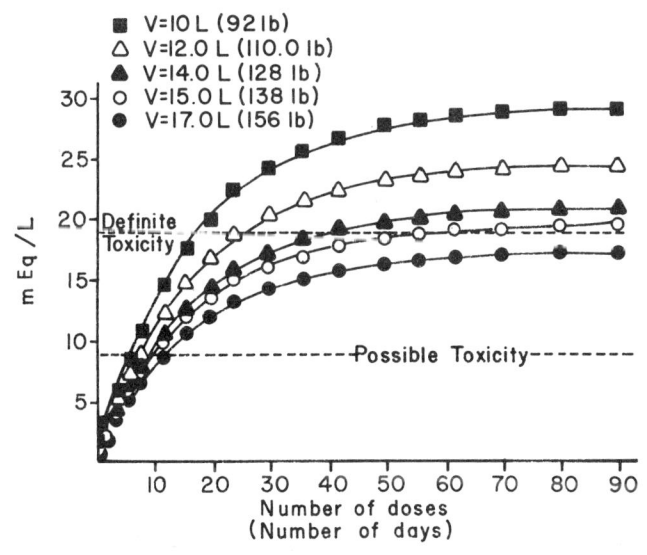

Figure 2-2. Maximum bromide blood levels versus the number of doses, showing the effect of the volume of distribution on the rate of approach to the toxic levels for adults taking 16.5 mEq of bromide/day, the maximum recommended dose (number of doses = number of days). (Reprinted from *Amer. J. Hosp. Pharm.*, 30:717, Aug., 1973.)

clearance to the elimination of procainamide was shown (Fig. 2-3) by Weily and Genton.[183] Numerous practical formulas have been developed to calculate dosages of drugs for patients with renal disease[16,61,99] which are useful in meeting therapeutic objectives and avoiding adverse effects.

Hepatic function has not consistently been found to be as important a factor as renal function in predisposing patients to adverse drug reactions. The reasons for this are not entirely clear, since metabolism of many drugs has been shown to be impaired significantly in the presence of liver disease. A major problem in this area is that there are no convenient tests available for the clinician to predict the capacity of the liver to metabolize drugs.

A number of heritable factors can affect an individual's response to a drug. A typical example is the hemolytic anemia resulting from a genetically determined glucose-6-phosphate dehydrogenase deficiency of erythrocytes.[95]

Other heritable features have been associated with increased susceptibility to adverse drug effects (Table 2-1). Kalow has characterized many of these genetic disorders.[92] Drug responses studied in large numbers of persons usually reveal a unimodal frequency distribution curve for any particular drug action. The unimodal distribution curves characteristic of biological variability are usually attributable to multifactorial inheritance. Several drugs, such as

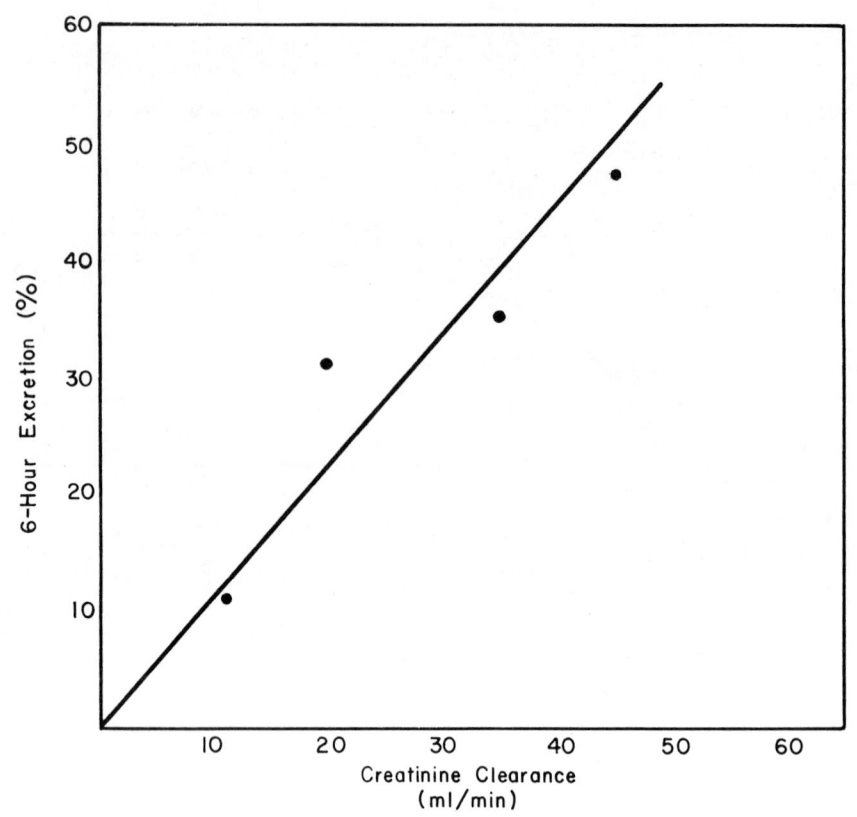

Figure 2–3. Relationship between 6-hour procainamide excretion and creatinine clearance in 4 patients with renal impairment. (From Weily, H. S., and Genton, E.: Arch. Intern. Med., 130:368, 1972.)

succinylcholine and isoniazid, have shown a discontinuous variation characteristic of bimodal or trimodal distribution. Such responses are attributable to single heritable determinants, and have been shown to result from modifications in the metabolism of drugs, which are usually associated with a specific enzyme deficiency. This may lead to adverse drug effects following genetic patterns.

Drugs taken during pregnancy or while breast-feeding infants may predispose the fetus or the infant to adverse reactions and variations in the pharmacologic action of drugs. Thalidomide is a well-known example of a teratogenic drug.[168] When this drug was administered to women between the 35th and 50th days of pregnancy, it produced dramatic embryopathies. Many prescription and non-prescription medications given to pregnant women may have adverse but unrecognized effects upon the fetus. Unless a drug produces an easily recognizable anatomic or physiologic abnormality, the effect may be unnoticed at birth and its association with a drug taken by the mother during pregnancy may be undetected. For example, a defect which manifests itself as a learning or behavioral disorder in a school-aged child would be very difficult to associate with a particular drug taken by the mother during pregnancy.

Major anatomic deformities of the fetus are more likely to occur

TABLE 2-1. Hereditary Characteristics Causing Increased Risks to Drug Reactions

INHERITED FACTOR	INCREASED RISK OF DRUG REACTIONS	EFFECT	REFERENCE
Abnormal plasma pseudocholinesterase	Succinylcholine	Prolonged apnea	91 102
Enzyme deficiency (erythrocyte) Glucose-6-phosphate dehydrogenase	Primaquine, Sulfonamides	Hemolysis	95
6-Phosphogluconic dehydrogenase	Sulfones		28
Glutathione reductase	Nitrofurans		138
Methemoglobin reductase (diaphorases)	Sulfonamides Acetanilid, nitrites Amines	Methemoglobinemia	29
Hemoglobin variants			
Hemoglobin H	Sulfonamides, nitrites	Hemolysis	143
Hemoglobin Zurich	Sulfonamides, primaquine	Hemolysis	55
Hepatic glucuronyl transferase (Crigler-Najjar syndrome)	Salicylates, menthol Corticosteroids	Decreased conjugation of these drugs	93
Hepatic porphyria	Barbiturates	Increased porphyrin synthesis	173
Glaucoma (certain types)	Corticosteroids	Exacerbation of disease	4
Slow acetylators Decreased ability of hepatic acetylation	Isoniazid	Prolonged half-life of drug	52
	Phenelzine		51
	Hydralazine		137
	Sulfamethazine		50
	Dapsone		139
Blood groups A, B, AB	Digoxin	Greater risk of arrhythmias in patients with A, B, and AB vs. O	84
	Oral contraceptives	Greater risk of developing venous thromboembolic disease in patients with A, B, and AB vs. O	85
Unknown	Nortriptyline	Increased plasma levels of drug	1

when drugs are given during the first trimester of pregnancy.[133] After the first trimester, the adverse effects of drugs on the fetus are not likely to result in such severe abnormalities. Prenatal use of an antidepressant drug (nortriptyline) has resulted in a case of urinary retention in a neonate for 17 hours after birth.[157] Since the newborn may not readily metabolize these drugs, their half-life will be prolonged, and therefore the fetus may have a more prolonged exposure to them than the mother.

Bleyer and Breckenridge studied the effects of prenatal aspirin on hemostasis in the newborn.[20] Three of 14 infants exposed to aspirin during the week prior to birth had recognizable defects in hemostasis or clotting functions at birth. Platelet aggregation was defective in all neonates exposed to aspirin, while platelet function was normal in 17 neonates not exposed to aspirin in utero.

Numerous drugs have been reported to adversely affect the fetus or neonate (Table 2–2). Until the safety of a drug can be firmly established, the use of drugs during pregnancy should be restricted to those that are absolutely necessary or are known to have no deleterious effects upon the fetus.

The newborn infant may be an unintended recipient of drugs contained in the mother's breast milk. Numerous reports have described pharmacologic responses to drugs in the newborn when mothers who were breast-feeding their infants were using various drugs. Table 2–3 lists examples of drugs known to be excreted in breast milk.

DETERMINANTS OF ADVERSE DRUG REACTIONS IN SICK PERSONS

Consider a depressed elderly patient requiring treatment with an antidepressant, such as amitriptyline. In addition to its antidepressant action, this drug has atropine-like actions, it inhibits the membrane-pump mechanism responsible for the uptake of norepinephrines, and it has been reported to produce arrhythmias, including prolongation of

TABLE 2–2. Common Drugs Associated with Fetal Abnormalities

Drug	Malformation or Adverse Effect	Reference
Aminopterin	Cleft palate	19
Anticoagulants	Hemorrhage (fatal)	65
Diphenylhydantoin	Cleft gum, lip and palate	131
Methyltestosterone	Pseudohermaphrodism	70
Streptomycin	Otic damage	36
Tetracycline	Tooth discoloration	170
Thiouracil	Hypothyroidism and goiter	6

TABLE 2–3. Common Drugs Excreted in Breast Milk

Drug	Observed Effect on Infant	Reference
Anthroquinones (laxatives)	Increased bowel activity in infant	97
Bromides	Drowsiness and rashes	101
Diazepam	Lethargy, weight loss	136
Heroin	Withdrawal symptoms	34
Lithium carbonate	None observed	190
Penicillin	None observed	69
Phenindione	Increased prothrombin time and hematoma	47

conduction time. Anticholinergic effects of this drug may preclude its use in a patient with a history of urinary retention or angle-closure glaucoma. If the patient has hypertension and is being treated with guanethidine, amitriptyline will antagonize the action of the antihypertensive drug and interfere with control of the patient's blood pressure. Arrhythmias, such as intraventricular conduction defects, may be worsened by the drug.

Many drugs cause adverse reactions in patients that occur less frequently or not at all in healthy people. The problem of increased risks of drug reactions in patients with renal failure has already been described. Smith, et al. found that sedative and diuretic drugs produced adverse effects four times more often in patients with decreased renal function than in patients with normal renal function.[160] Goodfriend has described a number of pathologic conditions which affect responses to drugs.[63]

A history of a previous adverse drug reaction has been found to be associated with an increased frequency of the occurrence of subsequent drug-induced disease.[79] Patients admitted to a hospital with an adverse drug reaction are much more likely to develop another reaction in the hospital than other patients.[56] Patients with active ulcer, neoplastic, or inflammatory gastrointestinal diseases may be predisposed to allergic reactions to orally administered drugs.[33] Infectious mononucleosis predisposes patients to severe cutaneous reactions when they are treated with ampicillin.[135]

PHARMACOLOGIC DETERMINANTS OF ADVERSE REACTIONS

Adverse pharmacologic effects of drugs are influenced by size of dose, rate of absorption (except when drugs are administered by the intravenous route), distribution, and elimination. Factors that influence the concentration of active (unbound) drugs in the plasma are depicted in Figure 2–4.[67]

First, the drug must be absorbed either from the gastrointestinal tract or from any other site to which it was administered. Once the

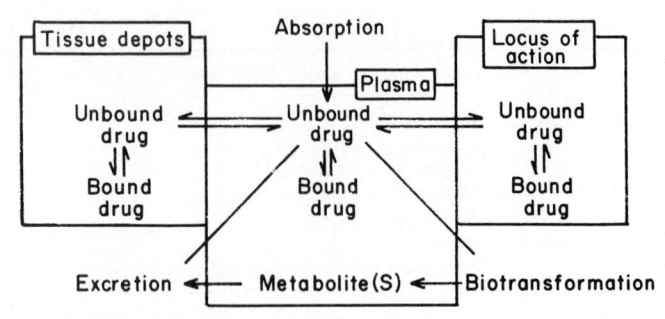

Figure 2-4. Factors influencing the concentration of a drug in the plasma and hence its locus of action. (From Gourley, D. R. H., *In:* Fulton, W. F. M., ed., Modern Trends in Pharmacology and Therapeutics, London, Butterworth, 1967, p. 2.)

drug is absorbed, it may be bound to proteins and other macromolecules, while the unbound drug in the plasma is in equilibrium with tissue depots and sites of action. This equilibrium is constantly changing as a result of excretion of unchanged drug molecules or of drug metabolites following biotransformation.

The physical and chemical properties of a drug also will influence its absorption, its distribution in the body, and its excretion patterns. Pharmacologic action and adverse effects, therefore, are influenced by a drug's kinetics, dosing schedule, method of administration, and formulation.

Absorption and Distribution

The lipid solubility, dissociation constant, and molecular weight of a drug affect its absorption, distribution and excretion. Most pharmacologically important, lipid soluble drugs cross biologic membranes by simple diffusion, and the drug moves from a region of high drug concentration to a region of low drug concentration. The rate of diffusion is partially dependent upon the drug's degree of lipid solubility, expressed as the partition coefficient. The partition coefficient of a drug is determined by its distribution and equilibration in a two-phase system of water and lipid. The ratio of its concentration in the lipid phase to its concentration in the aqueous phase is the lipid/water partition coefficient.[149]

An excellent example of the effect of a high lipid/water partition coefficient on distribution of a drug is seen with glutethimide. When this drug is injected intravenously, it is distributed in a pattern similar to that of thiopental; concentration in the brain and other highly vascular tissue rises rapidly and then falls as the drug is redistributed to poorly perfused tissues.[94] As a result of its high partition coefficient, dialysis of this drug in overdosed patients must be accomplished with oil rather than with an aqueous solution.[3]

The degree of ionization of a drug also has a significant effect on its diffusion across biologic membranes, and therefore on its absorption from the site of administration, or reabsorption in the renal tubules. Biologic membranes, such as the gastrointestinal epithelium, are composed of lipid and allow the passive absorption of lipid-soluble drug molecules. The majority of drugs are weak organic acids or bases which form ions in aqueous solutions. The undissociated or un-ionized form of the drug has the greater lipid solubility, and therefore is more readily absorbed. Degree of ionization of a drug depends on the pH of the solution in which it is placed and the dissociation constant (pKa) of the drug. The pH yielding the largest percentage of un-ionized molecules in solution will, therefore, enhance absorption.[13]

The effect of pKa and gastric pH on absorption of drugs is illustrated in Table 2-4.[151] To a large extent, these same factors determine the magnitude of reabsorption of drugs in the renal tubules. Many drugs can alter the pH of body fluids and thereby change the absorption and excretion patterns of other drugs, as described later in this section.

There is a barrier limiting the access of many drugs to the brain and affecting their transfer from the blood to the cerebrospinal fluid. The blood-brain and blood-cerebrospinal fluid barriers are highly resistant to the passage of completely ionized substances. Drugs which are largely un-ionized in plasma penetrate into the brain at rates determined by their lipid/water partition coefficient.[24,53] These same factors apparently control the extent of the passage of drugs into the lipoid-like placental barrier. For example, drugs with moderate to

TABLE 2-4. Effect of Drug pKa and Gastric pH on Absorption of Weak Acids and Bases from the Rat Stomach°

		PER CENT ABSORBED IN 1 HOUR	
DRUG	PKA	pH 1	pH 8
Acids			
5-Sulfosalicylic	2.0	0	0
Phenolsulfonphthalein	2.0	2	2
Salicylic	3.0	61	13
Acetylsalicylic	3.5	35	—
Secobarbital	7.9	30	—
Bases			
Caffeine	0.8	24	—
Antipyrine	1.4	14	—
Quinine	8.4	0	18
Mecamylamine	11.2	0	—

° Modified from Schanker, L. S., Shore, P. A., Brodie, B. B., and Hogben, C. A. M.: Absorption of drugs from the stomach. I., The rat. J. Pharmacol. Exp. Ther., 120: 528, 1957. Copyright © 1957, The Williams & Wilkins Co., Baltimore.[151]

high lipid solubility, such as anesthetic gases, barbiturates and meperidine, appear rapidly in fetal blood after administration to the mother, while lipid-insoluble substances, such as inulin, dextran, and many quarternary ammonium ions, do not.[150]

Protein Binding

The interaction of drugs with proteins can have a profound effect on their distribution in body tissues, as well as on their rate of elimination.[66]

Several plasma proteins interact with inorganic or organic drug molecules, but binding to serum albumin is the most important factor affecting a drug's pharmacologic action. Putnam has described the types of molecules which are bound to different plasma proteins[141] (Fig. 2–5). The rate of transfer of a drug from blood into tissue by means of diffusion across capillary membranes depends upon the concentration gradient of the unbound drug. The higher the proportion of a drug bound to serum proteins, the lower its proportion in the

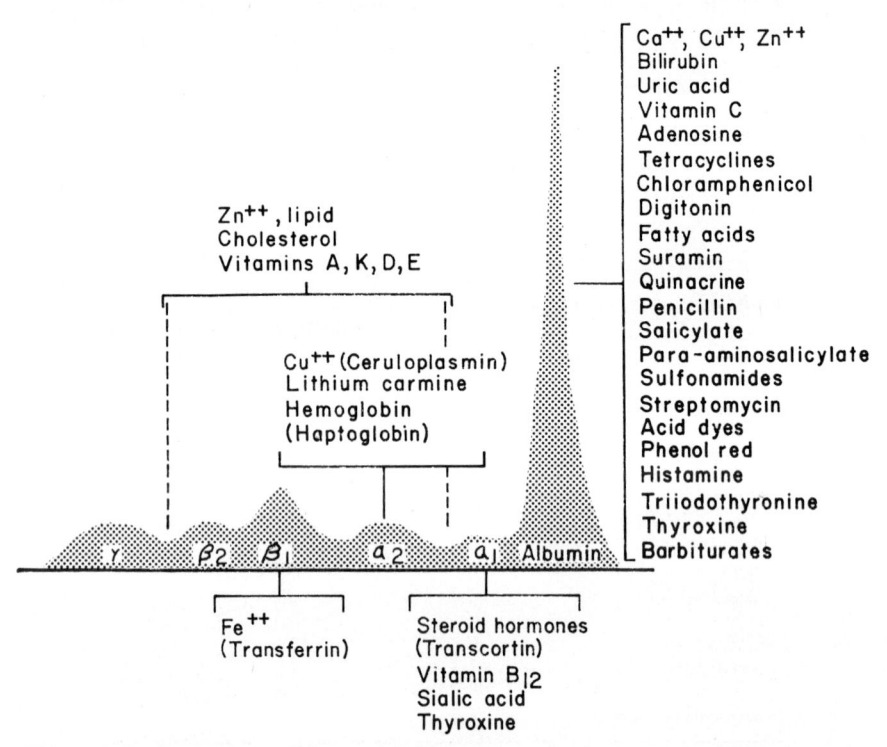

Figure 2–5. Interaction of drugs and chemicals with plasma proteins. Plasma proteins are depicted according to their relative amounts (y-axis). (Adapted from Putnam, F. W., Structure and Function of the Plasma Proteins. In: Neurath, H., ed., The Proteins, vol. 3, 2nd ed., New York, Academic Press, Inc., 1965.)

extravascular tissues, and the slower its rate of disappearance from the blood. For example, warfarin is approximately 98 per cent bound to albumin, leaving only 2 per cent of free unbound drug with pharmacologic activity. Anything which decreases the degree of binding of drug to serum albumin will increase the per cent of unbound, pharmacologically active drug. The bond of drug to albumin, however, is weak, reversible, and equilibrated with the amount of unbound drug.

The level of serum albumin can affect drug response. Patients receiving diphenylhydantoin, and having varying concentrations of serum albumin, will respond differently to the drug. Given standard doses of the drug, the patients with lower levels of serum albumin are three times as likely as those with higher serum albumin to develop adverse reactions. Hypoalbuminemic patients apparently have increased circulating levels of unbound diphenylhydantoin and a correspondingly increased risk to drug toxicity.[167]

Pharmacokinetics[180]

Increasing the dose of a drug will increase both the intensity and duration of the pharmacologic action, and may produce undesired effects. Therefore, amount and frequency of dose are factors influencing the therapeutic and deleterious effects of drugs.

When a drug is administered, only a proportion of that dose actually contributes to its concentration at an active site. The amount of the drug which is pharmacologically effective is dependent upon the rate and extent of its absorption, its tissue distribution, and its biotransformation and excretion. The time course of drug action can be separated into three phases: (1) latency, or the time of onset of action, (2) the time to peak effect, and (3) the duration of action (see Fig. 2-6).[104]

Time of onset of drug effect is that interval between administration and the first measurable sign of response. Time to peak effect is the interval between administration and the point where response to the drug is maximal. Duration of drug action is the period from the time of onset of an effect to termination of that effect. These time intervals are affected by rates of absorption, distribution, and elimination of the drug. In some instances, time of onset of action may be dependent on biotransformation of the drug from an inactive to an active form.

Most drugs move across biologic membranes by diffusion and at a rate proportional to their concentration gradient. Therefore, as the absorption process proceeds, the total amount of drug available at the administration site decreases and the concentration gradient also decreases. In this absorptive process, a constant fraction of the total amount of drug present is transported in equal units of time. This

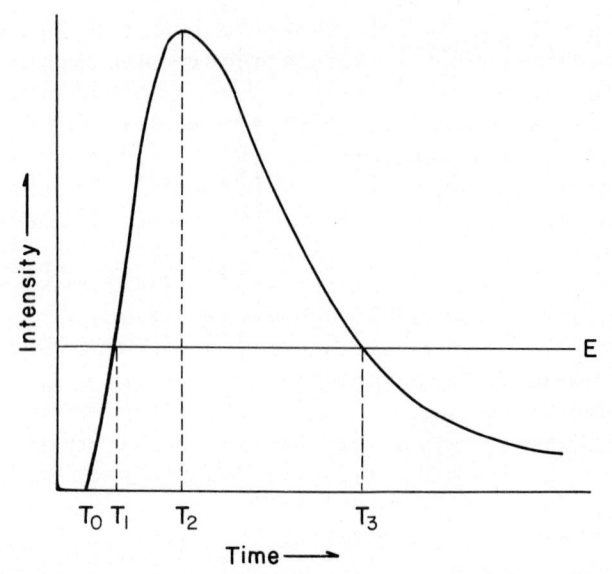

Figure 2-6. Intensity of effect as a function of time. Drug administered at Time 0 (T_0). (E = minimum level of measurable response; T_0 to T_1 = time for onset of drug effect; T_0 to T_2 = time to peak effect; T_1 to T_3 = duration of action.) (From Levine, R. R., Pharmacology: Drug Actions and Reactions, Boston, Little Brown and Co., 1973, p. 201.)

follows the kinetics of a first-order reaction (i.e., a reaction where velocity is proportional to the concentration of a single reactant). However, for many other drugs, the rate of absorption is constant and independent of the amount of drug available. One example of this type of absorption is active transport, a process whereby materials are transported against a concentration gradient. These two types of absorption are illustrated in Figure 2-7.[60]

For most drugs, their disappearance from the body is proportional to their concentration, and therefore, like absorption, elimination follows the principle of first-order kinetics. The rate at which a drug disappears from the body also is dependent on the rate of its biotransformation into inactive products and on its rate of excretion. The rate of elimination of a drug can be described by its biologic half-life or half-time for elimination, $T^{1}/_{2}$. This is the time necessary for the amount of unchanged drug in the body to be reduced to one-half its value after distribution equilibrium has been attained.[180]

The calculation of the half-life of a drug can be used to determine the frequency with which multiple doses can be safely administered. Biologic half-life is an inherent property of a drug, and it is not dependent on the manner in which the drug is administered; however, it may be altered in patients with a disease which alters processes of drug distribution, biotransformation, or elimination. As will be described later, many drug interactions result from one drug altering the half-life of another administered concurrently.

Drug Dosage

Since most drugs are eliminated according to first-order kinetics, the duration of action will increase as the logarithm of the dose increases. This means that to prolong the duration of action one half-life, the dose of the drug must be doubled.[107] This relationship is shown in Figure 2-8. For a drug with a 4-hour half-life and a minimal effective concentration of 1 unit per ml of plasma, the dose to produce a plasma concentration of 2 units per ml correspondingly increases the duration of action by 4 hours.

The method of prolonging action by doubling the dose may be totally unacceptable for highly toxic drugs. A more acceptable method would be to administer the initial therapeutic dose, followed by half that dose at intervals equal to the half-life of the drug. Even this regimen would be clinically unsuitable for drugs such as penicillin, which has a very short half-life (30 minutes), or bromide, which has a very long half-life (12 days). To prolong drug action using this method would require giving penicillin every 30 minutes, and bromide every 12 days. The technique commonly employed to overcome these problems is to replace the quantity of the drug lost during the dosing interval. By repeating this dose at appropriate intervals, adequate blood levels of the drug can be insured. The maintenance dose necessary, therefore, can be determined by the difference between the initial dose and the amount of the drug remaining at the end of the dosing interval.[148] By following this approach, the dosing in-

Figure 2-7. Absorption rate as a function of drug concentration at absorption site in passive absorption (Curve A) and active transport (Curve B). (From Gibaldi, M., Introduction to Biopharmaceutics, Philadelphia, Lea & Febiger, 1971, p. 10.)

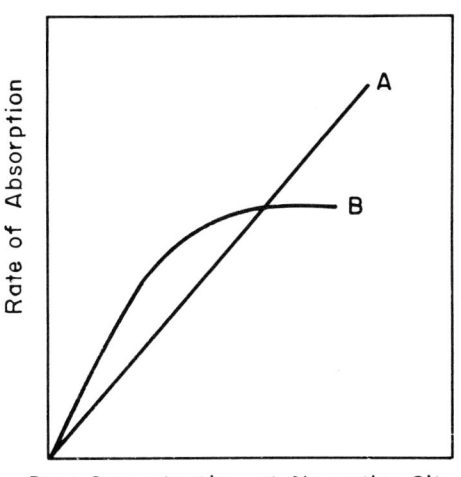

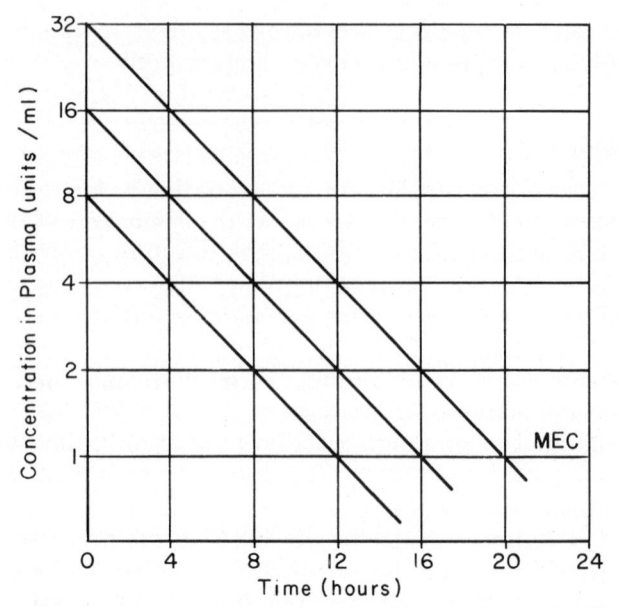

Figure 2-8. Relationship between duration of action and dose for a drug eliminated by first-order kinetics. Biologic half-life is 4 hours. If action lasts until the drug remaining in the body is reduced to the minimal effective concentration (MEC, shown in graph as 1 unit), then the duration of action increases as the logarithm of the dose increases. (Note that the units along the ordinate are on a geometric scale.) (From Levine, R. R., Pharmacology: Drug Actions and Reactions, Boston, Little, Brown and Co., 1973, p. 219.)

terval and the maintenance dose necessary to maintain a pharmacologically effective concentration of a drug can be determined.

Drugs are eliminated by an exponential process. Some of the drug remains in the body following the initial dosing, and at the time of the next dose. Therefore the amount of drug in the body will accumulate until the quantity excreted in the dosage interval is equal to the amount administered. Drug accumulations, therefore, may occur and result in adverse consequences. This problem has been illustrated with the use of bromide.[171] The bromide ion has a volume of distribution equivalent to the extracellular fluid. Its rate of excretion is slow because it is filtered at the glomerulus and extensively reabsorbed in the renal tubules, resulting in a half-life of 12 days. Repeated dosing, therefore, may cause bromism.

Pharmacologic Properties

Few drugs have restricted, precise, and narrow ranges of action. For example, salicylates have multiple pharmacologic actions, including: (1) local irritant effects to mucosa, (2) changes in the EEG,

(3) direct stimulation of respiration, (4) increased volume of bile, (5) reduced plasma prothrombin levels, (6) increased urinary excretion of urates, (7) decreased aggregation of thrombocytes, (8) negative nitrogen balance in large doses, (9) alteration of acid-base balance, and (10) uncoupling of oxidative phosphorylation with inhibitory action of many ATP dependent reactions.

Drugs with a small therapeutic/toxic ratio, or with multiple pharmacologic effects, therefore, are most likely to produce adverse reactions. A comparison of risks of several common drugs is presented in Table 2–5.

The incidence of side effects of a particular drug may be greatly altered by changing the route of administration. For example, hypotension is a common side effect when quinidine is given parenterally, but is rarely observed when the drug is given orally.[128] This may be attributable to higher peak blood levels and differences in metabolism of the drug when it is given parenterally.

Epidemiologic studies have indicated those drugs that are frequently associated with adverse reactions (Table 2–6), but detailed pharmacologic study is required before such effects can be verified or explained.

Bioavailability

Among approximately 3000 drugs evaluated recently, only 12 had been studied in humans under controlled conditions to determine bioavailability.[179] There were differences in bioavailability in the preparations of 7 of these 12 drugs marketed by different manufacturers. These seven drugs included riboflavin, aspirin, p-aminosalicylic acid, chloramphenicol, diphenylhydantoin, tetracycline, and oxytetracycline.

The oral administration of four different chloramphenicol preparations showed wide variations in resulting blood levels.[62] In this study

TABLE 2–5. *Comparison of Risks of Adverse Effects by Drug*

Drug	Type of Reaction	Incidence of Adverse Effect (Per Cent of Patients Reacting)	Reference
Amphotericin B	Chills, fever, nausea, vomiting, malaise	75	176
5-Fluorouracil	Gastrointestinal, blood, skin	77	129
Cephaloglycin	Gastrointestinal, central nervous system	40	172
Digoxin	Gastrointestinal, arrhythmias	18	156
Prednisone	Psychiatric, gastrointestinal	17	22

TABLE 2-6. High-Risk Drugs

Investigator	Type of Study	Drugs Studied
Caranasos et al.[27]	Drug reactions leading to hospitalization (adult patients, nonsurgical)	Most common drug(s) causing reactions leading to hospitalization Aspirin Digoxin Warfarin Hydrochlorothiazide Prednisone
Miller[125]	Drug reactions occurring in hospitalized patients	Drugs with highest adverse reaction rate Heparin Prednisone Spironolactone Hydrochlorothiazide Digoxin
McKenzie et al.[121]	Drug reactions occurring in hospitalized patients (pediatric patients, nonsurgical)	Drugs most frequently causing adverse reactions Prednisone Ampicillin Vincristine Dextrose/Water Digoxin

subjects were given a single 500 mg oral dose of chloramphenicol, and one product produced plasma levels nearly twice as high as those of a product made by a different manufacturer. Variations in the biologic availability of digoxin prepared by four manufacturers has also been shown.[109] In a cross-over study, identical doses of digoxin from different manufacturers were administered to patients. Significant differences in serum digoxin levels were achieved, with one product producing peak serum levels seven times those obtained with another product. Significant variations were also observed among different lots of the same manufacturer's product.

In view of these reported differences, particularly with clinically important drugs having a narrow therapeutic/toxic ratio, and those requiring precise blood concentrations to achieve desired effects, bioavailability data or pharmaceutical data shown to indicate bioavailability of each product must be obtained to avoid adverse effects.

OTHER DETERMINANTS OF ADVERSE DRUG REACTIONS

Factors examined earlier which play a role in the development of adverse drug reactions may not be related to the inherent characteristics of a single drug or to patient variations. Medication errors, drug interactions, and multiple-drug therapy also can play a significant role in drug-induced disease.

Medication Errors by Outpatients

At the University of Florida, an unfortunately large number of patients are admitted to the medical service with adverse drug reactions resulting not from a drug's inherent toxic property or an idiosyncratic effect, but from improper use of the drug. Failure to take or administer a drug properly, therefore, is a determinant of adverse drug reactions. The percentage of patients who commit errors in the self-administration of prescribed medications, with few exceptions, ranges from 25 to 59 per cent. Studies of medication errors are summarized in Table 2-7. In one study of diabetic patients, 7 out of 34 patients measured either half or double the prescribed dose of insulin by using the wrong scale on the U40-U80 syringe. In another study, cardiac patients were interviewed shortly after discharge from the hospital to determine if they were taking the prescribed medication, and it was found that 92 per cent had continued to use digoxin, 83 per cent had continued to use hydrochlorothiazide, but only 60 per cent had continued to use a potassium-chloride supplement.[25]

Mazzullo has described several nonpharmacologic therapeutic principles which might decrease medication errors in ambulatory patients.[118] He feels that look-alike medications should not be prescribed for the same patient because of the possibility of confusion. He recommends that when possible, medication should be prescribed on the basis of pharmaceutical characteristics such as size, shape, and color

*TABLE 2-7. Medication Error Studies**

Authors	Patient Type (Diagnosis)	No. of Patients Monitored	Per Cent of Patients Making Errors	Drug Studied	Type of Institution	Classification of Patient
Schwartz[152]	Mixed	178	59 26, serious errors	Mixed	General medical clinic, New York Hospital	Not stated
Malahy[115]	Mixed	40	36 to 90	Mixed	University (outpatient clinic)	Not stated
Watkins et al.[181]	Diabetes mellitus	115	58	Insulin	Two university metabolism clinics	Not stated
		47	26	Oral hypoglycemic		
Clinite and Kabat[32]	Mixed	30		Mixed	Veterans hospital	Veteran
Latiolais and Berry[103]	Eye, ear, nose and throat General medical Circulatory Surgical Obstetrics-gynecology Psychiatry	180	42.8	Mixed	University clinics	Indigent
Libow and Mehl[108]	Mixed	20	25	Placebo	Mt. Sinai Hospital	Elderly

* From Stewart, R. B. and Cluff, L. E.: A review of medication errors and compliance in ambulant patients, Clin. Pharmacol. Ther., 13:463-468, 1972.[163]

of the preparations, as well as on the basis of their pharmacologic action and therapeutic purpose.

Inpatient Medication Errors

The problem of medication errors is not peculiar to ambulatory patients. There have been numerous studies of medication errors in hospitals. In a study in 1962, Barker and McConnell found that the average nurse made one error for every six medications given.[10] While most of these errors were due to omission of drug administration, errors in dosage calculation and drug selection were also found. The development of a system of preparing unit doses in hospitals represents an attempt to reduce such errors. In this system, medications are processed in a package for individual patient use and delivered to the nursing station prior to the time for drug administration. Careful studies have demonstrated that the unit-dose system results in significantly fewer medication errors than traditional methods of drug distribution.[81] Installing this type of drug-distribution system in hospitals is one approach to preventing adverse drug reactions. As a result of the demonstrated effectiveness of the unit-dose system, the government is now encouraging its use in its hospitals.[166]

Multiple-Drug Therapy

Patients often are given many diagnostic and therapeutic agents which may cause an adverse reaction or interact to produce reactions. Hospitalized patients studied who had experienced adverse effects from drugs had received an average of 14 drugs.[153] In a study of drug utilization in six hospitals, Jick et al. found the average number of exposures to be 8.4 drugs.[87]

The rate of adverse effects increases disproportionately with an increase in the number of drugs given. Smith et al. observed an adverse reaction rate of 40 per cent in patients given 16 to 20 drugs, compared with a rate of 7 per cent in those given 6 to 10 drugs[160] (Fig. 2-9). The frequency of adverse reactions to drugs has been directly related to the number of drugs administered.[57] Decreasing the number of drug exposures is an effective and relatively simple method to decrease adverse drug reactions.

History of Previous Drug Reactions

Approximately 50 per cent of patients seen in a hospital outpatient clinic have reported intolerance to one or more drugs.[165] The predisposition of patients who have experienced one adverse drug reaction to additional reactions to different drugs is known. This identifies one determinant of such reactions which, at the moment, is largely unexplained.

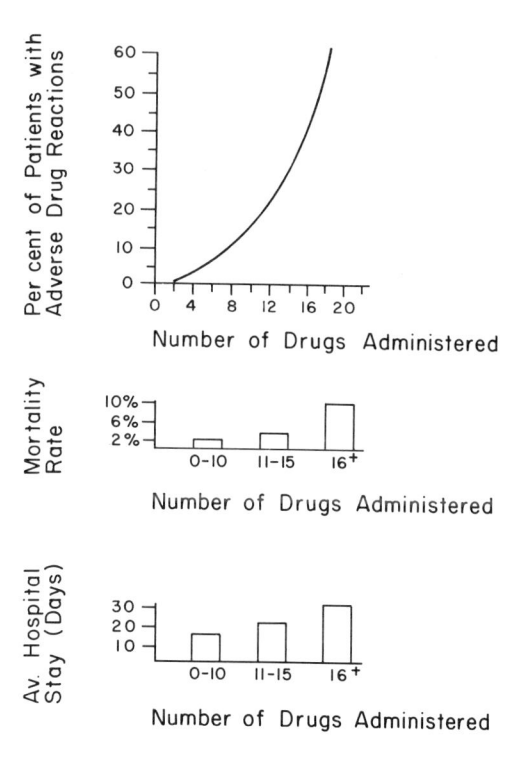

Figure 2-9. The relationship of rate of adverse drug reactions to (1) number of drugs administered, (2) mortality rate, and (3) duration of hospitalization. (Findings of Smith, J. W., Seidl, L. G., and Cluff, L. E.: Ann. Intern. Med., 65:631, 1966.)

Drug Interactions

The possibility that one drug may affect the activity of a concurrently administered agent has long been recognized.[111] These interactions may cause an increased or diminished activity of drugs, and may be desirable or undesirable. Systematic investigation of drug interaction, however, has been difficult, and recognition of certain effects has most often been a result of unplanned observation.

The importance of adverse drug interactions as a public health problem has not been clearly established, but the increasing number of different prescription and nonprescription drugs used by patients, and the increasing frequency of reports of clinically significant drug interactions suggest they may be common. Further study is required to identify drug interactions which represent serious problems in medical management.

Many publications reporting drug interactions have appeared in the past few years.[72,75,80] Some of these have attempted to clarify the subject, but many simply list hundreds of reports of drug interactions. A major portion of the literature deals with theoretical predictions of possible interactions, animal studies, and in vitro reports. Recognizing the multiplicity and variable clinical validity of studies on drug interactions, in 1973 the American Pharmaceutical Association published

44   PHARMACOLOGIC MECHANISMS

Evaluations of Drug Interactions, an attempt to present the available data on the subject in a clear and coherent manner.[48]

Drug interactions result from alterations by one drug in the absorption, distribution, metabolism, pharmacologic action, and excretion of other drugs. These mechanisms of interactions are depicted in Figure 2-10. Understanding these mechanisms is essential in predicting, detecting, and preventing adverse interactions between drugs taken by patients.

Alterations of Absorption

Clinical response to a medication can be altered by changing either the rate of drug absorption or the total amount of drug absorbed. Changing the rate of absorption or total quantity of drug absorbed significantly alters its concentration in the blood. Decreasing the total amount of drug absorbed is equivalent to decreasing the dose given. Decreasing the rate of drug absorption may result in ineffective drug blood levels. In addition, onset of pharmacologic effect may be greatly delayed, a significant factor to consider when speed of action is important.[11]

Nonionized drugs are more readily absorbed than the ionized form. In general, acidic drugs, such as aspirin and sulfonamides, are more readily absorbed from the stomach, where they exist in a non-

FATE OF DRUGS IN THE BODY AND SITES OF DRUG INTERACTIONS

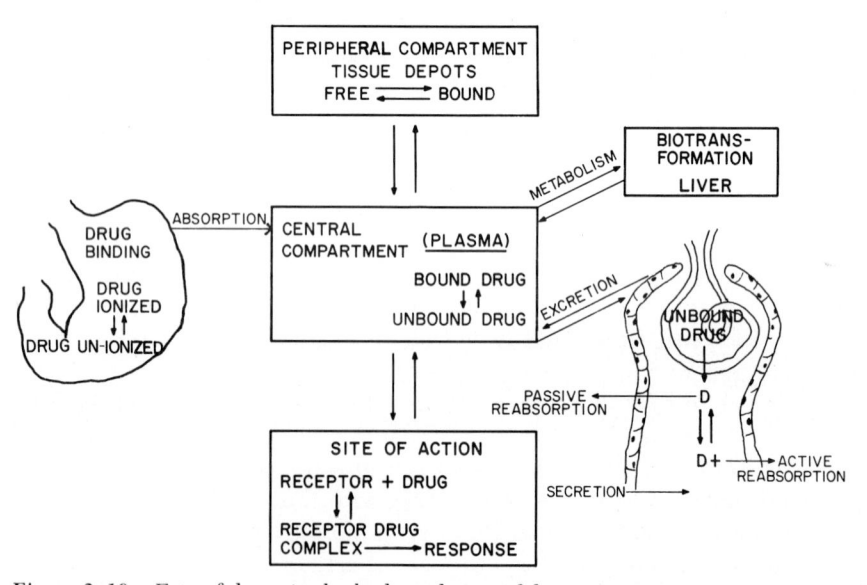

Figure 2-10. Fate of drugs in the body and sites of drug interactions.

ionized form, while basic drugs are absorbed from the small intestine. In theory, any drug which can change the pH of the gastrointestinal lumen could also alter the rate or amount of absorption of a concurrently administered medication. Clinically, however, these changes may have little effect on the response of a patient to a drug.[48] For example, Ambre and Fischer were unable to demonstrate that aluminum hydroxide caused any significant alteration in the absorption of warfarin when those drugs were administered concurrently to human subjects.[2]

Binding of one drug by another in the gastrointestinal tract is another mechanism of altering drug absorption. A widely known example of drug-drug binding is the interaction between tetracycline derivatives and divalent or trivalent metals such as aluminium, calcium, or magnesium. A chelate forms between these two agents and retards absorption of the antibiotic.[100] Sodium bicarbonate administered concurrently with tetracycline also decreases absorption, but this may be brought about by a different mechanism.[12] Reduction (40 to 85 per cent) of oxytetracycline, methacycline, and doxycycline blood levels has been associated with chelation of these drugs with ferrous sulfate given concomitantly.[130]

Chelation of toxic substances by drugs has been used therapeutically to control intoxications. A universal antidote consisting of activated charcoal, magnesium oxide, and tannic acid has been employed to bind and neutralize such ingested toxic substances. Desferrioxamine has a specific ability to chelate iron, and can be used to treat acute iron intoxication.[82] Similar applications have been used in treating intoxication from phosphorus.[185] Charcoal and kaolin can be very effective in treating drug overdoses by reducing the amount of drug absorbed.[78] However, this same effect may be undesirable if it interferes with a prescribed therapeutic regimen. For example, Figure 2–11 shows how a kaolin-pectin mixture can interfere with absorption of lincomycin.[178] A significant portion of the antibiotic is apparently absorbed on kaolin and passes through the gastrointestinal tract.

Ion-exchange resins, cholestyramine, and sodium polystyrene sulfonate have been used orally to prevent intestinal absorption and thereby facilitate elimination of certain materials. In one investigation, cholestyramine, when administered concomitantly with warfarin, was found to significantly decrease mean levels of warfarin in the plasma.[147] These findings suggest that interaction of other drugs with ion-exchange resins is probable, and until further studies are completed administration of ion-exchange resins with other drugs should be avoided.

Relatively minor changes in the formulation of a product can have a major effect on its rate of absorption. In Australia, a manufacturer changed the excipient in diphenylhydantoin-sodium capsules, and this resulted in increased blood levels of diphenylhydantoin and

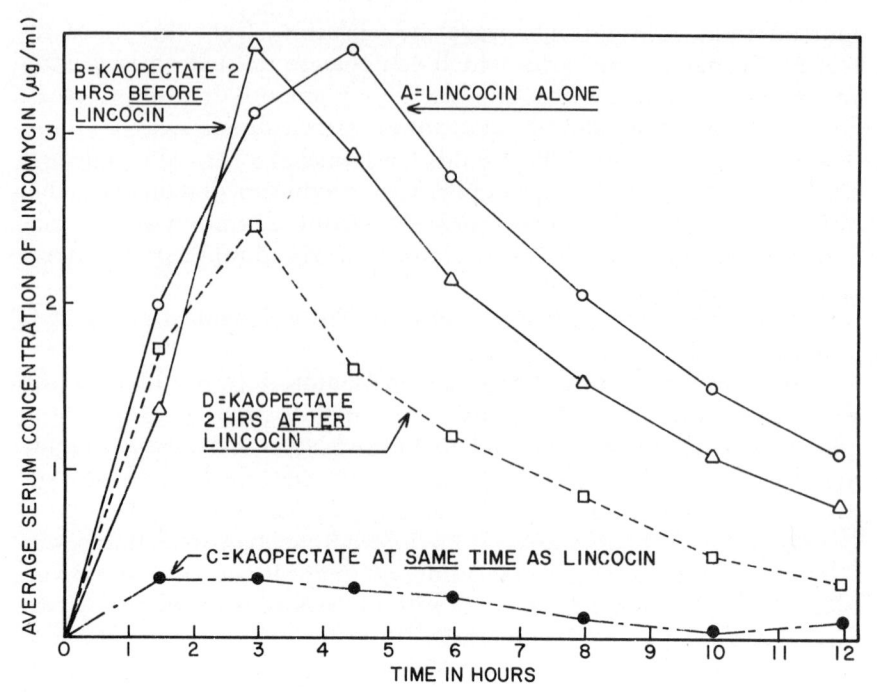

Figure 2–11. Average serum concentrations of lincomycin observed in a 4-way crossover study with light subjects. (From Wagner, J. G.: Design and data analysis of biopharmaceutical studies in man, Canad. J. Pharm. Sciences, 1:55–68, 1966.)

intoxication. All patients affected were taking one brand of 100 mg diphenylhydantoin capsules. The intoxications were attributed to changing the excipient from calcium sulfate dihydrate to lactose, which produced increased drug absorption.[174]

Changes in peristaltic movement also can affect the total amount of drug absorbed, particularly of slowly and incompletely absorbed agents such as digoxin and tetracyclines. Drugs such as atropine or parasympatholytics will increase gastric pH, delay gastric emptying time, and may decrease the total amount or rate of drug absorption. Prolongation of gastric emptying time may decrease absorption of drugs such as penicillin and erythromycin, which are degraded in acid conditions of the stomach. Tricyclic antidepressants have been shown to have sufficient anticholinergic activity to retard the intestinal absorption of other drugs.[41,42] Conversely, it has been suggested that cathartics may speed passage through the gastrointestinal tract, thereby reducing drug absorption.[7]

A common drug combination (chlorpromazine and trihexyphenidyl) used in treatment of psychiatric patients has recently been found to result in ineffective therapeutic blood levels of chlorpromazine. It was found that trihexyphenidyl results in significant lowering of plasma chlorpromazine levels. This mechanism may be due to the anticholinergic effect of trihexyphenidyl, resulting in decreased gastric emptying and slower transit of chlorpromazine, and thus allowing for increased metabolism of the drug in the intestine.[144]

Alteration of Drug Distribution

During the transport and distribution of drugs via the blood, drugs may be reversibly bound to tissues. The ratio of free drug to bound drug depends upon the properties of the drug, the physiological state of the patient, and the presence of other drugs in the tissue.

Albumin accounts for approximately 50 per cent of total serum protein and plays a major role in drug binding. At normal plasma pH (7.4) albumin has a net negative charge, but it may interact with anions as well as cations. The number of binding sites for a specific drug on an albumin molecule is usually very small and is dependent upon the drug's structure. Most drugs are reversibly bound to albumin. The bound drug is not free to diffuse to receptor sites and is, therefore, inactive. The bound portion is in equilibrium with the unbound free and active form of the drug. Several factors determine the fraction of total drug bound to plasma protein: drug concentration in plasma, plasma-protein concentration, number of binding sites on the protein, and the equilibrium-affinity constant. The fraction of bound drug decreases as the total plasma concentration of drug increases or as the concentration of protein decreases.

When two or more drugs are given to a patient, the binding of one drug may be affected by another, particularly if they are bound at the same sites. Displacement of drug from plasma protein will initially result in an increase of unbound drug in the plasma, and in turn an increased concentration at receptor sites. Owing to an increased level of free drug, elimination rates from the body may actually be increased, since more drug is available to the liver for metabolism and a higher concentration is presented to the glomerulus for filtration.

Alteration in drug-protein interaction can be a cause of toxic reactions or unexpected responses to a drug. The effect of drug-protein displacement is particularly hazardous in the case of anticoagulants such as warfarin and dicumarol. At effective plasma concentrations, these agents exhibit a high degree of binding to albumin. Concomitant use of drugs with an affinity for the same binding sites on albumin (see Table 2-8) will lead to an increased concentration of unbound drug, which may result in increased levels of the anticoagulant and unexpected increases in prothrombin time. Sellers and Koch-Weser found that chloral hydrate increased plasma levels of free warfarin when administered to subjects given anticoagulants.[154] Displacement of one drug by the other is believed to occur, since chloral hydrate is metabolized to trichloroacetic acid, a substance possessing strong affinity for binding sites on serum albumin. Potentiation in the form of displacement of coumadin by phenylbutazone from binding sites has been reported to lead to serious bleeding episodes.[77] It has also been reported that the antineoplastic drug methotrexate will be displaced by drugs such as salicylates and sulfonamides when they are used concomitantly.[140]

Simultaneous administration of any two drugs listed in Table 2-8 may result in increased blood levels of either or both drugs, particularly when those drugs with a high degree of binding are given in high doses. In their interaction with plasma protein, drugs may also affect other substances. Bilirubin, which is bound to plasma protein, can also be displaced by these drugs. Kernicterus has been precipitated in icteric premature infants who have been treated with sulfonamides; this results from redistribution of bilirubin bound to protein and tissues, and subsequent high levels of bilirubin in the blood.[158]

When dealing with this type of drug interaction, it is desirable for the physician to have information on the relative binding capacities of drugs being prescribed (i.e., whether or not drug A will displace drug B). Unfortunately, this type of information is not presently available. Sellers and Koch-Weser have used an in vitro method to determine the relative potency of displacing agents.[155] Competitive binding of warfarin to human albumin was studied by equilibrium dialysis. Relative displacement potency of drugs was, in decreasing order: mefenamic acid, ethacrynic acid, diazoxide, and nalidixic acid. A method has also been described by Solomon and Thomas to estimate constants of drug-albumin affinity in human plasma.[161] Whether or not these studies adequately predict in vivo binding is not clear. Until more complete information is available, physicians should recognize the potential hazards of combination therapy with these agents, and exercise particular care in monitoring for undesirable effects.

TABLE 2-8. Representative Drugs Reported to Bind to Albumin

Clofibrate (Atromid-S)
Diphenylhydantoin (Dilantin)
Phenylbutazone (Butazolidin)
Oxyphenbutazone (Tandearil)
Salicylates
Indomethacin (Indocin)
Chloral Hydrate
Diazoxide
Sulfonamides

Interaction of Drugs at Receptor Sites

Binding sites or receptors of cell membranes are involved in drug action, and agents which facilitate or antagonize the interaction of a drug with a receptor site may correspondingly affect drug action.[189] Binding sites on serum proteins are not directly involved in drug action and are referred to as secondary receptors, silent receptors, or storage sites.

A drug that combines with receptors and stimulates a biological response is said to have affinity and intrinsic activity, and is termed an agonist. Conversely, a drug that combines with the same receptor site but does not initiate a biological response and lacks intrinsic activity acts as a competitive antagonist.

There are varying degrees of agonists and antagonists. A partial agonist is one that produces a smaller effect than other drugs acting on the same receptor. Antagonists can be classified as competitive when they combine reversibly with the same binding sites as the active drug but can be displaced from these sites by an excess of the agonist. An antagonist is said to be noncompetitive when its effects cannot be overcome by increasing concentrations of the agonist. This competitive or noncompetitive binding of drugs to receptors is the mechanism responsible for most drug interactions on receptor sites. For example, atropine has a higher affinity-constant for receptors than acetylcholine. As a result, it displaces acetylcholine from the receptor site and decreases cholinergic effects. The blocking action of atropine can be reversed by administration of a cholinesterase inhibitor such as neostigmine, which will raise the level of acetylcholine, thus displacing atropine from binding sites. Naloxone acts as a competitive antagonist in the binding of morphine and similar narcotics to receptor sites, and is used to treat respiratory depression in morphine intoxication. Naloxone, when administered by itself, has essentially no effect on respiration.[83]

Thyroxine is believed to increase the anticoagulant effect of warfarin by noncompetitive binding to receptor sites of cells. It potentiates the effect of coumarins on prothrombin time, but has no detectable effect on plasma half-life or plasma-protein binding of the anticoagulants.[162]

Drugs may also interact by modifying enzymes which block the uptake or facilitate the release of active compounds at the site of action. Probably the most widely known example of enzyme inhibition is of monoamine oxidase (MAO). Monoamine oxidase metabolizes catecholamines and, when it is inhibited, levels of norepinephrine increase within the adrenergic neuron. Since large amounts of norepinephrine are stored, substances stimulating its release can result in an exaggerated sympathetic response. It was through this mechanism that MAO inhibitors, such as phenelzine (Nardil) and tranylcypromine (Parnate), produced headaches, hypertensive crises, and cardiac arrhythmias in patients using sympathomimetic amines such as amphetamine. Tricyclic antidepressants such as desipramine and amitriptyline (Elavil) reportedly inhibit the uptake of guanethidine into the adrenergic neuron, inhibiting the antihypertensive effect. Desipramine has been shown to inhibit the antihypertensive effect of guanethidine even after use of the antidepressant has been discontinued.[127]

Alterations in Metabolism

The smooth endoplasmic reticulum or microsomal fraction of the liver cells is the major site for the biotransformation of drugs, involving hydroxylation, dealkylation, and glucuronide conjugation. Drugs can alter biotransformation by stimulating or influencing microsomal enzymes, and can thereby influence the duration and intensity of action of those drugs metabolized by liver microsomes.

Enzyme induction increases the rate of metabolism of many drugs, and a variety of drugs induce an increase in microsomal enzymes.[40] Several hundred compounds, including hypnotics, anticonvulsants, and antihistamines, are known to stimulate metabolism of drugs when administered to animals, but few investigations have been carried out in human beings (Table 2-9). Enzyme induction by a drug is often recognized in patients by the exaggerated, depressed, or adverse effect of another drug administered concurrently. For example, phenobarbital, when administered simultaneously with warfarin and bishydroxycoumarin, has led to a decrease in the plasma levels and anticoagulant activity of these agents.[44,113] If an enzyme-inducing hypnotic drug is given to a patient at the same time he is being titrated with warfarin he may hemorrhage when the hypnotic drug is discontinued, unless the dose of the anticoagulant is reduced.

Environmental agents such as insecticides can also produce enzyme induction. For example, the half-life of antipyrine in subjects exposed to insecticides averaged 7.7 hours in contrast to a half-life of 13.1 hours in others who had not been exposed.[98]

In 1954, rats pretreated with an investigational compound, SKF 525-A, slept five times longer after being treated with hexobarbital

TABLE 2-9. *Enzyme Inducers*

Barbiturates	Nikethamide
Glutethimide	Diphenylhydantoin
Phenylbutazone	DDT
Chloral hydrate	Lindane
Meprobamate	Griseofulvin
Ethanol	

than those receiving hexobarbital alone.[37] The effects of meperidine, methadone, phenobarbital and other drugs were also enhanced.[38] The enhanced activity of these drugs resulted from an inhibitory effect of SKF 525-A on liver microsomal enzymes.[43]

Chloramphenicol retards the metabolic transformation of tolbutamide, diphenylhydantoin and dicumarol in human beings. When two grams per day of chloramphenicol are given to patients receiving these drugs, a considerable elevation in their serum levels results.[30] Allopurinol or nortriptyline can similarly inhibit the metabolism of antipyrine and bishydroxycoumarin.[175]

Alterations in Excretion

Numerous drugs have been shown to alter the excretion of concurrently administered drugs by several different mechanisms. In general, interactions affecting renal excretion of drugs will be clinically significant only when this is the primary route of elimination for the drug or its active metabolite. For example, digoxin is eliminated primarily by the kidneys; therefore, another drug which decreases elimination by this route may result in digitalis intoxication. On the other hand, digitoxin elimination is not greatly affected by decreased renal excretion because alternative elimination pathways are available to this drug.[142]

The drug fraction not bound to plasma proteins appears in the ultrafiltrate in the glomerulus. Reabsorption by passive diffusion into the renal tubule depends primarily upon the lipid solubility of the drug and the fraction of the drug in a nonionized state. As discussed before, a weakly acidic drug, such as aspirin or phenylbutazone, may be rapidly excreted in alkaline urine whereas a weakly basic drug, such as quinidine or amphetamine, may be more readily excreted in an acid urine. The half-life of certain drugs in serum, therefore, can be significantly altered by changes in urine pH. Those characteristics of drugs which can be affected by these changes include weak acids (with a pKa of 3 to 7) or weak bases (with pKa 7 to 11); the high partition coefficient of the un-ionized drug; and rate of excretion when there is significant elimination (greater than 20 per cent) by the renal route.[126,146] Alteration of urine pH by drugs can similarly change the half-life and pharmacologic action of simultaneously administered agents. There are many drugs which will alkalinize the urine (e.g., sodium bicarbonate, acetazolamide) and many that will acidify it (e.g., ammonium chloride, sodium biphosphate). Many commonly available agents such as ascorbic acid (vitamin C) and cranberry juice will also greatly acidify the urine.[119] The renal clearance of quinidine is reduced to one-tenth the normal level when urinary pH is increased from 6.0 to 7.5.[59] Similarly, the half-life of amphetamine can be doubled when the urinary pH is increased from 5 to 8. Weak acids such as salicylic acid, phenobarbital, and nalidixic acid have also been shown to exhibit pH-dependent urinary excretion.[126]

Interfering with active secretion across the renal tubular epithelium is yet another mechanism by which drugs may interact. Many acidic drugs, such as penicillins, salicylic acid, indomethacin, and thiazide diuretics, are transported from blood across the proximal tubular cell into tubular urine by an active secretory process.[184] A useful application of this interaction has been the use of probenecid to increase blood levels of penicillin. The renal excretion of labelled indomethacin also is inhibited by probenecid, and blood levels of indomethacin may be greatly increased in patients using both drugs concurrently.[159]

Interactions of Parenteral Medications

Many drugs are chemically or physically incompatible in solution and cannot be safely admixed for intravenous administration. Detection of this interaction is complicated because physical evidence of incompatibility, such as precipitation, need not be present to cause pharmacologic inactivation.

Several different drugs have been found to decompose when admixed prior to intravenous administration, without visual changes in solution.[134] Potassium penicillin G is most stable in the pH range of 6 to 7 and inactivation will result when it is mixed with acidic agents such as vitamin C. In one study the loss in potency from this mixture was 37 per cent in six hours.[123]

A review of incompatibilities involving intravenous admixtures can be found in publications of Bair, Fowler, and Webb.[8,54,182] To prevent the occurrence of this type of interaction, drugs should not be mixed prior to infusion whenever possible. In an effort to prevent these interactions, in many institutions responsibility for admixing drugs for intravenous use has been assumed by pharmacists. Centralizing this responsibility insures better control of these preparations.

REFERENCES

1. Alexanderson, B., and Sjoquist, F.: Individual differences in the pharmacokinetics of monomethylated tricyclic antidepressants: Role of genetic and environmental factors and clinical importance. Ann. N.Y. Acad. Sci., *179*:739–751, 1971.
2. Ambre, J. J., and Fischer, L. J.: Effect of coadministration of aluminum and magnesium hydroxides on absorption of anticoagulants in man. Clin. Pharmacol. Ther., *14*:231–237, 1973.
3. Arena, J. M.: Poisoning. 2nd ed., Springfield, Charles C Thomas, Publisher, 1970, p. 50.
4. Armaly, M. F., and Becker, B.: Intraocular pressure response to topical costicosteroids. Fed. Proc., *24*:1274–1278, 1965.
5. Armaly, M. F.: Genetic factors related to glaucoma. Ann. N.Y. Acad. Sci., *151*:861–875, 1968.

6. Asper, S. P., and Liss, R.: Fetal thyroid growth, In Barnes, A. C., ed., Intra-uterine Development. Philadelphia, Lea & Febiger, 1968.
7. Azarnoff, D. L., and Hurwitz, A.: Drug interactions. Pharmacol. Physicians, 4:2, 1970.
8. Bair, J. N.: A brief review of drug compatibility and stability literature. Am. J. Hosp. Pharm., 23:344–346, 1966.
9. Barker, K. N.: The demonstration and evaluation of an experimental medical system for U.A.M.C. hospital. In Barker, K. N., ed., Drug Systems Research, vol. 1, Little Rock, University of Arkansas Medical Center, 1967.
10. Barker, K. N., and McConnell, W. E.: How to detect medication errors. Mod. Hosp., 99:95–106, 1962.
11. Barr, W. H.: Factors involved in the assessment of systemic or biological availability of drug products. Drug Inform. Bull., 3:27–45, 1969.
12. Barr, W. H., Adir, J., and Garrettson, L.: Decrease of tetracycline absorption in man by sodium bicarbonate. Clin. Pharmacol. Ther., 12:779–784, 1971.
13. Bates, T. R., and Gibaldi, M.: Gastrointestinal absorption of drugs. In Swarbrick, J., ed., Current Concepts in Pharmaceutical Sciences: Biopharmaceutics, Philadelphia, Lea & Febiger, 1970.
14. Beckett, A. H., and Rowland, M.: Urinary excretion kinetics of amphetamine in man. J. Pharm. Pharmacol., 17:628–639, 1965.
15. Bennett, W. M., Singer, I., and Coggins, C. H.: A practical guide to drug usage in adult patients with impaired renal function. J.A.M.A., 214:1468–1475, 1970.
16. Bennett, W. M., Singer, I., and Coggins, C. H.: Guide to drug usage in adult patients with impaired renal function. J.A.M.A., 223:991–997, 1973.
17. Bergman, H. D., Aoki, V. S., Black, H. J., Leaverton, P. E., Dick, R. W., and Wilson, W. R.: A new role for the pharmacist in the detection and evaluation of adverse drug reactions. Am. J. Hosp. Pharm., 28:343–350, 1971.
18. Bergmann, C. L.: Dilantin (diphenylhydantoin); its effect on the gingival tissue. Dent. Dig., 73:63–70, 1967.
19. Blattner, R. J., Williamson, A. P., Simonsen, L., and Robertson, G. G.: Teratogenesis with cancer chemotherapeutic agents. J. Pediat., 56:285–293, 1960.
20. Bleyer, W. A., and Breckenridge, R. T.: Studies on the detection of adverse drug reactions in the newborn. II. The effects of prenatal aspirin on newborn hemostasis. J.A.M.A., 213:2049–2053, 1970.
21. Boger, W. P.: Non-allergic toxicity of sulfonamide drugs. Antibiot. Chemother., 87:255–265, 1960.
22. Boston Collaborative Drug Surveillance Program: Acute adverse reactions to prednisone in relation to dosage. Clin. Pharmacol. Ther., 13:694–698, 1972.
23. Oral contraception and depression. Br. Med. J., 4:380–381, 1969.
24. Brodie, B. B.: Physico-chemical factors in drug absorption. In Binns, T. B., ed., Absorption and Distribution of Drugs, Edinburgh, E. & S. Livingstone, Ltd., 1964, p. 199.
25. Brook, R. H., Appel, B. A., Avery, C., Orman, M., and Stevenson, R. L.: Effectiveness of inpatient follow-up care. N. Engl. J. Med., 285:1509–1514, 1971.
26. Canada, A. T., Jr., and Burka, E. R.: Aplastic anemia after indomethacin. N. Engl. J. Med., 278:743–744, 1968.
27. Caranasos, G., Stewart, R. B., and Cluff, L. E.: Adverse drug reactions leading to hospitalization. J.A.M.A., 228:713–717, 1974.
28. Carson, P. E.: Hemolysis due to inherited erythrocyte enzyme deficiencies. Ann. N.Y. Acad. Sci., 151:765–776, 1968.
29. Cawein, M., Behlen, C. H., Lappat, E. J., and Cohn, J. E.: Hereditary diaphorase deficiency and methemoglobinemia. Arch. Intern. Med., 113:578–585, 1964.
30. Christensen, L. K., and Skovsted, L.: Inhibition of drug metabolism by chloramphenicol. Lancet, 2:1397–1399, 1969.
31. Cline, M. J.: Cancer chemotherapy. In Smith, L. H., Jr., ed., Major Problems in Internal Medicine, vol. 1, Philadelphia, W. B. Saunders Co., 1971.
32. Clinite, J. C., and Kabat, H. F.: Prescribed drugs. Errors during self-administration. J. Am. Pharm. Assoc., 9:450–452, 1969.
33. Cluff, L. E.: Epidemiology of adverse reactions. M.C.V. Quart., 3:72–76, 1967.
34. Cobrinik, R. W., Hood, T., and Chusid, E.: The effect of maternal narcotic addiction on the newborn infant. Pediatrics, 24:288, 1959.

35. Cohen J. J.: Geriatric drug dosages. N. Engl. J. Med., 285:1152, 1971.
36. Conway, N., and Birt, B. D.: Streptomycin in pregnancy: Effect on the foetal ear. Br. Med. J., 2:260, 1965.
37. Cook, L., Macko, E., and Fellows, E. J.: The effect of B-diethylaminoethyldiphenylpropylacetate hydrochloride on the action series of barbiturates and C.N.S. depressants. J. Pharmacol. Exp. Ther., 112:382–386, 1954.
38. Cool, L., Navis, G., and Fellows, E. J.: Enhancement of the action of certain analgetic drugs by B-diethylaminoethyldiphenylpropylacetate hydrochloride. J. Pharmacol. Exp. Ther., 112:473–479, 1954.
39. Conney, A. H., and Gelboin, H. V.: Antagonism and potentiation of drug action. In Meyler, L., and Peck, H. M., eds., Drug-Induced Diseases, vol. 4, Amsterdam, Excerpta Medica Foundation, 1972, p. 184.
40. Conney, A. H.: Pharmacologic implications of microsomal enzyme induction. Pharmacol. Rev., 19:317–366, 1967.
41. Consolo, S., Morselli, P. L., Zaccala, M., and Garattini, S.: Delayed absorption of phenylbutazone caused by desmethylimipramine in humans. Eur. J. Pharmacol., 10:239–242, 1970.
42. Consolo, S., and Garattini, S.: Effect of desipramine on intestinal absorption of phenylbutazone and other drugs. Eur. J. Pharmacol., 6:322–326, 1969.
43. Cooper, J. R., Axelrod, J., and Brodie, B. B.: Inhibitory effects of B-diethylamenoethyldiphenylpropylacetate on a variety of drug metabolic pathways in vitro. J. Pharmacol. Exp. Ther., 112:55–63, 1954.
44. Cucinell, S. A., Conney, A. H., Sansur, M., and Burns, J. J.: Drug interactions in man. I. Lowering effect of phenobarbital on plasma levels of bishydroxycoumarin (Dicumarol) and diphenylhydantoin (Dilantin). Clin. Pharmacol. Ther., 6:420–429, 1965.
45. D'Arcy, P. F., and Griffin, J. P.: Iatrogenic Diseases. London, Oxford University Press, 1972, p. 95.
46. Dettli, L., Spring, P., and Habersang, R.: Drug dosage in patients with impaired renal function. Postgrad. Med. J. Suppl., 32–35, Oct., 1970.
47. Eckstein, H., and Jack, B.: Breast feeding and anticoagulant therapy, Lancet, 1:672–673, 1970.
48. Evaluations of Drug Interactions. Washington, D.C., American Pharmaceutical Association, 1973.
49. Ewy, G. A., Kapadia, G. G., Yao, L., Lullin, M., and Marcus, F. I.: Digoxin metabolism in the elderly. Circulation, 39:449–453, 1969.
50. Evans, D. A. P., and White, T. A.: Human acetylation polymorphism. J. Lab. Clin. Med., 63:394–403, 1964.
51. Evans, D. A. P., Davison, K., and Pratt, R. T. C.: The influences of acetylator phenotype on the effects of treating depression with phenelzine. Clin. Pharmacol. Ther., 6:430–435, 1965.
52. Evans, D. A. P., Manley, K. A., and McKusick, V. A.: Genetic control of isoniazid metabolism in man. Br. Med. J., 2:485–491, 1960.
53. Fenstermacher, J. D., and Rall, D. P.: Physiology and pharmacology of cerebrospinal fluid. In Carpi, A., ed., International Encyclopedia of Pharmacology and Therapeutics: Pharmacology of the Cerebral Circulation, New York, Pergamon Press, 1972.
54. Fowler, T. J.: Some incompatibilities of intravenous admixtures. Am. J. Hosp. Pharm., 24:450–457, 1967.
55. Frick, P. G., Hitzig, W. H., and Betke, K.: Hemoglobin zurick I. A new hemoglobin anomaly associated with acute hemolytic episodes with inclusion bodies after sulfonamide therapy. Blood, 20:261–271, 1962.
56. Gainesville Drug Study Group—Unpublished Data, University of Florida, 1974.
57. Gardner, P., and Cluff, L. E.: The epidemiology of adverse drug reactions: A review and perspective. Johns Hopkins Med. J., 126:77–87, 1970.
58. Gardner, P., and Watson, L. J.: Adverse drug reactions: A pharmacist-based monitoring system. Clin. Pharmacol. Ther., 11:802–807, 1970.
59. Gerhardt, R. E., Knouss, R. F., Thyrum, P. T., Luchi, R. J., and Morris, J. J.: Quinidine excretion in aciduria and alkaluria. Ann. Intern. Med., 71:927–933, 1969.
60. Gibaldi, M.: Introduction to Biopharmaceutics. Philadelphia, Lea & Febiger, 1971, p. 70.
61. Gingell, J. C., and Waterworth, P. M.: Dose of gentamycin in patients with normal renal function and renal impairment. Br. Med. J., 2:19–22, 1968.

62. Glazko, A. J., Kindel, A. W., Alegnani, W. C., and Holmes, E. L.: An evaluation of the absorption characteristics of different chloramphenicol preparations in normal human subjects. Clin. Pharmacol. Ther. 9:472–483, 1968.
63. Goodfriend, T. L.: Pathologic conditions affecting responses to drugs. Wisc. Pharm. Exten. Bull., 12:2–4, 1969.
64. Goodwin, F. K., Murphy, D. L., Brodie, K. H., and Bunney, W. E.: Levodopa: Alterations in behavior. Clin. Pharmacol. Ther., 12:383–396, 1971.
65. Gordon, R. R., and Dean T.: Foetal deaths from antenatal anticoagulation therapy. Br. Med. J., 2:719, 1955.
66. Gourley, D. R. H.: Biological responses to drugs. In Burger, A., ed., Medicinal Chemistry, 3rd ed., New York, Wiley-Interscience, 1970, p. 39.
67. Gourley, D. R. H.: Factors modifying drug action in the body. In Fulton, W. F. M., ed., Modern Trends in Pharmacology and Therapeutics, London, Butterworth, 1967, p. 2.
68. Graham, J. R.: Fibrosis associated with methysergide therapy. In Meyler, L., and Peck, H. M., eds., op. cit., vol. 3, Amsterdam, 1968, p. 249.
69. Greene, H. J., Burkhart, B., and Hobby, G. L.: Excretion of penicillin in human milk following parturition. Am. J. Obstet. Gynecol., 51:732–733, 1946.
70. Grunwaldt, E., and Bates, T.: Non-adrenal female pseudohermaphrodism after administration of testosterone to a mother during pregnancy: Report of a case. Pediatrics, 20:503, 1957.
71. Hansen, J. M., Kampmann, J., and Laursen, H.: Renal excretion of drugs in the elderly. Lancet, 1:1170, 1970.
72. Hansten, P. D.: Drug Interactions. 2nd ed., Philadelphia, Lea & Febiger, 1973.
73. Ibid., p. 24.
74. Ibid., p. 257.
75. Hartshorn, E. A.: Handbook of Drug Interactions. Cincinnati, Don Franke, 1970, p. 74.
76. Herbst, A. L., Ulfelder, H., and Poskanzer, D. C.: Adenocarcinoma of the vagina: Association of maternal stilbesterol therapy with tumor appearance. N. Engl. J. Med., 284:878–881, 1971.
77. Hoffbrand, B. I., and Kininmonth, D. A.: Potentiation of anticoagulants. Br. Med. J., 2:838–839, 1967.
78. Holt, E. L., and Holz, P. H.: The black bottle. J. Pediatr., 63:306–314, 1963.
79. Hurwitz, N.: Predisposing factors in adverse reactions to drugs. Br. Med. J., 1:536–539, 1969.
80. Hussar, D. A.: Drug interactions—A review of the mechanisms by which they develop. Hosp. Form. Manage., 5:16–28, 1970.
81. Hynniman, C. E., Conrad, W. F., Urch, W. A., Rudnick, B. R., and Parker, P. F.: A comparison of medication errors under the University of Kentucky unit dose system and traditional drug distribution systems in four hospitals. Am. J. Hosp. Pharm., 27:802–814, 1970.
82. Jacobs, J., Greene, H., and Gendel, B. R.: Acute iron intoxication. N. Engl. J. Med., 273:1124–1127, 1965.
83. Jasinski, D. R., Martin, W. R., and Haertzen, C. A.: The human pharmacology and abuse potential of N-allylnoroxymorphone (naloxone). J. Pharmacol. Exp. Ther., 157:420–426, 1967.
84. Jick, H., and Slone, D.: Relation between digoxin arrhythmias and ABO blood groups. Circulation, 45:352–357, 1972.
85. Jick, H., and Slone, D.: Venous thromboembolic disease and ABO blood type. Lancet, 1:539–542, 1969.
86. Jick, H., Slone, D., Borda, I. T., and Shapiro, S.: Efficacy and toxicity of heparin in relation to age and sex. N. Engl. J. Med., 279:284–286, 1968.
87. Jick, H., Miettinen, O. S., Shapiro, S., Lewis, G. P., Sisking, V., and Slone, D.: Comprehensive drug surveillance. J.A.M.A., 213:1455–1460, 1970.
88. Jick, H., Slone, D., Shapiro, S., et al.: Psychiatric side effects of nonpsychiatric drugs. Semin. Psychiat., 3:406–420, 1971.
89. Johnson, H. D.: Therapy of acute poisoning. J. Am. Pharm. Assoc., NS 9:214–231, 1969.
90. Johnson, P., Kickon, A. H., Lowther, C. P., and Turner, R. W. D.: Treatment of hypertension with methyldopa. Br. Med. J., 1:133–137, 1966.
91. Kalow, W.: Pharmacogenetics: Heredity and the Response to Drugs. Philadelphia, W. B. Saunders Co., 1962, p. 83.

92. Ibid., p. 96.
93. Ibid., p. 154.
94. Keberle, H., Hoffman, K., and Bernhard, K.: The metabolism of glutethimide. Experientia, *18*:105-111, 1962.
95. Kirkman, H. N.: Glucose-6-phosphate dehydrogenase variants and drug induced hemolysis. Ann. N. Y. Acad. Sci., *151*:753-764, 1968.
96. Klein, F.: Hypotensive drugs. *In* Meyler, L., and Herxheimer, A., eds., Side Effects of Drugs, vol. 7, Amsterdam, Excerpta Medica Foundation, 1972, p. 301.
97. Knowels, J. A.: Excretion of drugs in milk—A review. J. Pediatr., *66*:1068-1082, 1965.
98. Kolmodin, B., Azarnoff, D. L., and Sjoqvist, F.: Effect of environmental factors on drug metabolism: Decreased plasma half-life of antipyrine in workers exposed to chlorinated hydrocarbon insecticides. Clin. Pharmacol. Ther., *10*:638-642, 1969.
99. Kunin, C. M.: A guide to use of antibiotics in patients with renal disease: A table of recommended doses and factors governing serum levels. Ann. Intern. Med., *67*:151-158, 1967.
100. Kunin, C. M., and Finland, M.: Clinical pharmacology of the tetracycline antibiotics. Clin. Pharmacol. Ther., *2*:51-69, 1961.
101. Kwit, N. T., and Hatcher, R. A.: Excretion of drugs in milk. Am. J. Dis. Child., *49*:900, 1935.
102. La Du, B. N.: Pharmacogenetics. Med. Clin. North Am., *53*:839-855, 1969.
103. Latiolais, C. J., and Berry, C. C.: Misuse of prescription medications by outpatients. Drug Intel. Clin. Pharm., *3*:270-277, 1969.
104. Levine, R. R.: Pharmacology: Drug Actions and Reactions. Boston, Little, Brown and Company, 1973, p. 201.
105. Ibid., p. 185.
106. Ibid., p. 199.
107. Ibid., p. 219.
108. Libow, L. S., and Mehl, B.: Self-administration of medications by patients in hospitals or extended care facilities. J. Am. Geriatr. Soc., *18*:81-85, 1970.
109. Lindenbaum, J., Mellow, M. H., Blackstone, M. O., and Butler, V. P.: Variation in biologic availability of digoxin from four preparations. N. Engl. J. Med., *285*:1344-1347, 1971.
110. Livingston, S., and Livingston, H. L.: Diphenylhydantoin gingival hyperplasia. Am. J. Dis. Child., *117*:265-270, 1969.
111. Loewe, S.: The problem of synergism and antagonism of combined drugs. Arzneim. Forsch., *3*:285-290, 1953.
112. Lowe, C. U.: Pediatric pharmacology. J. Clin. Pharmacol., 8:31-40, 1968.
113. MacDonald, M. G., Robinson, D. S., Sylvester, D., and Jaffe, J. J.: The effects of phenobarbital, chloral betaine and glutethimide administration of warfarin plasma levels and hyproprothrombinemic responses in man. Clin. Pharmacol. Ther., *10*:80-84, 1969.
114. Maher, J. F.: Nephrotoxicity of drugs and chemicals. Pharmacol. Physicians, *4*:1-5, 1970.
115. Malahy, B.: The effect of instruction and labeling on the number of medication errors made by patients at home. Am. J. Hosp. Pharm., *23*:283-292, 1966.
116. Manten, A.: Antibiotic drugs. *In* Meyler, L., and Herxheimer, A., eds., op. cit., vol. 6, 1968, p. 263.
117. Martelo, O. J., Katims, R. B., and Yunis, A. A.: Bone marrow aplasia following propylthiouracil therapy: Report of a case with complete recovery. Arch. Intern. Med., *120*:587-590, 1967.
118. Mazzullo, J.: The nonpharmacologic basis of therapeutics. Clin. Pharmacol. Ther., *13*:157-158, 1972.
119. McDonald, D. F., and Murphy, G. P.: Bacteriostatic and acidifying effects of methionine, hydrolyzed casein and ascorbic acid on the urine. N. Engl. J. Med., *261*:803-804, 1959.
120. McIntosh, H. A., and Storey, E.: Tetracycline-induced tooth changes: Discoloration and hypoplasia induced by tetracycline analogues. Med. J. Aust., *57*:114-119, 1970.
121. McKenzie, M., Stewart, R. B., Weiss, C. F., and Cluff, L. E.: A pharmacist-based

study of the epidemiology of adverse drug reactions in pediatric medicine patients. Am. J. Hosp. Pharm., 30:898–903, 1973.
122. Medical Intelligence: Neurologic syndromes associated with antipsychotic-drug use. N. Engl. J. Med., 289:20–23, 1973.
123. Continuous versus intermittent intravenous antibiotics. Med. Lett. Drugs Ther., 10:57, 1968.
124. Meyler, L.: Drug-induced diseases. In Meyler, L., and Peck, H. M., eds., op. cit., vol. 3, 1968, p. 1.
125. Miller, R. R.: Drug surveillance utilizing epidemiologic methods. Am. J. Hosp. Pharm., 30:584–592, 1973.
126. Milne, M. D.: Influence of acid-base balance on efficiency and toxicity of drugs. In Symposium on interaction between drugs. Proc. R. Soc. Med., 58:955–960, 1965.
127. Mitchell, J. R., Arias, L., and Oates, J. A.: Antagonism of the antihypertensive action of guanethidine sulfate by desipramine hydrochloride. J.A.M.A., 202:973–975, 1967.
128. Moe, G. K., and Abildskov, J. A.: Antiarrhythmic drugs. In Goodman, L. S., and Gilman, A., eds., The Pharmacological Basis of Therapeutics, 4th ed., New York, The Macmillan Company, 1971, p. 716.
129. Moore, G. E., Bross, I. D. J., Ausman, R., Nadler, S., Jones, R., Slack, N., and Rimm, A. A.: Effects of 5-fluorouracil (NSC-19893) in 389 patients with cancer. Cancer Chemother. Abstr., 52:641, 1968.
130. Neuvonen, P. J., Gothoni, G., Hackman, R., and Bjorksten, K.: Interference of iron with the absorption of tetracycline in man. Br. Med. J., 4:532–534, 1970.
131. Monson, R. R., Rosenberg, L., Hartz, S. C., Shapiro, S., Heinonen, O. P., and Slone, D.: Diphenylhydantoin and selected congenital malformations. N. Engl. J. Med., 289:1049–1052, 1973.
132. Nickerson, M.: Drugs inhibiting adrenergic nerves and structures innervated by them. In Goodman, L. S., and Gilman, A., eds., op. cit., p. 570.
133. Palmisano, P. A., and Polhill, R. B.: Fetal pharmacology. Pediatr. Clin. North Am., 19:3–20, 1972.
134. Parker, E. A.: Solution additive chemical incompatibility study. Am. J. Hosp. Pharm., 24:434–439, 1967.
135. Patel, B. M.: Skin rash with infectious mononucleosis and ampicillin. Pediatrics, 40:910–911, 1967.
136. Patrick, M. J., Tilstone, W. J., and Reavey, P.: Diazepam and breast-feeding. Lancet, 1:542–543, 1972.
137. Perry, H. M., Jr., Sakamoto, A., and Tan, E. M.: Relationship of acetylating enzyme to hydralazine toxicity. J. Lab. Clin. Med., 70:1020–1021, 1967.
138. Peters, J. H.: Genetic factors in relation to drugs. Annu. Rev. Pharmacol., 8:427–452, 1968.
139. Peters, J. H., Gordon, G. R., Gelber, R., Levy, L., and Glazko, A. J.: Polymorphic acetylation of dapsone (4,4,-diaminodiphenylsulfone-DDS) in man. Fed. Proc., 29:803, 1970.
140. Prescott, L. F.: Pharmacokinetics drug interaction. Lancet, 2:1239–1243, 1969.
141. Putnam, F. W.: Structure and function of the plasma proteins. In Neurath, H., ed., The Proteins, vol. 3, 2nd ed., New York, Academic Press, Inc., 1965.
142. Rasmussen, K., Jervell, J., Strostein, L., and Gjerdrum, K.: Digitoxin kinetics in patients with impaired renal function. Clin. Pharmacol. Ther., 13:6–14, 1972.
143. Rigas, D. A., and Koler, R. D.: Decreased erythrocyte survival in hemoglobin H disease as a result of the abnormal properties of hemoglobin H: The benefit of splenectomy. Blood, 18:1–17, 1961.
144. Rivera-Calimlim, L., Castaneda, L., and Lasagna, L.: Effects of mode of management on plasma chlorpromazine in psychiatric patients. Clin. Pharmacol. Ther., 14:978–986, 1973.
145. Rosenberg, J. M., and Mann, K.: Factors that modify drug activity and patient response. Drug Intel. Clin. Pharm., 7:346–350, 1973.
146. Ritschel, W. A.: pKa values and some clinical applications. In Frank, D., and Whitney, H. A. K., eds., Perspectives in Clinical Pharmacy, Hamilton, Illinois, Drug Intelligence Publications, 1972.
147. Robinson, D. S., Benjamin, D. M., and McCormack, J. J.: Interaction of warfarin

and non-systemic gastrointestinal drugs. Clin. Pharmacol. Ther., *12*:491–495, 1971.
148. Rowland, M.: Drug administration and regimens. *In* Melmon, K. L., and Morrelli, H. F., eds., Clinical Pharmacology: Basic Principles in Therapeutics, New York, The Macmillan Company, 1972, p. 51.
149. Schanker, L. S.: On the mechanism of absorption of drugs from the gastrointestinal tract. J. Med. Pharm. Chem., *2*:343–359, 1960.
150. Schanker, L. S.: Physiological transport of drugs. *In* Harper, N. J., and Simmonds, A. B., eds., Advances in Drug Research, London, Academic Press, Inc., 1964, pp. 71–106.
151. Schanker, L. S., Shore, P. A., Brodie, B. B., and Hogben, C. A. M.: Absorption of drugs from the stomach. I., The rat. J. Pharmacol. Exp. Ther., *120*:528–539, 1957.
152. Schwartz, D., Wang, M., Zeitz, L., and Goss, M. E.: Medication errors made by elderly chronically ill patients. Am. J. Public Health, *52*:2018–2029, 1962.
153. Seidl, L. G., Thornton, G. F., Smith, F. W., and Cluff, L. E.: Studies on the epidemiology of adverse drug reactions. Bull. Johns Hopkins Hosp., *119*:299–315, 1966.
154. Sellers, E. M., and Koch-Weser, J.: Oral anticoagulant therapy. Can. Med. Assoc. J., *106*:302, 1972.
155. Sellers, E. M., and Koch-Weser, J.: Displacement of warfarin from human albumin by diazoxide and ethacrynic, mefenamic, and nalidixic acids. Clin. Pharmacol. Ther., *11*:524–529, 1970.
156. Shapiro, S., Slone, D., Jick, H., and Lewis, G. P.: Epidemiology of digoxin. J. Chronic Dis., *22*:361–371, 1969.
157. Shearer, W. T., Schreiner, R. L., and Marshall, R. E.: Urinary retention in a neonate secondary to maternal ingestion of nortriptyline. J. Pediatr., *81*:570–572, 1972.
158. Silverman, W. A., Andersen, D. H., Blanc, W. A., and Crozier, D. N.: Difference in mortality rate and incidence of kernicterus among premature infants allotted to two prophylactic antibacterial regimens. Pediatrics, *18*:614–625, 1956.
159. Skeith, M. D., Simkin, P. A., and Healey, L. A.: The renal excretion of indomethacin and its inhibition by probenecid. Clin. Pharmacol. Ther., *9*:89–93, 1968.
160. Smith, J. W., Seidl, L. G., and Cluff, L. E.: Studies on the epidemiology of adverse drug reactions. V: Clinical factors influencing susceptibility. Ann. Intern. Med., *65*:629–640, 1966.
161. Solomon, H. M., and Thomas, G. B.: A rapid method for estimation of drug-affinity constants in human plasma. Clin. Pharmacol. Ther., *12*:445–448, 1971.
162. Solomon, H. M., and Schrogie, J. J.: Change in receptor site affinity: A proposed explanation for the potentiating effect of D-thyroxine on the anticoagulant response to warfarin. Clin. Pharmacol. Ther., *8*:797–799, 1967.
163. Stewart, R. B., and Cluff, L. E.: A review of medication errors and compliance in ambulant patients. Clin. Pharmacol. Ther., *13*:463–468, 1972.
164. Stewart, R. B., and Cluff, L. E.: Gastrointestinal manifestations of adverse drug reactions. Am. J. Dig. Dis., *19*:1–7, 1974.
165. Stewart, R. B., and Cluff, L. E.: Studies on the epidemiology of adverse drug reactions. VI: Utilization and interactions of prescription and nonprescription drugs in outpatients. Johns Hopkins Med. J., *129*:319–331, 1971.
166. Comptroller General of the United States: Study of Health Facilities Construction Costs, Report to the Congress. U.S.G.P.O. 86-379-0, Washington, D.C., 1972, p. 69.
167. Swett, C., Jr., and Jick, H.: Diphenylhydantoin side effects and serum albumin levels. Clin. Pharmacol. Ther., *14*:529–532, 1973.
168. Taussing, H. B.: A study of the German outbreak of phocomelia: The thalidomide syndrome. J.A.M.A., *180*:1106, 1962.
169. Tester, W. W.: Final Report. A study of patient care involving a unit dose system. U.S.P.H.S. Grant HM 00238-01, University of Iowa, 1967.
170. Toaff, R., and Ravid, R.: Tooth discoloration due to tetracyclines. *In* Meyler, L., and Peck, H. M., eds., op. cit., vol. 3, 1968, pp. 117–133.
171. Torosian, G., Finger, K. F., and Stewart, R. B.: Hazards of bromides in proprietary medication. Am. J. Hosp. Pharm., *30*:716–718, 1973.
172. Trafton, H. M., and Lind, H. E.: The treatment of urinary tract infections with a new antibiotic cephaloglycin. J. Urol., *101*:392–395, 1969.

PHARMACOLOGIC MECHANISMS

173. Tschudy, D. P.: Clinical aspects of drug reactions in hereditary hepatic porphyria. Ann. N.Y. Acad. Sci., *151*:850–860, 1968.
174. Tyrer, H. H., Eadie, M. J., Sutherland, J. M., and Hooper, W. D.: Outbreak of anticonvulsant intoxication in an Australian city. Br. Med. J., *4*:271–273, 1970.
175. Vesell, E. S., Passananti, G. T., and Greene, F. E.: Impairment of drug metabolism in man by allopurinol and nortriptyline. N. Engl. J. Med., *283*:1484–1488, 1970.
176. Utz, J. P.: Current concepts in therapy: Chemotherapeutic agents for the systemic mycoses. N. Engl. J. Med., *268*:938–940, 1963.
177. Wagner, J. G.: Biopharmaceutics and Relevant Pharmacokinetics. Hamilton, Illinois, Drug Intelligence Publications, 1971, p. 237.
178. Wagner, J. G.: Design and data analysis of biopharmaceutical studies in man. Canad. J. Pharm. Sci., *1*:55–68, 1966.
179. Wagner, J. G.: Generic equivalence and inequivalence of oral products. Drug Intel. Clin. Pharm., *5*:115–128, 1971.
180. Wagner, J. G.: Half-life definitions. Am. J. Hosp. Pharm., *30*:667, 1973.
181. Watkins, J. D., Roberts, D. E., Williams, T. F., Martin, D. A., and Coyle, V.: Observation of medication errors made by diabetic patients in the home. Diabetes, *16*:882–885, 1967.
182. Webb, J. W.: A pH pattern for I.V. additives. Am. J. Hosp. Pharm., *26*:31–35, 1969.
183. Weily, H. S., and Genton, E.: Pharmacokinetics of procainamide. Arch. Intern. Med., *130*:366–369, 1972.
184. Weiner, I. M., and Mudge, G. H.: Renal tubular mechanisms for excretion of organic acids and bases. Am. J. Med., *36*:743–762, 1964.
185. Welt, L. G., and Blythe, W. B.: Anions: phosphate, iodide, fluoride, and other anions. *In* Goodman, L. S., and Gilman, A., eds., op. cit.
186. Wichmann, H. M., Rind, H., and Gladtke, E.: Die Elimination von Bromsulphalein biem Kind. Zschr. Kinderheilk., *103*:262–276, 1968.
187. Winston, F.: Oral contraceptives and depression. Lancet, *1*:1209, 1969.
188. Woodbury, D. M.: Analgesics, antipyretics, anti-inflammatory agents, and inhibitors of uric acid synthesis. *In* Goodman, L. S., and Gilman, A., eds., op. cit., p. 314.
189. Woodbury, D. M., and Fingl, E.: General principles. *In* Goodman, L. S., and Gilman, A., eds., op. cit., p. 17.
190. Woody, J. N., London, W. I., and Wilbanks, G. D.: Lithium toxicity in newborns. Pediatrics, *47*:94–96, 1971.

CHAPTER 3

IMMUNOLOGIC MECHANISMS

DRUGS AS ANTIGENS

Today, most drugs are synthetic chemicals of low molecular weight (<1000 mol wt), and induce an immunologic response only when linked as haptens to protein carriers. Some polypeptides with mol wts of about 3500, such as calcitonin, gastrin, oxytocin, glucagon, and adrenocorticotropin, are weakly antigenic, but become more strongly antigenic when conjugated to a carrier protein.[8] Substances with higher molecular weights may be fully antigenic without conjugation to a carrier. Immunologic reactions to drugs, however, are related largely to the role of drugs as haptens.

Drugs and Protein Carriers

Since Landsteiner's[26] pioneering immunologic studies of antigenic determinants, it has been recognized that simple chemicals, such as drugs, must bind covalently, or irreversibly, with a carrier molecule (usually a protein) in order to become immunogenic. Such conjugates are thought to form by interaction of the drug with an autologous protein. The evidence supporting this interpretation is based upon several observations[30]: (1) There is a direct relationship between the formation of hapten-protein amide bonds and the ability of the hapten to induce an immunologic response. (2) Drugs and other simple chemicals may induce immunologic responses specific for the hapten and protein carrier, rather than for the unconjugated drug. (3) Oligopeptides capable of causing an immunologic response usually are composed of at least seven amino acids.[45] (4) Reversible binding of a drug to a protein, as with binding to serum albumin, usually does not make the drug antigenic. However, the binding of a hapten by noncovalent reversible bonds to antigenic foreign or denatured proteins or bacteria, referred to as "schlepper," may induce an immunologic response to a hapten.[49] Conceivably, during the course of microbial infection or tissue death, as in infection, the microorganism or altered tissue proteins may serve as "schlepper" carriers for drugs and lead to an immunologic response to the hapten, but this possibility has not been investigated.

Drug Interaction with Cell Membranes

Penicillin can bind covalently to the membranes of lymphocytes and erythrocytes, producing immunologic stimulation.[14,43] The antigenicity of drugs bound to cell membranes, however, has only been investigated recently, even though interactions of drugs with cell membranes related to pharmacologic action have been studied intensively. Nevertheless, drugs adsorbed to blood cells may be responsible for immunologic reactions, resulting in hemolysis and thrombocytopenia, indicating the importance of interactions of haptens with cell membranes in drug allergy.[44,56] Whether or not other hapten-cell membrane interactions are responsible for immunological responses is not yet completely defined.

Cell membranes generally consist of a bimolecular layer of lipid sandwiched between layers of protein.[47] Substances soluble in lipid may dissolve freely in the cell membrane and be transferred passively into the cell. Inorganic ions and some small molecules which are not lipid soluble may also penetrate cell membranes, presumably through small pores or channels.[23] Most drugs are either weak acids or bases and may exist in both ionized and un-ionized forms, in a ratio dependent upon pH. A weak acid or base most readily penetrates the cell membrane at the pH at which it is least ionized. Certain strong organic acids or bases are ionized over a wide range of pH, have low lipid solubility, and are poorly incorporated in or absorbed across cell membranes.

The incorporation into and transfer across cell membranes of some substances may occur by means of their complexing with a "carrier" or "receptor" component.[54] The "carrier" or "receptor" concentration may be limited, and the amount of the drug or other substance which may be complexed or bound is correspondingly limited. Different drugs may be complexed by the same "carrier" or "receptor" of the cell membrane and may compete with one another for the same receptor sites, in much the same way as drugs bind competitively to serum proteins.

Once in the blood plasma, most drugs must pass through the lipid cell membrane of the capillary endothelium to reach their site of action, to enter the extravascular space, and to enter the lymphatic system. This process is affected by the drug's molecular weight, its binding to serum protein, its complexing with cell membranes of circulating blood cells, and its lipid solubility. Drugs bound to blood-plasma protein or blood-cell membranes will not pass through the capillary endothelium. Patients who have hypoalbuminemia may have less of a drug bound to serum protein, and a larger proportion of the drug may be available to complex with other proteins and cell membranes. The low albumin content of the blood could increase the possibility of drugs binding irreversibly to other proteins or cell membranes, making them antigenic. No direct evidence exists to support this possibility, but the basis for advancing it seems sound and worthy of study.

Drug Distribution, Metabolism, and Excretion

Drugs vary in their concentration or sequestration in different tissues,[23] and this may affect their antigenicity and the manifestations of allergic drug reactions. Pathological changes in tissues or organs also can influence drug distribution, the immunogenicity of antigens, and the allergic reactions they induce. For example, drugs do not penetrate so freely into certain fractions of the extracellular water, such as cerebrospinal, lymphatic, synovial, pericardial, peritoneal, and pleural fluids, which constitute less than 5 per cent of the extracellular water. In the presence of inflammatory disease, however, the penetration of drugs, even though they are bound to serum protein, may increase in these fluids or affected tissues. Stimulation of an immunologic response thus may be facilitated, and the site of an allergic drug reaction also may differ from that expected under other conditions, since the tissues involved in allergic reactions are affected by antigen localization. In addition, abnormalities in drug excretion or metabolism of a drug attributable to renal or hepatic insufficiency, enzyme deficiencies, or heritable disorders may affect drug distribution and concentration, conceivably also influencing the immunogenicity of and allergic reactions to drugs.

Some drugs have a particular affinity for certain tissues, just as some drugs are bound to plasma proteins. This tissue affinity is not necessarily related to the site of a drug's pharmacologic action, but it may influence the drug's immunogenicity and also may play an important part in determining the site of tissue injury in allergic drug reactions.

The speed of elimination of a drug and its metabolic products is an important factor in the occurrence of drug allergy. Drugs may be degraded by the enzymes of normal intermediary metabolism. Enzymes, principally located in the liver, act on drugs containing hydroxyl, amino, or other reactive groups, resulting in their conjugation with glucuronic acid, acetic acid, sulphuric acid, glycine, ribose, and methyl groups (O-methyltransferase). In some instances, the conjugated drug, as in the case of acetylated sulfonamides, may be more soluble than the parent drug, and this may lead to adverse drug effects such as crystalluria. Such conjugates also may be less or more antigenic and less or more likely to result in allergic reactions in sensitized individuals.

Microsomes of liver cells can metabolize a variety of drugs, and are particularly active on drugs with high lipid solubility. These microsomal enzymes are dependent upon NADPH (nicotinamide-adenine dinucleotide phosphate), cytochrome P-450, and cytochrome reductase; they add hydroxyl groups to drug substrates making them more polar and water soluble, and, therefore, less able to penetrate cell membranes, possibly influencing their immunogenicity and allergenicity. Apart from hydroxylation, microsomal enzymes may reduce some drugs, by substituting oxygen for sulfur and hydrolyzing certain esters and amides. This renders them suitable for conjugation and more likely to bind covalently to protein carriers. The products of the metabolism of drugs, therefore, may be less active or more active, less toxic or more toxic, and less immunogenic or more immunogenic than the original substances. The metabolic products of penicillin, for example, appear to be the major determinants of penicillin allergy (including penicilloic, penamaldic, and penicillenic acids), have a greater propensity to form covalent bonds with proteins, and may bind irreversibly to cell membranes.[29,42] It is very likely that allergic reactions to many drugs are attributable to degradation, or the metabolic products of the drug, rather than to the parent drug itself, but this has not been adequately investigated. It is also possible that the susceptibility of some persons to developing drug allergy is attributable, in part, to heritable or acquired differences in the metabolism of drugs rather than to differences in immunologic responsiveness.

Drug Interaction with Lymphoid Tissue

The route of administration and the dose of antigens or haptens or drugs may have an important influence upon the type of immunologic response induced. Although the foreign substance may be distributed widely and in varying concentrations in different tissues, only a small proportion of the antigen or hapten may be captured and retained in lymphoid tissues responsible for the immunologic response. After cutaneous application the hapten may bind to proteins in skin, and be concentrated in draining lymph nodes, even though the greatest amount of hapten or antigen will be distributed systemically. After entering the blood, haptens will be variously distributed in tissues, as discussed before, but the spleen and other lymphoid tissues also will retain antigen and are important in the immunologic response. The sequestration of soluble antigen or hapten in lymphoid tissue is not related to its particle size, but is related to its immunogenicity, possibly to its affinity for conjugating to cell membrane, and to the presence of specific antibodies.

In lymph nodes antigen is predominantly associated with cells in the peripheral and medullary sinuses.[12,34] In the spleen, stellate macrophages in the red pulp and in the marginal zone of the white pulp or near central arterioles contain antigen. Follicular localization of antigens in lymphoid tissues is dependent upon the presence of circulating antibodies.[34] Recent evidence suggests, therefore, that antigens may not need to enter the precursors of antibody-producing cells in the nonimmune animal and very little, if any, antigen is concentrated in mature antibody-producing cells. This may seem inconsistent with any direct instructional theory of antibody production, but the possibility remains that antigen may be responsible for formation of messenger RNA which either alters or codes for a portion of the immunoglobulin chains. Whether antigen itself or some induced messenger substance is responsible for causing an immunologic response by lymphoid cells remains to be determined. It is also not known whether or not induction of the immunologic response by the cell requires intact antigen or a "processed" antigen.[34]

Cells stimulated in draining lymph node follicles are usually T-lymphocytes responsible for delayed hypersensitivity or cellular immunity, while those in the spleen and paracortical areas of lymph nodes usually are B-lymphocytes responsible for antibody production.[51] The responses of the B- and T-lymphocytes are modulated by each other, and antibodies produced by B-cells may enhance the immunologic response of T-cells.

Drug Interaction with Specific Antibody and Sensitized Lymphocytes

The immunologic reactivity of haptens is dependent upon the conjugation of haptens to specific antibody or specific lymphocyte membrane receptor sites.[40] The reactions of antigens with antibodies involve weak, short-range forces, resulting in reversible binding, as contrasted with the irreversible binding of hapten to carrier protein required for sensitization. The effective forces are electrostatic or hydrogen bonds, Van der Waals forces and hydrophobic forces. This necessitates proper alignment of combining groups on the antibody molecules, allowing interaction with those of the antigen. The interacting groups of the combining regions must be arranged in a complementary manner, so that they are enabled to come in close contact. Hapten alone, or conjugated to carrier protein, may react with these antibodies. The structural features important in the interaction of haptens and antibodies include closeness of fit, charge, configuration and conformation, hydration, and flexibility. The factors influencing the interaction of haptens and antibodies, however, are those involved in any biologic interaction, including that between enzyme and substrate.

The combining site of the antibody has been shown to be in the Fab fragment. This component of both heavy (H) and light (L) chains of immunoglobulins contributes to the binding site.

Immunologic cross-reacting haptens related antigenically to the specific inducing antigen will be less complementary to the combining sites of specific antibodies.[40] However, interaction of specific antibodies with a cross-reacting antigen may occur. Reduced avidity or tightness of fit of the antigen and antibody usually reduces the likelihood that an allergic reaction will develop.

In addition, antigen-specific antibody molecules are not necessarily identical, and even though they may be directed against the same antigenic site, they may have different kinds of combining regions. Furthermore, the complementariness of the antigen for the antibody is limited by the ability of the antibody molecule to orient around the antigenic structure. These factors influence the biologic or clinical implications of antibodies and antigens specifically interacting with one another.

Unconjugated haptens may combine with lymphocyte membrane or antibody receptor sites of specifically stimulated or immune animals,[14,34] as mentioned before. If an excess of unconjugated haptens is added to cells or antibody from specifically immunized or sensitized animals, competition with the binding of conjugated hapten by these cells and antibody ensues, causing a state of immunologic inhibition.[35,36] This inhibition is attributable to competition between inducer (hapten conjugate) and inhibitor (free hapten) for receptor sites on immunologically reactive cells or antibodies. Such competitive binding may inhibit the biologic effects of the antigen-antibody interaction if free hapten occupies the receptor site and is incapable of eliciting an allergic reaction, particularly one caused by delayed hypersensitivity or cellular immunologic reactions.

Free haptens such as penicillin may be better stimulators of sensitive lymphocytes than preformed hapten conjugates, but may exert their effect upon lymphocytes only after conjugation to cell membrane. Prior hydrolysis of the hapten (penicillin to penicilloic acid) may prevent lymphocyte stimulation.[14] In addition, monovalent haptens may inhibit anaphylactic reactions, and may not stimulate sensitized lymphocytes in vitro when concentration of the monovalent hapten exceeds that of the polyvalent hapten.[14] This occurs when receptor sites on antibody and cell membranes are occupied by monovalent haptens which inhibit binding of polyvalent haptens and thereby prevent allergic reactions with the more stimulatory polyvalent antigens. This observation has important implications for preventing and terminating allergic reactions to drugs, in that administration of monovalent simple chemicals may prevent or terminate reactions to polyvalent haptens.

Drug Impurities

Impurities in drug preparations, rather than the drugs themselves, may be responsible for allergic reactions.[14,55] Impurities in drug preparations which may be implicated in these allergic reactions include preservatives or additives, side products of drug synthesis, proteins originating in the course of preparing drugs biologically, or contaminants (i.e., other drugs) incorporated during the course of manufacturing or dispensing drugs. Sometimes synthetic formulation of a drug may result in the unintentional addition of a substance which serves as a hapten carrier, and renders the drug antigenic. Carboxymethylcellulose (CMC), for example, may be included in some formulations containing penicillin, and penicillin may bind to CMC, forming a conjugate capable of eliciting allergic reactions in sensitized patients.[43]

IMMUNOLOGIC REACTIONS TO DRUGS

Immunologic reactions to drugs are attributable to specific classes of antibodies or to delayed cellular hypersensitivity (cellular immunity), and the clinical manifestations associated with drug allergy are attributable largely to release of chemical mediators responsible for tissue injury.[5,7] The pathogenesis of diseases produced by immunologic reactions to drugs is no different from that produced by reactions to other antigens, except that it is influenced by the manner of administration, absorption, distribution, metabolism, elimination, and immunogenicity of the responsible drugs.

REACTIONS CAUSED BY ANTIBODIES

Five major classes of immunoglobulin comprise the human antibodies responsible for allergic or hypersensitivity reactions and immunity.[32,37] These immunoglobulin classes are termed IgA, IgE, IgG, IgM, and IgD. They are alike in that they contain similar or identical L (light) polypeptide chains, linked by disulfide bonds to dissimilar H (heavy) polypeptide chains. Immunoglobulin molecules in the different classes may be further subclassed on the basis of structural differences in the H and L chains detectable by immunologic methods. In addition to structural and immunologically detectable differences between the immunoglobulin classes, they also have different biologic properties, and can mediate different kinds of allergic reactions.

Those most importantly related to allergy to drugs and other environmental antigens are IgE, IgG, and IgM, although recently IgD also has been implicated in an allergic reaction to penicillin.[9] Some of the characteristics of these immunoglobulins and their probable involvement in different allergic reactions are listed in Table 3-1.

ANAPHYLAXIS. Anaphylaxis is often attributable to the drug-specific IgE antibody (reagin, skin-sensitizing antibody—SSA).[3,25] IgE binds firmly to the surface of tissue mast cells and basophils. Interaction of the antigen with the cell-bound (cytotropic) IgE-specific antibody triggers the release of histamine and other chemical mediators which act upon smooth muscle and vascular tissue.[4] These mediators are responsible for the manifestations of an anaphylactic reaction. The reactions involving specific cytotropic antibody (IgE) and antigen do not produce irreversible changes in the target cell (the cell to which IgE is bound), and the chemical mediators of the allergic reaction are probably secreted by these cells.

Anaphylaxis also may be attributed to aggregates of antigen with specific IgG antibody, in which sensitization or binding of the antibody to cell surfaces is not involved.[4] Aggregates, however, can activate the complement system and lead to release of anaphylatoxin, a peptide capable of releasing histamine from mast cells. In addition to histamine, other highly active mediators which may be involved in producing anaphylaxis, whether it is attributable to antigen-

TABLE 3-1. Characteristics of Immunoglobulins Associated with Drug Allergy

Characteristic	IgE	IgG	IgM
Molecular weight	200,000	150,000	900,000
Concentration in normal serum mg/100 ml	0.0005	12	2
Heat lability	+	−	−
Agglutination of drug-sensitized RBC (e.g., penicillin)	−	+	+
Complement fixation	−	+	+
Placental passage	+	+	−
Skin sensitization (Prausnitz-Küstner reaction)	+	−	−
Allergic reaction	Anaphylaxis urticaria	Serum sickness Hemolytic anemia Thrombocytopenia Blocking antibody Fever	Hemolytic anemia Exanthem Thrombocytopenia

antibody aggregates or cytotropic antibody and antigen, include serotonin, kinin, and slow-reacting substances (SRSA).

Histamine is released from white blood cells and lung tissue of allergic individuals. Reactions to administered histamine are characterized by pruritus, erythema, urticaria, angioedema, hypotension, and retrosternal oppression, with little evidence of bronchoconstriction. Intradermal injection of antigen, including drugs, to which an individual is allergic, and reaction with specific IgE antibody, causes wheal and erythema attributable to the release of histamine, and this sensitivity can be passively transferred to a nonallergic person with serum obtained from a person allergic to the antigen (Prausnitz-Küstner reaction). Such skin-test reactions to drugs occur irregularly and unpredictably in the allergic person injected with the conjugated or unconjugated drug or product of drug degradation, even though such testing by skin inoculation of drugs may cause anaphylaxis. In humans, SRSA has been isolated from the lung, and bronchoconstriction has been demonstrated following exposure to an antigen to which the individual is specifically allergic. Passive sensitization of a normal human lung with cytotropic IgE antibody also results in the release of histamine and SRSA upon antigenic challenge. At present, however, the role of SRSA in systemic anaphylaxis in human beings is uncertain. In addition, as yet, there is no definitive data that shows serotonin to be implicated in anaphylaxis. The isolated human bronchiole is insensitive to serotonin, and is devoid of the amine. Kininogen levels have been shown to fall during anaphylaxis to penicillin, and kinins have no action when administered as an aerosol. Therefore the exact role of kinin in human anaphylaxis is unclear.

SERUM SICKNESS. Serum sickness is recognized as an allergic reaction to several drugs as well as to other antigens.[3,25] Specific skin-sensitizing (IgE) and IgG antibodies, as well as delayed hypersensitivity to the responsible antigen, have been found in patients with serum sickness, but immune complexes (antigen-IgG antibody) are probably responsible for this allergic reaction. Most of our understanding of the pathogenesis of serum sickness is derived from studies of this allergic reaction in experimental animals and studies of reactions to foreign proteins in man. There are similarities in the pathologic and immunologic features of serum sickness, systemic lupus erythematosus, and polyarteritis nodosa, suggesting that the latter two also may be caused, at least in part, by immune complexes. Two classes of immunoglobulins, IgG and IgE, may be implicated in producing manifestations of serum sickness. IgG-antigen complexes, usually associated with complement components, have been found in the pathological lesions of serum sickness, particularly in those characterized by vasculitis and glomerulonephritis. In addition, there is a relationship between rising IgG antibody titers, the specific responsible antigen, and the appearance of manifestations of serum sickness, which is also associated with falling or declining serum complement titers. Experimental evidence indicates that serum sickness develops as specific antibodies appear while there is excess antigen in the blood. *Urticaria* frequently accompanies serum sickness, and it is likely that this allergic reaction is attributable to antigen-specific IgE antibodies, rather than to IgG antibodies. *Glomerulonephritis* also is an occasional feature of serum sickness, and appears in patients who develop this allergic reaction to drugs such as methicillin and penicillin. However, it probably is attributable to complexes of the hapten conjugate with antigen-specific IgG antibody.

Cutaneous Manifestations[46]

These manifestations of drug allergy are variable and protean, and for many of them the immunologic mechanism or mechanisms involved are not known. Urticaria[4] is most readily associated with the IgE or cytotropic drug-specific antibody, and possibly with the antigen-specific IgG antibody. This reaction is associated with the release of chemical mediators, particularly histamine, by mast cells, by the same mechanisms which occur in anaphylaxis. *Morbilliform* or *maculopapular* rashes may be attributable to drug-specific IgM antibodies, but also may be produced by delayed hypersensitivity reactions. Not all rashes, however, are due to immunologic mechanisms. Some may be related to a drug's pharmacologic action (e.g., ampicillin). *Erythema multiforme* and Henoch-Schönlein *anaphylactoid purpura* are often accompanied by arthralgia, fever, and other manifestations of serum sickness, and may be related to drug- or antigen-specific IgG antibodies and immune complexes, although there is insufficient evidence to characterize the immunologic mechanism of these reactions.

Hematologic Manifestations

Hematologic manifestations of reactions to drugs may be attributable to either immunologic or nonimmunologic mechanisms,[56] and these are not always easily differentiated. Thrombocytopenia, hemolytic anemia, and agranulocytosis, however, have been identified as allergic reactions to drugs.

THROMBOCYTOPENIA.[21] Thrombocytopenia caused by drugs has been associated with serum antiplatelet factors which can agglutinate the patient's platelets, as well as compatible normal platelets, in vitro in the presence of drug. Interaction of the complement system, the specific drug, and the specific serum antiplatelet factor also may cause platelet lysis. When plasma from a patient with thrombocytopenia associated with a specific drug is infused into a normal recipient, it will not alter the platelet count unless the recipient also has been given the drug. In most instances, the serum factor or antibody appears to combine with the drug, followed thereafter by adsorption of the complexes to platelet membranes. The adsorption of drug-specific antibody complexes to platelets is not inhibited by excess drug, suggesting that the platelet-drug complex is not the antigen, although it also has been proposed that the antigen may be formed by conjugation of the drug to platelet membrane. If the drug-platelet membrane conjugate were the antigen, however, excess drug might be expected to inhibit binding of the drug-antibody complex to platelets. The suggestion also has been made that drugs bound to platelets may alter platelet cell membrane, rendering it autoantigenic. In this case the antibody induced would be reactive not only with the drug but also with autologous platelet membranes.

IMMUNOLOGIC HEMOLYTIC ANEMIA.[19,28] This anemia has been associated with reactions to several drugs, and may develop by means of one of four different mechanisms: (1) irreversible binding of a drug to red-cell membranes, with the drug functioning as a hapten and inducing an immunologic response; (2) injury to erythrocyte membranes caused by immunologic reactions not specifically directed toward red-cell antigens or erythrocyte-drug complexes, the erythrocyte being involved indirectly; (3) alteration of erythrocyte membrane by a drug (e.g., alpha methyldopa or mefenamic acid) rendering the red cell autoantigenic; (4) nonimmunologic binding of plasma proteins to erythrocytes induced by drugs (e.g., cephalothin).

Irreversible binding of a drug (hapten) to red-cell membranes may induce an immunologic response with the development of hapten-specific IgG antibody, immunologic hemolysis, and anemia. This process of drug-induced anemia may be associated with a positive response to Coombs' test of red cells in the presence of a drug.[13] Affected erythrocytes may hemolyze or they may have a shortened life span in vivo, each process leading to anemia. In addition to IgG antibody, drug-specific IgM or IgA antibody may be induced by the binding of hapten to red-cell membranes. IgM antibody readily fixes complement in the presence of antigen and may cause hemolysis, as does IgG. IgA antibody, however, probably is not responsible for hemolysis, but could shorten the life span of red cell-drug conjugates.

Drug-antibody complexes in plasma may adsorb to erythrocytes and produce hemolysis without the erythrocyte membrane binding the drug and serving as the responsible antigen. In this instance, the drug has a primary affinity for the antibody and the erythrocyte is involved secondarily. Complement activation by the drug-antibody complex may occur after adsorption of the complex to the red cell, leading to cell lysis. The binding of the drug-antibody complex to the erythrocyte may be transitory, and dissociation of the drug-antibody complex from erythrocytes may be followed by adsorption to other cells and lead to further immunologically induced injury. The transitory adsorption of antibody to erythrocytes in immunologic hemolysis is responsible for the fact that affected persons ordinarily have a negative reaction to the Coombs test, since the test serves to detect immunoglobulin on erythrocyte membranes. Affected patients, however, may have complement attached to red cells as a result of the transitory adsorption of antibody-drug complexes, and this may be responsible for erythrocyte agglutination by anticomplement testing serum.

Drugs acting upon red-cell membranes may make membrane components autoantigenic, inducing an immunologic response responsible for "autoimmune" hemolytic anemia. In these instances the drug does not function as a hapten or serve as an antigenic determinant of the immunologic response or induced antibody. These erythrocyte autoantibodies resemble "warm" reactive IgG immunoglobulins occurring in idiopathic immunologic hemolytic anemia. The erythrocyte membrane component which is "unmasked" or rendered "autoantigenic" by the drug usually shows Rh-system specificity.

Administration of cephalothin to some patients is associated with development of a positive direct Coombs test, which is not attributable to demonstrable immunologic responses to the drug or to erythrocyte antigens. Drug-induced nonspecific adsorption of plasma protein, particularly immunoglobulin, to erythrocyte membranes appears to be responsible for the positive Coombs test in this process. The nonspecific adsorption of immunoglobulin to erythrocytes has not been associated with hemolysis, although the affected patients may be anemic.

AGRANULOCYTOSIS. The immunologic mechanisms associated with instances of drug-induced agranulocytosis have not been completely worked out. In some instances leucocyte agglutinins have been found in the serum of patients with drug-induced agranulocytosis, suggesting that drugs may bind to leucocyte membranes in the same way that they may bind to erythrocytes, and serve as haptens responsible for an immunologic response.

FEVER. Fever as a manifestation of immunologic reactions was established in the early studies on serum sickness, and is now recognized as a feature of allergic reactions to certain drugs.[10,48] Fever also may be attributable to the therapeutic action of a drug (e.g., Jarisch-Herxheimer reaction), to drug-induced tissue injury, to drug effects upon tissue metabolism, to drug-induced vasoconstriction with decreased heat loss, to action of drugs upon the hypothalamus, and to contamination by bacterial pyrogens.

The immunologic mechanisms involved in causing fever have been studied extensively, and have been related to circulating antigen-specific antibody and to delayed hypersensitivity or cellular immunity. IgG, IgE, and IgM antigen-specific antibodies probably are responsible for febrile reactions.

Drug fever may occur as the only demonstrable feature of an

allergic reaction, or may be associated with rash, vasculitis, hemolysis, thrombocytopenia, hepatic disorder, or other manifestations.

The pathogenesis of drug fever probably is the same as that of most other types of fever, and is related to the elaboration of pyrogens from granulocytes and possibly lymphocytes. These endogenous or leucocytic pyrogens act upon the thermoregulatory centers of the brain to decrease heat loss and cause temperature elevation.

CELLULAR IMMUNE OR DELAYED HYPERSENSITIVITY REACTIONS[52]

CONTACT DERMATITIS. This dermatitis is the classic manifestation of reactions to drugs attributable to delayed hypersensitivity, and some rashes or fever caused by drugs also may be attributable to this immunologic mechanism.[6,53] Experimentally, contact sensitization of skin can be induced readily by a number of simple chemicals. It is not known whether or not the skin contact sensitization originates in the epidermis or dermis, but the drug or chemical probably combines as a hapten to proteins in the skin to induce an immunologic response by the T-cells of draining lymph nodes. In the skin, conjugation of drugs or chemicals to the lysine or cystine sulfhydryl reactive sites of dermal protein probably is most important in rendering the drug or chemical immunogenic.[16,18]

Delayed hypersensitivity to haptens conjugated to dermal protein results in specific sensitization to the protein as well as to the drug, and reactions can be elicited only by the conjugate and not by the unconjugated drug or chemical. In contrast with antibody-mediated reactions, therefore, in which the hapten alone reacts with the specific immunoglobulin, delayed hypersensitivity reactions occur when molecules (carrier and hapten) induce the initial immunologic response. Certain unusual haptens, however, may induce hapten-specific sensitization irrespective of the carrier protein.

Although contact dermatitis may be the principal manifestation of delayed hypersensitivity induced by application of chemicals to the skin, this immunologic response can be demonstrated in other tissues as well, if they have contact with the hapten conjugate. If the antigen to which sensitization occurs enters the blood, a systemic reaction (e.g., fever) may develop, or if it is injected into tissues other than skin, a delayed hypersensitivity reaction may develop at the injection site.

Mononuclear cells or lymphocytes are principally involved in producing the manifestations of delayed hypersensitivity reactions, and are prominently seen in the perivenous inflammation characteristic of these reactions. Increased vascular permeability, "invasive destruction," and granulomatous lesions affecting parenchymatous tissues occur in delayed hypersensitivity reactions, and are possibly attributable to the release of chemical mediators from lymphocytes and macrophages.[27]

In the presence of specific antigen, sensitized lymphocytes undergo blast transformation, release a protein substance known as the macrophage inhibitory factor (MIF), increase the multiplication and maturation of mononuclear cells, demonstrate increased pinocytotic activity, cause enzyme changes of macrophages, and can cause cell injury or death. In addition, antigenic stimulation of sensitized lymphocytes can result in the release of endogenous pyrogen and interferon. Delayed hypersensitivity or cellular immunity can be transferred from allergic to nonallergic individuals only by lymphoid cells or by a transfer factor derived from lymphocytes of sensitized persons. T-lymphocytes in draining lymphoid tissues and blood are responsible for delayed hypersensitivity reactions, and the transfer factor derivable from these cells is a dialyzable material with a mol wt of $< 10,000$ which is neither a protein nor a globulin fragment, and is resistant to desoxyribonuclease, ribonuclease, and trypsin.

IMMUNOLOGIC DIAGNOSTICS

Laboratory or technical procedures which demonstrate allergic reactions to drugs are often unavailable, unreliable, or misleading. The major reasons for the inadequacy of the tests presently available are an insufficient understanding of the reactive derivatives and the immunologic mechanisms responsible for drug allergy. Furthermore, even if reliable tests were available, it would be impractical to employ them regularly prior to each drug administration. This does not discount the importance of developing effective diagnostic tests, but in a routine screening of patients directed at avoiding the occurrence of allergic reactions to drugs, the patient's drug history is most important. Unfortunately, physicians usually are not skilled in or do not give sufficient emphasis to eliciting a patient's drug history, and therefore, they frequently are not aware of medications their patients take, or of any past history of a patient's adverse reactions to drugs.

Patient Drug History

Most patients take a varying number of nonprescription or OTC and prescription drugs. In one study of general medical adult clinic patients, it was found that the patients interviewed had taken on the average of about three different OTC and three different prescription drugs in the 30 days prior to being seen by the physician, and about one-third gave a seemingly reliable history of at least one adverse drug reaction in the past.[11] Reactions to penicillin or penicillin-like antibiotics accounted for the largest proportion of allergic reactions to drugs. A comparative evaluation of such histories obtained from interviews conducted by a skilled clinical pharmacist and several physicians revealed that physicians were able to detect only one-third of the drugs taken and one-third of the adverse reactions to drugs which were detected by the pharmacist. It is important to know what drugs a patient is taking in order to avoid administering duplicative drugs, to avoid adverse interactions, to provide guidance to the patient in appropriate use of OTC drugs, and to detect drugs possibly responsible for illness.

When they first see a physician patients should be asked to bring with them all medications taken in the previous 30 days, and these should be identified and noted in the patient's record. At times patients may not identify as drugs OTC medications which they have taken regularly or for cosmetic purposes, such as laxatives, antihistamines, oral contraceptives, and lotions or creams. Reciting common symptoms to patients, such as headache, constipation, diarrhea, menstrual pain, hay fever, etc., will often remind them of problems for which they have taken medications that they have neglected to mention. Verification of prescription and OTC drugs used may require consultation with other physicians caring for the patient and with the pharmacist dispensing drugs to the patient. Maintenance of a regularly updated drug profile on patients is important to provide full information on the medications a patient takes, and also serves as an aid in identifying untoward drug reactions when they occur.

Allergic manifestations during illness should always be investigated to see if they have been induced by drugs the patient has taken recently. Familiarity with the more common adverse reactions attributable to the drugs a patient has been receiving is necessary in order to identify the drug most likely implicated. The tables in the final section of this book may be useful in this regard. It is important to appreciate that the patient's interpretation of harmful drug effects in the past may be inaccurate. A patient's claim of a previous allergic reaction to a drug cannot be accepted as a valid observation without further evaluation and confirmation. For example, recently a patient was seen in consultation because of a history she had given of an allergic reaction to penicillin a few years before. The physician caring for the patient wanted to prescribe penicillin for her for a current illness, but was reluctant to do so because of her reported history. Further questioning of the patient revealed that when she had been given penicillin earlier for sinusitis, she had returned to the physician after five days of treatment, and he had indicated that the inflammation had not responded well to the medication. From this, the patient interpreted that she had penicillin allergy. After the misinterpretation was explained to her, she was treated with penicillin, and no adverse reaction developed. If the previous experience had in fact been an allergic reaction to penicillin, the patient's historical account would have been essential in deciding whether or not to administer penicillin again. In such a case, no laboratory test can be as useful as the drug history.

The development of an allergic reaction while a patient is receiving a drug manifests certain characteristics which are helpful in its recognition. A period of five to ten days of sensitization or drug administration is required before the manifestations of an allergic reaction appear, and these signs become progressively more severe or apparent over a few days. Readministration of the responsible drug to the previously sensitized patient often results in an accelerated reaction which usually appears within the first few hours after the drug is given, and it may appear abruptly, as in anaphylaxis. This sequence of events is often the principal evidence that the reaction is attributable to immunologic rather than pharmacologic mechanisms. Adverse reactions attributable to the pharmacologic action of a drug are closely related to dose of the drug, sensitization is not required, and upon readministration of the drug the accelerated reactions do not occur.

Laboratory or Technical Procedures

Three major types of tests are used in the diagnosis of drug allergy. These are (1) skin tests, (2) serological tests, and (3) passive sensitization of cells or tissues.

SKIN TESTS. The most valuable and readily available skin test for recognizing drug allergy is the patch test, which detects the incriminated agent in patients with contact dermatitis attributable to delayed hypersensitivity. These reactions become positive 24 to 48 hours after application of the skin test, producing erythema and induration.

Scratch, prick, or intradermal tests with drug solutions may detect skin sensitivity, or cytotropic or IgE antibodies, but their usual failure to demonstrate drug allergy is explained by the inability to identify the reactive drug product for inoculation. As mentioned before, a particular drug-protein conjugate or specific degradation products of the metabolism of drugs, rather than the drug administered, may be required to elicit an allergic reaction. If the drug conjugates to a protein different than that serving as a carrier and inducer of the immunologic response, these tests may fail to produce a skin reaction in individuals with contact dermatitis due to delayed hypersensitivity. If the drug injected into the skin is not metabolized to form the specifically reactive degradation product, the skin test will be negative. Irritant effects of the drug may also elicit an acute inflammatory reaction, and this may not be easily distinguishable from an allergic reaction. Even when such tests are positive and produce immediate wheal and flare or delayed hypersensitivity reaction, they do not invariably indicate that the patient will develop a reaction when the drug is given therapeutically. Furthermore, even when minute doses of a drug are used, skin tests may induce systemic reactions which can be hazardous to the patient. In addition, negative tests do not indicate that the patient will not develop an allergic reaction following administration of a therapeutic dose of the drug. If the reactive drug product is known and can be conjugated to a nonimmunologic oligopeptide as a carrier, skin tests of allergic reactivity to a drug can be performed more safely and reliably. Development of penicilloyl-polylysine as a test agent for penicillin allergy has demonstrated the effectiveness of this procedure. However, penicillin-degradation products other than the penicilloyl derivative are recognized as responsible for some instances of penicillin allergy, and in these cases testing with the penicilloyl derivative is not reliable.[20]

SEROLOGIC TESTS. These tests for immunologic reactivity of patients to drugs are notoriously deceptive and difficult to interpret, except for tests involving erythrocytes. Drugs binding covalently to erythrocytes on incubation in vitro, such as penicillin,[50] may be used in detecting serum antibody-producing hemagglutination. However, there is a limited correlation between such hemagglutinating antibodies and allergic reactions to drugs, even though such immunologic analyses allow determination of whether or not IgG or IgM antibodies are reactive with the penicillin conjugated to erythrocytes. In the case of penicillin, positive hemagglutination tests merely indicate that the patient has had prior exposure to penicillin, but they do not show whether or not the patient will have an allergic reaction to the drug when it is administered.[15] Most drugs, unlike penicillin, do not show covalent binding to erythrocytes, thereby further restricting the value of hemagglutination tests. Conjugates of other drugs with erythrocytes can be prepared, however, by the use of coupling reagents, but these conjugates have testing limitations similar to those of penicillin. Penicillin-erythrocyte conjugates formed in vivo in patients with IgG antipenicilloyl antibodies have been associated with hemolytic anemia following administration of large doses of penicillin,[31] but this reaction cannot be predicted by demonstration of hemagglutination with serum of erythrocyte-penicillin conjugates formed in vitro. Patients with penicillin-induced immuno-hemolytic anemia caused by penicilloyl-specific IgG antibody will have a positive Coombs test, as indicated before.

The difficulty of studying platelets in vitro has precluded the wide use of lysis or agglutination of platelet-drug conjugates by serum of patients with drug-induced thrombocytopenia as a diagnostic test.[1]

Histamine is released by blood leucocytes and basophils in the presence of antigen and specific antibody.[38] This test, however, has not been very useful in diagnosing drug allergy. Similarly, basophil degranulation, as a morphologic expression of antigen-antibody reactions, has been controversial and not always reproducible, but newer modifications may make this and other similar tests more useful.[39]

Serologic methods useful in studying protein and other complete antigens, including precipitation, immunodiffusion, and immunoelectrophoresis, have not thus far proved valuable in testing for drug allergy. Differential immunologic assays may be useful, but they have not been fully developed.

PASSIVE SENSITIZATION OF CELLS OR TISSUES. Lymphocyte reactivity in vitro in the presence of antigen, including blast transformation, detected by morphologic change, autoradiography, incorporation of DNA precursor, and elaboration of macrophage inhibitory factor may be demonstrated with cells of patients with delayed hypersensitivity reactions to drugs, but the results have been conflicting.[41] Many other cell and tissue tests to detect drug allergy have been investigated, but results have been contradictory or the procedure so complex as to preclude general applicability.

REFERENCES

1. Ackroyd, J. F.: The diagnosis of disorders of the blood due to drug hypersensitivity caused by an immune mechanism. In Ackroyd, J. F., ed., Immunological Methods, Oxford, Basil Blackwell, 1964.
2. Ada, G. L., Nossal, G. J. V., and Pye, J.: Antigens in immunity: III, Distribution of iodinated antigens following injection into rats via the hind footpads. Aust. J. Exp. Biol. Med. Sci., 42:295, 1964.
3. Arbesman, L. E., and Reisman, R. E.: Serum sickness and human anaphylaxis. In Samter, M., and Alexander, H. L., eds., Immunological Diseases, Boston, Little, Brown, and Company, 1971.
4. Austen, K. F.: Histamine and other mediators of allergic reactions. In Samter, M., and Alexander, H. L., eds., op. cit.
5. Austen, K. F., and Becker, E. L.: Biochemistry of the Acute Allergic Reaction. Oxford, Basil Blackwell, 1968.
6. Baer, R. L., and Harber, L. C.: Allergic eczematous contact dermatitis. In Samter, M., and Alexander, H. L., eds., op. cit.
7. Becker, E. L., and Henson, P. M.: In vitro studies of immunologically induced secretion of mediators from cells and related phenomena. Adv. Immunol., 17:93, 1973.
8. Butler, V. P., Jr., and Beiser, S. M.: Antibodies to small molecules: Biological and clinical applications. Adv. Immunol., 17:255–310, 1973.
9. Caldwell, J.: IgD antipenicillin antibodies in patients with penicillin reactions. Clin. Res., 21:56, 1973.
10. Cluff, L. E., and Johnson, J. E.: III, Drug fever. Progr. Allergy, 8:149, 1964.
11. Cluff, L. E., and Stewart, R. B.: Studies on the epidemiology of adverse drug reactions, VI, Utilization and interaction of prescription and non-prescription drugs in out-patients. Johns Hopkins Med. J., 129:319, 1971.
12. Coons, A. H., Leduc, E. H., and Kaplan, M. H.: Localization of antigen in tissue cells. J. Exp. Med., 93:173, 1951.
13. Croft, J. D., Jr., Swisher, S. N., Jr., Gilliland, B. C., et al.: Coombs' test positivity induced by drugs: Mechanisms of immunologic reactions and red cell destruction. Ann. Intern. Med., 68:176, 1968.
14. deWeck, A. L.: Immunochemical mechanisms in drug allergy. In Dash, C. H., and Jones, H. E. H., Mechanisms in Drug Allergy, Edinburgh and London, Churchill Livingstone, 1972.

15. DeWeck, A. L., and Blum, G.: Recent clinical and immunological aspects of penicillin allergy. Int. Arch. Allergy, 27:221, 1965.
16. Eisen, H. N., and Belman, S.: Studies of hypersensitivity to low molecular weight substances: Reactions of some allergenic substituted dinitrobenzenes with cysteine or cystine of skin proteins. J. Exp. Med., 98:533, 1953.
17. Eisen, H. N., Orris, L., and Belman, S.: Elicitation of delayed allergic skin reactions with haptens. J. Exp. Med., 95:473, 1952.
18. Eisen, H. N.: Hypersensitivity to simple chemicals. In Lawrence, H. S., ed., Cellular and Humoral Aspects of the Hypersensitive States, New York, Hoeber, 1959.
19. Erslev, A. J., and Wintrobe, M. M.: Detection and prevention of drug induced blood dyscrasias. J.A.M.A., 181:114, 1962.
20. Finke, S. R., Grieco, M. H., Connell, J. T., et al.: Results of comparative skin tests with penicilloyl-polylysine and penicillin in patients with penicillin allergy. Am. J. Med., 38:71, 1965.
21. Gardner, F. H.: Idiopathic thrombocytopenia purpura. In Samter, M., and Alexander, H. L., eds., op. cit.
22. Garvey, J. S., and Campbell, D. H.: The relation of circulating antibody concentration to localization of labeled antigen. J. Immunol., 72:131, 1954.
23. Goodman, L. S., and Gilman, A.: The Pharmacological Basis of Therapeutics. 4th ed., New York, The Macmillan Company, 1970.
24. Humphrey, J. H.: Receptors on lymphocytes. In Miescher, P. A., ed., Immunopathology, VIth International Symposium. New York, Grune & Stratton, Inc., 1970.
25. Ishijaka, K.: Experimental anaphylaxis. In Samter, M., and Alexander, H. L., eds., op. cit.
26. Landsteiner, K.: The Specificity of Serological Reactions. Cambridge, Mass., Harvard University Press, 1945.
27. Lawrence, H. S., and Landy, M.: Mediators of Cellular Immunity. New York, Academic Press, 1969.
28. Leddy, J. P., and Swisher, S. N.: Acquired immune hemolytic anemia. In Samter, M., and Alexander, H. L., eds., op. cit.
29. Levine, B. B.: Immunochemical mechanisms of drug allergy. Annu. Rev. Med., 17:23, 1966.
30. Levine, B. B.: Immunochemical mechanisms of drug allergy. In Miescher, P. A., and Muller-Eberhand, H. J., eds., Textbook of Immunopathology, vol. 1, New York, Grune & Stratton, Inc., 1968.
31. Levine, B. B., and Redmond, A. P.: Immunochemical mechanisms of penicillin induced Coombs' positive and hemolytic anemia. Int. Arch. Allergy, 21:594, 1967.
32. Merler, E., ed.: Immunoglobulins. Washington, D.C., National Academy of Sciences, 1970.
33. Antigen cell interaction and the control of antibody synthesis. In Miescher, P. A., ed., Immunopathology, VIth International Symposium, New York, Grune & Stratton, Inc., 1970.
34. Miller, J. L. III: Localization and fate of foreign antigens. In Samter, M., and Alexander, H. L., eds., op. cit.
35. Mitchison, N. A.: Antigen recognition responsible for the induction inhibit of the secondary response, Cold Spring Harbor symposium. Quant. Biol., 32:431, 1967.
36. Mitchison, N. A.: Suppression of immune responses by antigen. In Samter, M., and Alexander, H. L., eds., op. cit.
37. Natvig, J. B., and Kunkel, H.: Human immunoglobulins: Classes, subclasses, genetic variants and idiotypes. Adv. Immunol., 16:1, 1972.
38. Osler, A. G., Lichtenstein, L. M., and Levy, D. A.: In vitro studies of human reagin in allergy. Adv. Immunol., 8:183, 1968.
39. Perelmutter, L., and Khera, K.: Basophil degranulation and IgE antibody. Int. Arch. Allergy, 39:27, 1970.
40. Pressman, D.: The nature of antigen and antibody combining regions. In Samter, M., and Alexander, H. L., eds., op. cit.
41. Sarkany, I.: Lymphocyte transformation in drug hypersensitivity. Lancet, 1:743, 1967.
42. Schneider, C. H., and deWeck, A. L.: Immunogenic penicillin conjugates. Immunochemistry, 7:157, 1970.
43. Schneider, C. H., deWeck, A. L., and Stauble, E.: Carboxymethylcellulose addi-

tives in penicillin and the elicitation of anaphylactic reactions. Experientia, 27:167, 1971.
44. Sela, M.: Antigenicity: Some molecular aspects. Science, 166:1365, 1969.
45. Sherman, W. B., ed.: Allergic reaction patterns of skin. In Samter, M., and Alexander, H. L., eds., op. cit.
46. Shulman, N. R.: Immunoreactions involving platelets. J. Exp. Med., 107:697, 1962.
47. Sjostrand, F. S.: The structure of cell membranes. Protoplasma, 63:248, 1967.
48. Snell, E. S.: Hypersensitivity fever. In Dash, C. H., and Jones, H. E. H., eds., op. cit.
49. Stupp, Y., Paul, W. E., and Benacerraf, B.: Structural control of immunogenicity. Immunology, 21:583, 1971.
50. Thiel, J. A., Mitchell, S., and Parker, C. W.: The specificity of hemagglutination reactions in human and experimental penicillin hypersensitivity. J. Allergy, 35:399, 1964.
51. Turck, J. L., Parker, D., and Poulter, L. W.: Interaction between B- and T-lymphocytes in chemical contact sensitization. In Dash, C. H., and Jones, H. E. H., eds., op. cit.
52. Vassalli, P., and McCluskey, R. T.: Delayed hypersensitivity. In Movat, H. Z., ed., Inflammation, Immunity and Hypersensitivity, New York, Harper & Row, 1971.
53. Waksman, B. H.: Delayed hypersensitivity: Immunologic and clinical aspects. Hosp. Pract., 3:22, 1968.
54. Waud, D. R.: Pharmacologic receptors. Pharmacol. Rev., 20:49, 1968.
55. Wilkinson, D. S.: Sensitivity to pharmaceutical additives. In Dash, C. H., and Jones, H. E. H., eds., op. cit.
56. Worlledge, S.: Drug allergy and blood pathology. In Dash, C. H., and Jones, H. E. H., eds., op. cit.

CHAPTER 4

CLINICAL MANIFESTATIONS

1. DERMATOLOGIC MANIFESTATIONS

Clinically, the skin is more often affected by adverse drug reactions than any other organ system. A drug eruption is defined as a cutaneous or oral mucosal lesion produced by a drug regardless of the route of administration. Almost any known skin disease may be mimicked by a drug reaction. Virtually all drugs have the potential of producing a cutaneous adverse effect.

The nature of the skin lesion does not necessarily identify the drug that has caused it, since similar reactions may be produced by different drugs. A given drug tends to produce the same reaction on repeated administration (e.g., fixed drug eruption from phenolphthalein), but it may produce different reactions at different times (e.g., penicillin may induce urticaria at one time and exfoliative dermatitis at another). Also, the same drug may produce different skin reactions in different individuals. A careful clinical history of the patient and observation of the patient after the drug has been administered are often necessary to identify the causative drug. Frequently, the offending agent may not be considered a drug by the patient, and may be a proprietary compound, such as aspirin, or a laxative containing phenolphthalein.

Drug eruptions may vary in severity from a mild asymptomatic rash or a few urticaria easily controlled with an antihistamine to a potentially fatal reaction (e.g., exfoliative dermatitis, Stevens-Johnson syndrome, or toxic epidermal necrolysis). A localized area of skin or virtually the entire cutaneous surface may be affected. Many reactions are confined to the skin, but other organs may be affected (e.g., drug-induced systemic lupus erythematosus).

The mechanisms of many drug eruptions are hard to define, but

CLINICAL MANIFESTATIONS

clinically the most common cause seems to be drug allergy. Allergic dermatoses, however, are less common in older people.

Most skin reactions abate when the offending drug is discontinued. Exceptions include some severe reactions, such as exfoliative dermatitis, which may progress to a fatal outcome, and late cumulative effects as seen in arsenical dermatitis. Intercurrent therapy may be required in some instances because of troublesome symptoms.[13,122,198,240]

The drug-induced dermatoses will be outlined in the sections which follow, and the most frequently implicated drugs will be listed. At times the drugs discussed may be mostly of historical interest (e.g., arsenicals). The most serious drug eruptions will be considered first.

SEVERE CUTANEOUS DRUG REACTIONS

Exfoliative Dermatitis

Exfoliative dermatitis (Fig. 4-1) may be produced by drugs, may result from other skin diseases (psoriasis, contact dermatitis, atopic

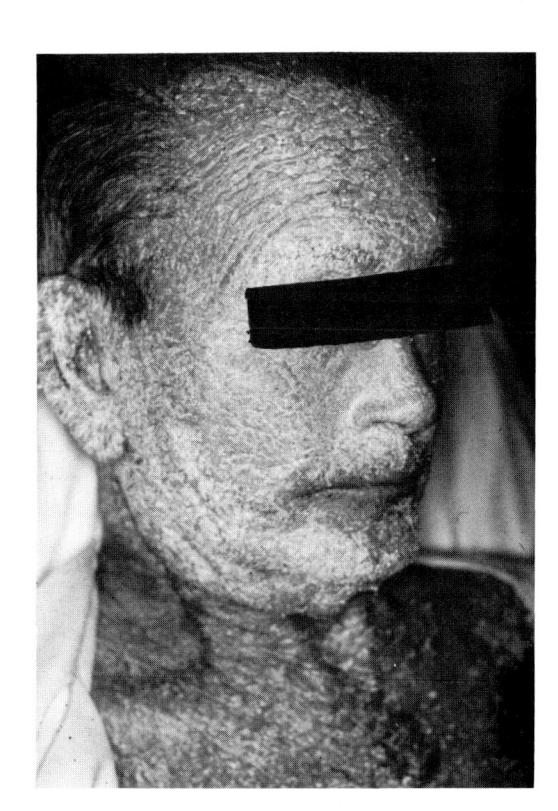

Figure 4-1. Exfoliative dermatitis with marked dryness and scaling of skin (courtesy of S. I. Cullen, M.D.).

dermatitis), or may be caused by lymphomas or unknown conditions. Symptomatically, most of the skin becomes erythematous, dry, and scaly. Itching often occurs. The hair and nails may be secondarily damaged and lost. The protective barrier of the skin is diminished, and fluid-electrolyte losses and secondary infection pose a serious threat to life.

Numerous drugs have been implicated in producing this disease (Table 4-1). Its clinical course is usually short if the responsible drug is discontinued and appropriate therapy is instituted. Good nursing care is mandatory, and the administration of parenteral fluids is usually necessary to maintain proper fluid and electrolyte balance. Application of triamcinolone cream (0.1 per cent) four times a day after moist compresses, and prednisone, 60 mg per day, help alleviate symptoms and shorten the course of the illness. Infections should be treated appropriately when they occur.[77,122,240,288]

Stevens-Johnson Syndrome

This serious form of erythema multiforme begins acutely with fever, painful erosions of the mouth and lips, and erythematous,

TABLE 4-1. *Drugs Known to Cause Exfoliative Dermatitis**

<u>Penicillin</u>
<u>Sulfonamides</u>
<u>Barbiturates</u>
<u>Hydantoins</u>: diphenylhydantoin, mesantoin
<u>Phenylbutazone</u>
<u>Arsenicals</u>
Gold salts
Mercurial diuretics
Antimony compounds
Iodides
Chloroquine
Quinacrine
Tetracyclines
Streptomycin
Para-aminosalicylic acid
Thiouracil
Griseofulvin
Phenothiazines
Salicylates
Phenacemide
Actinomycin D
Allopurinol
Chlorpropamide
Quinidine
Vitamin A

* Underlined drugs indicate frequent cause of reaction.

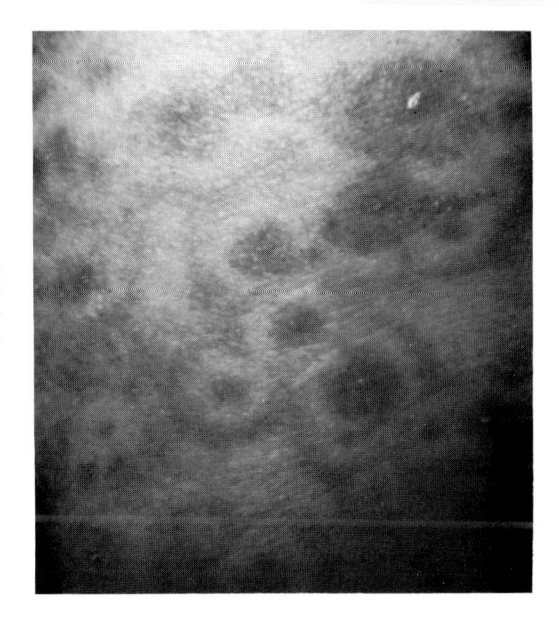

Figure 4-2. Stevens-Johnson syndrome (erythema multiforme). Typical target or iris lesions (courtesy of S. I. Cullen, M.D.).

bullous lesions of the skin with a typical target or iris appearance (Fig. 4-2). Another symptom, bilateral conjunctivitis, may result in varying degrees of blindness. Mortality rates in up to 25 per cent of patients have been reported.

This syndrome may also be associated with infections, pregnancy, food allergy, deep x-ray therapy, or with no discernible cause. Many drugs have been implicated in its etiology (Table 4-2). Penicillin is probably the most common of these, while sulfonamides are regarded as a less important etiologic factor.[30]

Therapy consists of stopping the offending drug, careful nursing care, general supportive measures, and administration of systemic corticosteroids. Prednisone should be begun promptly in doses of 80 to 100 mg per day, and tapered off as the illness improves. In some instances the illness may worsen despite corticosteroid therapy. Renal impairment may supervene, progressing to tubular necrosis. Eye complications should be treated by an ophthalmologist.[77,122,240]

Toxic Epidermal Necrolysis (Lyell's Syndrome)

This disorder is characterized by tender, erythematous, peeling areas of skin resembling a burn and is often termed the scalded skin syndrome (Fig. 4-3). In adults, this disease is usually associated with a drug reaction, while in children it mainly follows staphylococcal infections. Elements of the Stevens-Johnson syndrome may be present in the same patient. Death occurs in up to 40 per cent of patients, usually from shock secondary to fluid loss, from secondary

*TABLE 4-2. Drugs Known to Cause Stevens-Johnson Syndrome**

<u>Penicillin</u>
<u>Phenolphthalein</u>
Sulfonamides: sulfamethoxypyridazine (Kynex, Medicel), and short-acting sulfonamides
Sulfones
Diphenylhydantoin (Dilantin)
3-Ethyl–phenyl–ethyl hydantoin
Trimethadione (Tridione)
Phenobarbital
Aspirin
Phenylbutazone
Para-aminosalicylic acid
Antipyrine
Bromides
Iodides
Phenothiazines
Meprobamate
Gold salts
Chloramphenicol
Tetracyclines
Carbamazepine (Tegretol)
Griseofulvin
Hydralazine
Thiazides
Methandrostenolone
Digitalis
Chlorpropamide (Diabinese)
Amithiozone
Vaccines: diphtheria-pertussis, small pox, measles

* Underlined drugs indicate frequent cause of reaction.

bacterial infection, or, in rare cases, from disseminated intravascular coagulation.

The causative mechanism is felt to be an allergic reaction. The many drugs that have been implicated in toxic epidermal necrolysis are listed in Table 4-3. Therapy is similar to that for burns. Adequate intravenous fluids and electrolytes should be given to replace losses. Aseptic techniques should be used to avoid bacterial infection, which should be appropriately treated if it occurs. High doses of prednisone, from 100 to 150 mg per day, appear to be beneficial if given early in the course of the illness, and gradually decreased as the skin lesions heal.[77,122,240]

Systemic lupus erythematosus

Drug-induced systemic lupus erythematosus affects not only the skin but also multiple organs. It is discussed in the section on multisystem diseases.

CLINICAL MANIFESTATIONS 85

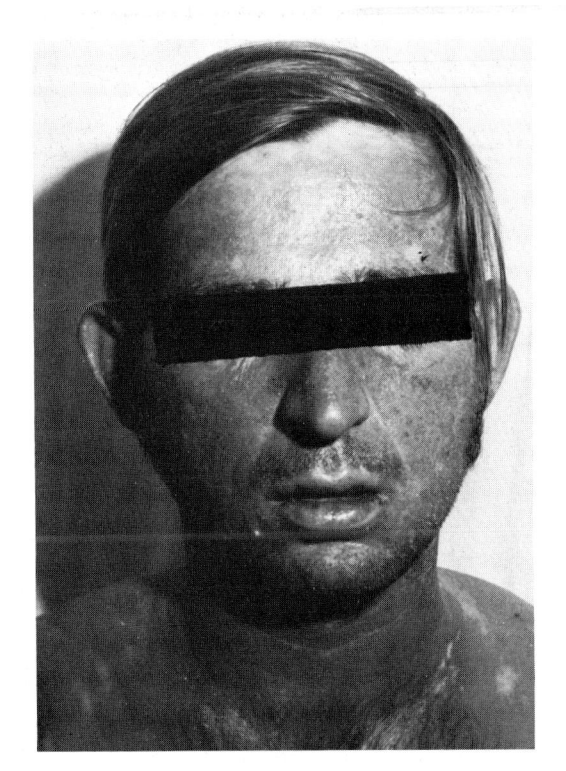

Figure 4-3. Toxic epidermal necrolysis (scalded skin syndrome). Skin changes resemble those of a burn (courtesy of S. I. Cullen, M.D.).

TABLE 4-3. Drugs Known to Cause Toxic Epidermal Necrolysis°

Phenylbutazone
Hydantoins: diphenylhydantoin
Sulfonamides
Dapsone
Acetazolamide
Aminopyrine
Antipyrine
Phenolphthalein
Penicillin
Nitrofurantoin
Tetracycline: demeclocycline (Declomycin)
Tolbutamide (Orinase)
Barbiturates
Brompheniramine (Dimetane)
Gold salts
Allopurinol
Tetanus antitoxin
Polio vaccine
Diphtheria inoculation

° Underlined drugs indicate frequent cause of reaction.

OTHER FORMS OF CUTANEOUS DRUG REACTIONS

ACNEIFORM OR FURUNCULOID ERUPTIONS. These eruptions are brought about by drugs and usually have an abrupt onset in individuals over age 25. They regress rapidly when the drug is stopped or the dose is reduced (Table 4-4). Acne is a frequent effect of ACTH (adrenocorticotropic hormone) or cortiscosteroid therapy, as well as of oral contraceptives, anabolic steroids, and androgens. Other drugs that may produce acne include bromides, iodides, isoniazid, ethionamide, cyanocobalamin (vitamin B_{12}), and haloperidol (Haldol).[122,240]

CONTACT DERMATITIS (ECZEMATOUS TYPE). This is a frequently encountered drug eruption which occurs less commonly in older people. The site of the rash may be a clue to the offending agent. A rash around the eyelids may be caused by pilocarpine eye drops. Eruptions on the upper lip and nostrils are produced by nose drops containing antihistamines, epinephrine, penicillin, or sulfonamides. A host of drugs may produce contact dermatitis. The drugs most frequently associated with the disease are listed in Table 4-5.[13,122]

Allergic contact dermatitis has been reported to be produced by clioquinol (Vioform), occurring after topical application of the drug and reappearing in the previously sensitized area of the body after ingestion of iodochlorhydroxyquin (Entero-Vioform).[97]

ERYTHEMA NODOSUM. An inflammatory skin disease, characterized by red nodules or lesions, usually on the shins, which is often caused by an allergic reaction to drugs (Table 4-6). Causative drugs include penicillin, sulfonamides, sulfonylurea oral hypoglycemics, bromides, iodides, salicylates, phenacetin, barbiturates, thiazide diuretics, codeine, thiouracil, anticonvulsants, and oral contraceptives.[122,240]

TABLE 4-4.° Drugs Known to Cause Acne

ACTH
Corticosteroids
Oral contraceptives
Anabolic steroids
Androgens
Bromides
Iodides
Isoniazid
Ethionamide
Cyanocobalamin (vitamin B_{12})
Haloperidol (Haldol)

° Underlined drugs indicate frequent cause of reaction.

TABLE 4–5. *Drugs that Commonly Cause Contact Dermatitis*

Antihistamines
Arsenicals
Bacitracin
Chloramphenicol (Chloromycetin)
Chlorpromazine (Thorazine)
Ephedrine
Formaldehyde
Hexachlorophene
Meprobamate
Mercurials
Merthiolate
Neomycin
Nitrofurazone (Furacin)
Novobiocin
Penicillin
Procaine and other local anesthetics
Promethazine (Phenergan)
Quinacrine (Atabrine)
Quinine
Resorcin
Streptomycin
Sulfonamides
Tetracycline
Thiamine

RASHES. Exanthematic (morbilliform and scarlatiniform) rashes may be caused by many drugs, among them ampicillin, allopurinol, barbiturates, sodium sulfobromophthalein (Bromsulphalein, or BSP), chlorothiazide (Diuril), gold salts, griseofulvin, hydantoins, insulin, isoniazid, meprobamate, mercurials, novobiocin, para-aminosalicylic acid, penicillin, phenothiazines, phenylbutazone (Butazolidin), quinacrine (Atabrine), salicylates, serums, streptomycin, sulfonamides, sulfones, tetracyclines, and thiouracil.[122,198]

TABLE 4–6. *Drugs Known to Cause Erythema Nodosum*

Penicillin
Sulfonamides
Sulfonylureas
Bromides
Iodides
Salicylates
Phenacetin
Barbiturates
Thiazide diuretics
Codeine
Thiouracil
Oral contraceptives
Diphenylhydantoin (Dilantin)
Trimethadione (Tridione)

88 CLINICAL MANIFESTATIONS

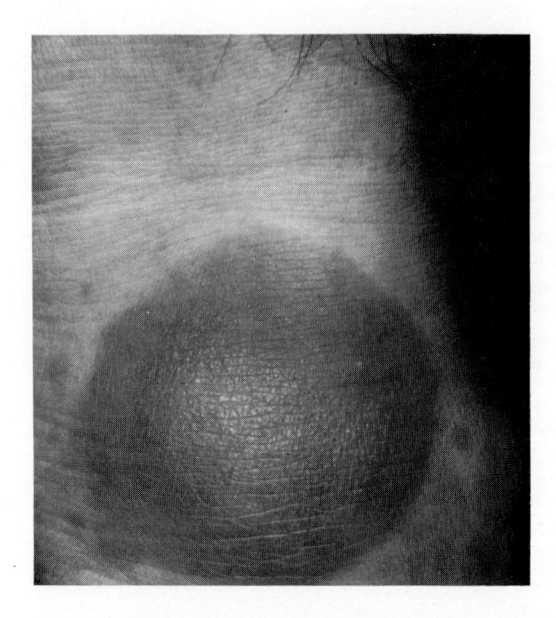

Figure 4-4. Fixed drug eruption on back of neck. Round, erythematous, edematous, solitary plaque with small satellite lesions (courtesy of S. I. Cullen, M.D.).

FIXED DRUG ERUPTIONS. These eruptions are caused by drugs administered systemically, and they are insufficiently recognized. The lesions which result may be round or oval, single or multiple; they are erythematous, edematous plaques varying in size from less than a centimeter to several centimeters in diameter, and are often accompanied by itching or burning (Fig. 4-4). They regress rapidly

TABLE 4-7. Drugs Known to Cause Fixed Drug Eruptions°

<u>Phenolphthalein</u>
<u>Phenacetin</u>
<u>Barbiturates</u>
<u>Sulfonamides</u>
<u>Salicylates</u>
Antihistamines
Anticonvulsants (Dilantin, Mesantoin, Paradione, Tridione)
Oral contraceptives
Antipyrine
Carisoprodol (Rela, Soma)
Gold salts
Meprobamate
<u>Penicillin</u>
Para-aminosalicylic acid
Phenylbutazone
<u>Quinidine</u>
Quinacrine (Atabrine)
Tetracyclines
Rauwolfia alkaloids

° Underlined drugs indicate frequent cause of reaction.

when the drug is stopped, and heal with some hyperpigmentation. Lesions recur at the same site if the drug is readministered. This disorder is felt to be brought about by drug allergy. The more frequently implicated drugs are shown in Table 4–7.[13,122,198,240]

GANGRENOUS LESIONS. These lesions may develop in distal parts of the body secondary to vasoconstriction, which is produced by large doses of ergot and its derivatives. Local skin necrosis has occurred from extravasation of intravenous norepinephrine (Levophed) and metaraminol (Aramine). Coumarin derivatives and phenindione (Danilone, Dindevan, Hedulin) have caused necrosis of the skin and subcutaneous tissues. Histologically, these lesions show vasculitis and thrombosis. Three to five days after anticoagulant therapy is begun, painful red patches appear and become necrotic, with hemorrhagic blisters and slough. Most instances have been found in obese women, with the lesions showing a preference for areas of subcutaneous fat: breasts, abdomen, buttocks, and thighs.[203]

FUNGAL INFECTIONS. Drug therapy may excite fungal infections of the skin. Monilial infections may appear after the administration of griseofulvin for dermatophyte infections. Monilial and dermatophyte infections also may follow corticosteroid therapy.[122]

Dry, rough, scaly skin changes similar to those of ichthyosis have been caused by haloperidol (Haldol), nicotinic acid, and triparanol.[13,122]

PHOTOSENSITIVE DRUG REACTIONS. These reactions (Fig. 4–5) appear after exposure to light (ultraviolet rays) of areas of skin in which the drug is present, whether it has been administered systemically or topically. Photodermatitis may resemble a severe sun-

Figure 4–5. Photodermatitis on back over area not shielded from sunlight by bathing suit (courtesy of S. I. Cullen, M.D.).

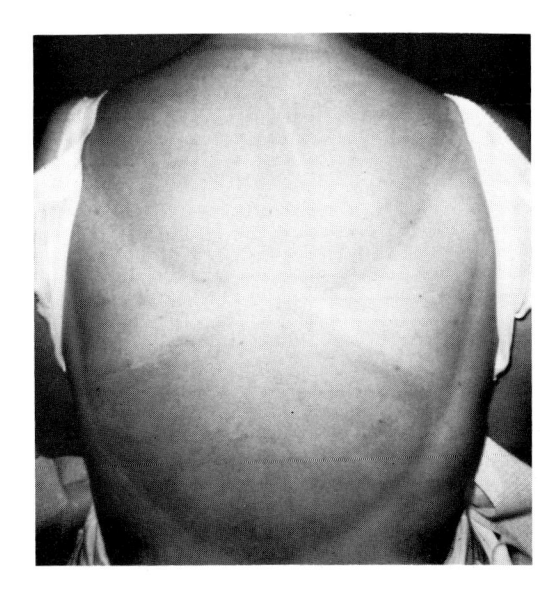

TABLE 4-8. Drugs Known to Cause Photodermatitis°

<u>Demeclocycline</u> (Declomycin)
<u>Griseofulvin</u>
<u>Sulfonamides:</u>
  Sulfisoxazole (Gantrisin)
Sulfonylureas:
  Tolbutamide (Orinase)
  Chlorpropamide (Diabinese)
Phenothiazines:
  Chlorpromazine (Thorazine)
  Prochlorperazine (Compazine)
  Promazine (Sparine)
  Promethazine (Phenergan)
  Trimeprazine (Temaril)
<u>Thiazides</u>:
  Chlorothiazide (Diuril)
  Hydrochlorothiazide (Hydrodiuril)
Haloperidol (Haldol)
Antimalarials
Chlordiazepoxide (Librium)
6-Mercaptopurine
Nalidixic acid
Antihistamines:
  Diphenhydramine (Benadryl)
  Carbinoxamine (Rondec)
Bithionol
Hexachlorophene
Halogenated salicylanilides
Psoralens
Coal tars

° Underlined drugs indicate frequent cause of reaction.

burn or be edematous, scaly, or urticarial, and the papules may be similar to those seen in lichen planus, or be eczematous. This type of reaction is of greater concern in sunny climates, but temperate zones have adequate sunlight to produce troublesome reactions. Demeclocycline (Declomycin) is probably the systemically administered drug most frequently implicated in photodermatitis. Photosensitive drug reactions also are produced by topical compounds such as hexachlorophene, and by halogenated salicylanilides used in antibacterial soaps.[177] Psoralens, which are used orally or topically to treat vitiligo or to hasten sun tanning, can also produce light eruptions. The many drugs known to cause photodermatitis are listed in Table 4–8.[122,240,244]

URTICARIA AND ANGIONEUROTIC EDEMA. Urticaria and angioneurotic edema are manifestations of acute allergic reactions, and are among the more common forms of adverse drug reactions. Acute urticaria (Fig. 4–6) may last for a few hours or for several weeks, while chronic urticaria, more often encountered in individuals over 50 years old, may last for months or years. Almost any drug is capable of causing urticaria, regardless of its route of administration. Both

CLINICAL MANIFESTATIONS

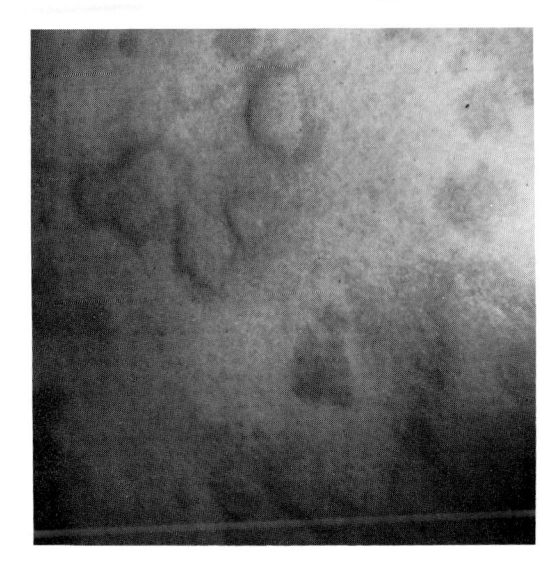

Figure 4-6. Urticaria. Elevated, edematous lesions with peripheral erythema (courtesy of S. I. Cullen, M.D.).

angioneurotic edema and urticaria may be associated with anaphylaxis. Inflammation and urticaria may occur at the injection sites of penicillin, insulin, or sera.

Therapy consists of discontinuing the offending drug. In mild cases antihistamines usually control symptoms. In more severe instances, especially with angioneurotic edema, corticosteroids may be required.

The more common drugs causing urticaria are listed in Table 4-9.[13,122,240]

VESICULOBULLOUS ERUPTIONS. Vesicular and bullous eruptions, besides those of the Stevens-Johnson syndrome, may be caused by drugs. These lesions vary in size, site, and extent. Among the more common causative drugs are antipyrine, arsenic, acetazolamide (Diamox), thiazide diuretics, barbiturates, bromides, iodides, mercurials, hydantoin anticonvulsants, penicillin, phenolphthalein, salicylates, streptomycin, and sulfonamides.

Salicylates may produce bullous urticaria, bullous erythema multiforme, and lesions resembling dermatitis herpetiformis. During treatment with nalidixic acid, photosensitivity reactions may progress to bullae. In acute barbiturate poisoning, about 6 per cent of patients develop large bullae either early or late in the course of their illness, which may be a clue to diagnosis. A vesicular epidermophytid eruption may appear in rare instances one to three days after griseofulvin therapy is begun for tinea pedis.[122,240,288]

HERXHEIMER REACTION. In the treatment of early syphilis, within a few hours after initiating therapy with parenteral penicillin (and' also previously with parenteral arsenicals), about half of the

TABLE 4-9. *Common Drugs Known to Cause Urticaria**

<u>Penicillin</u> and its congeners, especially ampicillin
<u>Chloramphenicol</u>
Erythromycin
Novobiocin
Streptomycin
Tetracyclines
Penicillinase
<u>Sulfonamides</u>
<u>Aspirin</u>, and other salicylates
<u>Barbiturates</u>
<u>Morphine</u>, meperidine, codeine, and other opiates
Propoxyphene (Darvon)
Adrenocorticotropic hormone (ACTH)
Atropine and belladonna
Insulin
Bromides and iodides
Sodium sulfobromophthalein (Bromsulphalein, BSP)
Oral contraceptives
Griseofulvin
Hydantoin anticonvulsants
Isoniazid
Nitrofurantoin
Nalidixic acid
Meprobamate
Mercurials
Phenolphthalein
Rauwolfia derivatives
Thiouracils
Serums
Enzymes
Liver extract
Dextran
Iodinated radiographic contrast media

* Underlined drugs indicate frequent cause of reaction.

patients develop exacerbated cutaneous lesions and concomitant fever, malaise, myalgias, and headache that last a few hours. This is termed a Herxheimer reaction, and is felt to be an allergic reaction caused by the release of treponemal products from the killed microorganism.[122]

HYPERPIGMENTATION

DIFFUSE VARIETIES

CHANGES IN SKIN COLOR. Skin pigmentation changes can be caused by many drugs in various ways. Diffuse hyperpigmentation may result from prolonged therapy with adrenocorticotropic hormone (ACTH). Use of busulfan and 6-mercaptopurine has led to a clinical syndrome resembling Addison's disease, with darkening of the skin, but usually sparing the mucous membranes, and electrolyte disturbances.

Phenothiazines, most often chlorpromazine (Thorazine), when taken in large doses for three or more years, may occasionally result in hyperpigmentation, primarily in women. Light-exposed areas become darker and may become slate gray or violet in color. This is due to a melanin-like pigment that tends to fade when the drug is discontinued.

HEMOCHROMATOSIS. Large doses of iron for prolonged periods, or multiple blood transfusions, particularly in patients with chronic hemolytic anemias, e.g., thalassemia, may result in hemochromatosis with hyperpigmentation owing to increased melanin and iron in the skin.

Prolonged exposure to arsenic, which is no longer used in medical therapy but is still a hazard from occupational sources, also can lead to diffuse hyperpigmentation.

HYPERVITAMINOSIS A. An excess ingestion of vitamin A produces not only dry, flaking, hyperkeratotic skin changes, but also may promote tanning of the skin. These changes are reversible when the drug is stopped.

A darkening of the skin may also follow the flush produced by nicotinic acid if the drug is used for prolonged periods.

REGIONAL VARIETIES

CHLOASMA, FACIAL MELASMA, OR MASK OF PREGNANCY. Drugs can also induce regional hyperpigmentation. Chloasma, facial melasma, or the mask of pregnancy occurs in some women with the use of oral contraceptives. Hyperpigmentation fades only slightly if these drugs are discontinued. A similar phenomenon may occur in males treated with hydantoin anticonvulsants.

Pigmentation of the breast areola has been produced in patients by phenothiazines and griseofulvin.

Sulfone therapy used in the treatment of leprosy can result in postinflammatory hyperpigmentation in the most severely affected parts of the skin.

CHRYSIASIS AND ARGYRIA. Gold and silver salts also can change skin color; these changes are termed chrysiasis and argyria, respectively. When given to a patient, large doses of gold, presently used in the treatment of rheumatoid arthritis, lead to the deposition of gold granules and melanin in the upper dermis. In light-exposed areas the skin changes to a violet or gray-brown color. Silver salts were used previously in nose drops, but now individuals with argyria are infrequently encountered. In this disease, silver granules are deposited in the skin, and a black color develops which may resemble cyanosis.

SKIN DISCOLORATION. The use of chloroquine and hydroxychloroquine can result in a grayish blue to black skin discoloration, especially on the face, the pretibial area, and the nail beds. The prolonged use of phenolphthalein may produce dark gray patches on the skin that are unrelated to a fixed drug reaction.

Quinacrine (Atabrine), and less often amodiaquine (Camoquin), produces a yellow skin color that mimics jaundice and that fades when the drug is discontinued. With prolonged use, however, a greenish to bluish-gray discoloration of the ears, nose, and nail beds may develop.

Drugs rarely cause lightening of the skin, but this reaction has been reported secondary to prolonged corticosteroid therapy, and from treatment with the alkylating agents triethylenemelamine (TEM) and thiotepa, as well as with triparanol.[122,240]

Lesions resembling psoriasis have been produced by antimalarials, arsenic, gold salts, and salicylates.[240]

Purpuric reactions may be thrombocytopenic or nonthrombocytopenic and will be discussed with hematologic reactions. Anaphylactoid purpura, which is associated with multiple organ involvement, is considered with multisystem diseases.

Existing rosacea may be aggravated by topical fluorinated corticosteroids and systemic iodides. Oral contraceptives, and infrequently, oral hypoglycemic agents, may incite this disorder.[240]

WARTY LESIONS. Bromides, and occasionally iodides, can produce warty lesions in patients, mostly on the extremities, which may persist for months after the drug is stopped. Arsenic may induce warty keratoses, usually on the palms of the hands and soles of the feet, which in rare cases may develop into basal cell carcinomas up to 30 years later.[122,240]

SPIDER ANGIOMATA. Spider angiomata may appear with the use of oral contraceptives or trihexyphenidyl (Artane).[198]

DRUG REACTIONS RELATED TO HAIR AND NAILS

ALOPECIA. Drugs may, on occasion, cause loss of hair (alopecia), hirsutism, or change in hair color. Alopecia brought about by cytotoxic drugs is dependent upon the dose given and is usually more marked in young patients because of more actively growing hair follicles. In most instances, hair loss is reversible. Thallium, which is still used as a rodent poison in some countries, produces marked alopecia. Heparin may cause transient hair loss weeks after it has been dis-

TABLE 4-10. *Drugs Known to Cause Alopecia*

Cytotoxic agents:
  Cyclophosphamide (Cytoxan)
  Melphalan (Alkeran)
  Vinblastine (Velban)
  Vincristine (Oncovin)
  5-Fluorouracil
  6-Mercaptopurine
  Methotrexate
Thallium
Heparin
Triparanol (discontinued drug)
Clofibrate (Atromid-S)
Colchicine
Trimethadione (Tridione)
Chloroquine
Quinacrine (Atabrine)
Oral contraceptives
Trichlormethiazide (Naqua)
Ethionamide (Trecator SC)
Vitamin A
Para-aminosalicylic acid
Mephenasin (muscle relaxant)
Nicotinyl Alcohol
Mepesulfate
Thiouracil

continued. Alopecia was one of the many troublesome side effects of triparanol, a drug used to lower cholesterol levels that is no longer available. Besides the drugs listed in Table 4-10 that have caused alopecia, radiation therapy can destroy hair follicles and produce permanent alopecia.[122,240]

HIRSUTISM. Drug-induced hirsutism has become increasingly more common (Table 4-11). Androgens, anabolic steroids, and oral contraceptives produce hirsutism concomitant with their masculinizing effects. Androgens (e.g., testosterone) result in varying degrees of hirsutism among women, even when given in equivalent doses. The progestogens in oral contraceptives and anabolic steroids are

TABLE 4-11. *Drugs Known to Cause Hirsutism*

With Masculinizing Effects:
  Androgens
  Anabolic steroids
  Oral contraceptives
Without Masculinizing Effects:
  ACTH
  Corticosteroids
  Diphenylhydantoin (Dilantin)
  Diazoxide
  Chlorpromazine (Thorazine)

also associated with hirsutism, but the incidence of these reactions is low.

ACTH and corticosteroids produce hirsutism without significant accompanying masculinization. Diphenylhydantoin and diazoxide produce generalized hypertrichosis of the face, the trunk, and the extremities. Chlorpromazine (Thorazine) can produce hirsutism in women in association with amenorrhea, weight gain, and increased sebaceous gland activity. Hexachlorobenzene, a fungicide added to wheat, caused an outbreak of poisoning in Turkey which led to the appearance of porphyria cutanea tarda with associated diffuse hirsutism, more marked in children than in adults.[240,260]

LOSS OF HAIR COLOR. Drugs that may result in a loss of hair color include chloroquine, haloperidol (Haldol), and mephenesin, a muscle relaxant. Triparanol has caused hyperpigmentation of the skin and discoloration of the hair.[240]

NAILS. A bluish discoloration of the proximal part of the nails may be produced in argyria, or silver salt poisoning, and can also be caused by quinacrine (Atabrine), phenolphthalein, and local application of mercury.[366]

Tetracyclines can cause a yellow discoloration of the nails, and busulfan can cause a brownish color. Demeclocycline (Declomycin) may lead to onycholysis as part of a photodermatitis. Thinning and coarsening of the nails is sometimes seen in hypervitaminosis A.[122]

2. HEMATOPOIETIC MANIFESTATIONS

Drug-induced hematologic changes occur often and may be trivial, or, in some instances, such as aplastic anemia, agranulocytosis, and thrombocytopenia, may have a fatal outcome. Drugs can produce changes in all elements of the blood, changes in the oxygen carrying capacity of hemoglobin, decreased numbers of white cells and platelets, coagulation defects, changes in lymphoid tissue, and perhaps leukemia and lymphomas. Drugs may affect a single cellular element (as in granulocytopenia), or may produce changes in more than one blood component (as in pancytopenia).

The types of clinical and laboratory changes usually noted are divided into 4 categories for discussion: Red blood cell diseases induced by drugs are examined first, followed by white blood cell diseases, bleeding disorders, and finally, other blood and lymph disorders in which drugs play a major causative role.

DRUG-INDUCED RED BLOOD CELL DISEASES

Aplastic Anemia (Pancytopenia)

Aplastic anemia, whether drug-induced or not, is a manifestation of bone-marrow failure expressed by pancytopenia. About half of the reported cases are produced by drugs, but there is no simple way to differentiate drug-induced from idiopathic aplastic anemia. A history of drug ingestion at the time of the onset of the disorder does not necessarily indicate a causal link. Symptoms of hemorrhage and ecchymoses are usually caused by accompanying thrombocytopenia, but pallor, weakness, and poor resistance to bacterial infections also occur often. Lymphadenopathy and splenomegaly do not occur. The bone marrow is usually hypocellular and fatty, but areas of hypercellularity may occur.

Therapy consists of immediately discontinuing all drugs. Recovery is generally slow, and about half of the patients die even with optimal care. Blood transfusions should be used only to prevent the symptoms of severe anemia. Platelet transfusions may be needed on occasion. Prophylactic antibiotics should not be used, since infections which occur are caused by resistant organisms. If bacterial infections appear, they should be treated promptly. Testosterone, prednisone, and splenectomy have been associated with remissions on occasion. Although aplastic anemia is an uncommon and unpredictable complication of drug therapy, individuals taking drugs known to cause this disorder (Table 4-12) should have periodic blood counts.[117]

Benzene, presently found in solvents and paint removers, was

TABLE 4-12. *Drugs Known to Cause Aplastic Anemia*°

Antineoplastic:
  Nitrogen mustard
  Busulfan
  Cyclophosphamide (Cytoxan)
  Methotrexate
  6-Mercaptopurine
  5-Flourouracil
  Melphalan (Alkeran)
  Cytosine arabinoside
  Vinblastine (Velban)
  Vincristine (Oncovin)

Antimicrobial:
  <u>Chloramphenicol</u>
  <u>Sulfonamides</u>
  Sulfisoxazole (Gantrisin)
  Sulfamethoxypyridazine (Kynex)
  Penicillin
  Methicillin
  Tetracyclines (oxytetracycline, chlortetracyclines)
  Streptomycin
  Ristocetin (Spontin)
  Thiosemicarbazone (tuberculostatic drug)
  Amphotericin B (Fungizone)

Analgesics:
  <u>Phenylbutazone</u> (Butazolidin)
  <u>Oxyphenbutazone</u> (Tandearil)
  Aspirin
  Phenacetin
  Indomethacin (Indocin)

Anticonvulsants:
  <u>Mephenytoin</u> (Mesantoin)
  <u>Trimethadione</u> (Tridione)
  <u>Diphenylhydantoin</u> (Dilantin)
  Primidone (Mysoline)

Heavy metals:
  <u>Organic arsenicals</u> (neoarsphenamine, sulfarsphenamine)
  <u>Gold compounds</u>
  Bismuth
  Mercury
  Colloidal silver

Phenothiazines:
  Chlorpromazine (Thorazine)
  Promazine (Sparine)
  Triflupromazine (Vesprin)

Tranquilizers:
  Meprobamate
  Chlordiazepoxide (Librium)

Oral hypoglycemics:
  Tolbutamide (Orinase)
  Chlorpropamide (Diabinese)
  Carbutamide

Diuretics:
  Acetazolamide (Diamox)
  Chlorothiazide (Diuril)

Antihistamines:
  Chlorpheniramine (Chlor-Trimeton)
  Tripelennamine (Pyribenzamine)

Table 4-12 *continued on opposite page.*

TABLE 4–12. Drugs Known to Cause Aplastic Anemia* (continued)

Antithyroid drugs:
  Thiouracil
  Methimazole (Tapazole)
  Carbimazole (Neo-mercazole)
  Perchlorate
  Thiocyanate
Antimalarials:
  Quinacrine (Atabrine)
  Pyrimethamine (Daraprim)
Other drugs:
  Colchicine
  Dinitrophenol
  Carbamazepine (Tegretol)
  Thorotrast (thorium dioxide)
Organic solvents:
  Benzene
  Carbon tetrachloride
Insecticides:
  Gamma-benzene hexachloride
  DDT
  Chlordane

* Underlined drugs are those implicated in more than 20 reported cases.

the first agent discovered to cause aplastic anemia. Subsequently, many drugs and some insecticides have been implicated, but chloramphenicol (Chloromycetin) has produced more cases of the disease than any other drug, and, therefore, has been most intensively studied. The incidence of aplastic anemia from chloramphenicol is estimated at about 1 in 60,000 individuals receiving the drug.[252] Two forms of bone marrow suppression occur. The first type is dose-related and leads to anemia and mild thrombocytopenia, but only rarely to leukopenia. There is no serious bone marrow hypoplasia, but maturation arrest with vacuolization of the cytoplasm of erythroid cells, and to a lesser extent, of myeloid precursor cells, is seen. Vacuolization is diminished by ingestion of phenylalanine. All changes are reversible when the drug is stopped. Symptoms may be due to the ability of chloramphenicol to inhibit RNA and DNA synthesis.[175,252,316]

The second type of bone marrow suppression produced by chloramphenicol is not dose-related, and occurs after variable amounts of the drug have been taken. Aplastic anemia often appears after drug administration has ceased. Cases frequently occur after the patient has had repeated drug exposure. Delayed hypersensitivity may be the underlying mechanism. The hematologic and clinical manifestations are severe, often irreversible, and may lead to death.

Table 4–12 lists drugs that are known to cause aplastic anemia.[86,252,315,364]

Most antineoplastic drugs are myelosuppressive and can produce dose-related pancytopenia, which is reversible when the drug is discontinued.

Besides chloramphenicol, the drugs most often implicated in causing aplastic anemia are phenylbutazone and oxyphenbutazone (Tandearil), a metabolite of phenylbutazone.[282] Aspirin, often regarded as an innocuous drug, may cause pancytopenia,[336] as may phenacetin and indomethacin.[50]

Anticonvulsants, and notably trimethadione (Tridione), are the next group of drugs most frequently implicated. Organic arsenicals, which were used in the treatment of syphilis in the past, produced aplastic anemia. Gold therapy for rheumatoid arthritis also can cause pancytopenia.

Phenothiazines, a rare cause of aplastic anemia, probably lead to this disorder by interfering with nucleotide synthesis. Propylthiouracil often produces granulocytopenia, produces agranulocytosis less often, and produces aplastic anemia rarely.

Quinacrine (Atabrine), which was widely used for malarial prophylaxis during World War II, caused aplastic anemia in about 3 of every 100,000 soldiers treated with the drug.[86]

Organic solvents and insecticides, although they are not drugs, are another important group of compounds that may cause aplastic anemia, and should be kept in mind as potential etiologic agents.

Hemolytic Anemias

Drug-induced hemolysis may be due to red cell defects (enzymatic deficiencies or unstable hemoglobins), immunologic factors, or mechanisms that are not well understood. Severe hemolysis may occur abruptly, with hemoglobinemia, pallor, and jaundice, or it may be more indolent, with resultant mild asymptomatic anemia.

GLUCOSE 6-PHOSPHATE DEHYDROGENASE (G-6-PD) DEFICIENCY. The most frequently encountered types of drug-induced hemolysis are due to erythrocyte enzymatic defects in the pentose-monophosphate-shunt, which make red blood cells susceptible to hemolysis from oxidant drugs. Glucose-6-phosphate dehydrogenase (G-6-PD) deficiency is the most common variety. This trait is X-linked and appears mostly in men. There are three major forms. About 10 per cent of American Negroes have depressed erythrocyte G-6-PD enzymatic activity, in the range of 10 to 15 per cent of normal. A variable incidence occurs in individuals of Mediterranean ancestry, in whom more severe hemolysis occurs because of only up to 5 per cent erythrocyte enzyme activity. A rare qualitative enzymatic defect is sporadically encountered in individuals of northern European background, which is believed to protect against falciparum malaria.[364]

CLINICAL MANIFESTATIONS

This disorder was initially recognized when the antimalarial primaquine was found to lead to hemolysis in certain individuals; hence, this disorder is often termed primaquine sensitivity. In a typical hemolytic episode, hemolysis begins on about the third day after taking the drug. Symptoms include malaise, occasional abdominal discomfort, anemia, and dark urine (hemoglobinuria). Heinz bodies appear in erythrocytes. Jaundice, mostly direct-reacting bilirubin, often supervenes. Older red blood cells are destroyed preferentially because of their lower G-6-PD content. A brisk reticulocytosis follows. The hematocrit will slowly return to normal levels, even if the drug is continued, as long as the bone marrow is capable of producing red blood cells at a rate equal to erythrocyte destruction. If the drug dose is increased, or if the drug is stopped for a few months and then reinstituted, a secondary hemolytic episode will

TABLE 4-13. Drugs Known to Cause Hemolysis in G-6-PD Deficiency

Antimalarials (8-aminoquinolines):
  Primaquine
  Pamaquin
  Quinacrine (Atabrine)
  Quinocide
Sulfonamides:
  Sulfanilamide
  Sulfapyridine
  Sulfisoxazole (Gantrisin)
  Sulfamethoxypyridazine
  Sulfacetamide
  Salicylazosulfapyridine (Azulfidine)
Nitrofurans:
  Nitrofurantoin (Furadantin)
  Nitrofurazone (Furacin)
  Furazolidone (Furoxone)
Sulfones:
  Dapsone
  Solapsone
Vitamin K (water soluble derivatives):
  Potassium menaphthosulfate
  Menazodine
  Menadiol sodium diphosphate (Synkayvite)
Cinchona alkaloids:
  Quinine
  Quinidine
Phenylhydrazine (formerly used as an antipyretic):
  Naphthalene
  Probenecid (Benemid)
  Chloroquine (mild hemolysis)
  Acetanilid
  Phenacetin
  Aspirin (mild hemolysis)
  Neoarsphenamine
  Nalidixic acid (NegGram)
  Chloramphenicol
  Methylene blue

occur. This "self-limited" course is typical of Negroes with this enzymatic defect, but not of Mediterraneans, who experience a sustained anemia because of lower erythrocyte enzyme levels.[28,54,86] Women who are heterozygous for this trait have an intermediate degree of hemolysis.

Hemolysis is dose-dependent. Mediterraneans usually require a smaller amount of a drug to produce hemolysis because of their greater lack of G-6-PD. Hemolysis also occurs with intercurrent illness, especially infections. Broad (fava) beans, when ingested or when their pollen is inhaled, can also incite hemolysis among Mediterraneans. The drugs that produce hemolysis in G-6-PD deficiency are oxidants that are innocuous in normal individuals. The many drugs that can produce hemolysis in susceptible individuals are listed in Table 4–13.[28,54,86,364]

GLUTATHIONE REDUCTASE DEFICIENCY. Other less common enzymatic defects within red blood cells can result in drug hemolysis. Glutathione reductase deficiency is sporadically found among whites, and appears to be inherited as an autosomal trait. In people with this deficiency, hemolysis is produced by quinine, primaquine, isopentaquine (an 8-aminoquinoline closely related to primaquine), and sulfoxone.[28,54]

Glutathione deficiency is a very rare autosomal recessive trait which leads to primaquine-induced hemolysis.[28,54]

6-PHOSPHOGLUCONIC DEHYDROGENASE (6-PDG) DEFICIENCY. This enzymatic defect is transmitted by an autosomal gene, and occurs equally as often in whites and Negroes. Primaquine can produce hemolysis in this disorder.[28,54]

GLUTATHIONE-PEROXIDASE DEFICIENCY. This most recently described abnormality leads to hemolysis when sulfonamides and nitrofurantoin (Furadantin) are administered.[339]

HEMOGLOBINOPATHIES. Certain hemoglobinopathies also predispose individuals to drug-induced hemolysis. Patients with hemoglobin Zurich or hemoglobin H who receive sulfonamides and primaquine experience hemolytic episodes.[28,86]

Immune Hemolysis

There are three types of drug-related immune hemolysis which produce a positive response on the Coombs test: (1) the hapten (penicillin) type, (2) the "innocent bystander" (quinine) type, and (3) the methyldopa type (Table 4–14).

HAPTEN TYPE. The hapten type is best exemplified by the hemolysis that is occasionally induced by penicillin. Antipenicillin antibodies occur in 1 to 8 per cent of patients treated with penicillin, but large doses of intravenously administered penicillin (10 million units or more) are required to produce hemolysis. In these patients, the results of the direct Coombs test are positive. Penicillin binds

CLINICAL MANIFESTATIONS

TABLE 4-14. Drugs Known to Cause Immune Hemolysis

Penicillin
Quinine
Quinidine
Stibophen (Fuadin)
Methyldopa (Aldomet)
Levodopa (Larodopa, Dopar)
Mefenamic acid (Ponstel)
Cephalothin (Keflin)
Cephaloridine (Loridine)
Melphalan (Alkeran)
Acetanilid-phenacetin
Sulfonamides
Amphotericin B
Para-aminosalicylic acid
Chlorpromazine (Thorazine)

tightly to red blood cells, and the presence of circulating IgG antipenicillin antibodies results in hemolysis. Both the drug, acting as a hapten, and IgG antibodies are requisite for hemolysis to occur. Hemolysis ceases when the drug is discontinued.[81,280,345]

"INNOCENT BYSTANDER" TYPE. In the "innocent bystander" type of hemolysis, erythrocytes are agglutinated by anti-C serum in the presence of the offending drug. A drug-antibody complex is formed, followed by complement binding to the red blood cell—the "innocent bystander"—and leading to complement fixation and destruction of the red cell. Quinine, quinidine, and stibophen (Fuadin) are drugs that may produce this type of hemolysis, which rapidly ceases when the drug is discontinued.[81]

METHYLDOPA TYPE. About 20 per cent of patients who take methyldopa (Aldomet), especially those receiving large doses, show a positive reaction to the direct Coombs test, but only a few develop hemolysis. The antibody does not react with methyldopa, but with red blood cell antigens of the Rh system. The role of the drug in this form of autosensitization is not clear. Levodopa and mefenamic acid (Ponstel) have produced similar reactions. Patients taking methyldopa may also develop a positive antinuclear factor. The presence of a positive reaction to the Coombs test does not indicate that methyldopa needs to be discontinued. Antibodies slowly disappear when the drug is stopped. If hemolysis does supervene, methyldopa should be discontinued. In treatment of severe hemolysis, corticosteroids may be helpful.[40,81,230]

Administration of cephalothin (Keflin) may produce a positive direct Coombs test in a patient which can cause difficulty in crossmatching blood. Cephalothin binds a normal nonantibody globulin.

In one study, cephalothin produced a positive response to the direct Coombs test in 75 per cent of the patients, which was more pronounced in azotemic patients.[257] On rare occasions, hemolytic anemia has resulted from the use of cephalothin and cephaloridine (Loridine).[187]

Melphalan (Alkeran) has been reported to have caused a hemolytic anemia in a patient with multiple myeloma who developed erythrocyte agglutinins.[118] Another case has been reported in which analgesic abuse of a proprietary compound containing acetanilid and phenacetin led to hemolysis which was difficult to diagnose because of the patient's denial that a "drug" was being taken.[11]

Although the precise mechanisms are not clear, sulfonamides, amphotericin B, para-aminosalicylic acid, and chlorpromazine (Thorazine) have been known to induce immune hemolysis.[35,118]

Megaloblastic Anemia

Megaloblastic anemia may result from drugs that are either folate antagonists or impair folate absorption (Table 4–15).[183,360,364,369] Antineoplastic drugs, such as 6-mercaptopurine, 5-fluorouracil, and cytosine arabinoside, produce megaloblastosis by blocking DNA synthesis without interfering with folic acid metabolism. Methotrexate, used as an antineoplastic drug and in the treatment of psoriasis, is a true folic acid antagonist. Pyrimethamine (Daraprim), used to treat chloroquine-resistant malaria and toxoplasmosis, may on occasion produce megaloblastic anemia.[361] Pentamidine, which is effective in treating *Pneumocystis carinii* pneumonia, and trimethoprim, when combined with sulfomethoxazole in the preparations Septra and Bactrim, can lead to megaloblastic anemia. Triamterene (Dyrenium), a potassium-conserving diuretic, has led to megaloblastic anemia in alcoholics with marginal folate stores.[225]

TABLE 4–15. Drugs Known to Produce Megaloblastic Anemia

Folic acid antagonists:
  Methotrexate
  Pyrimethamine (Daraprim)
  Pentamidine
  Trimethoprim
  Triamterene
Impair folate absorption:
  Diphenylhydantoin (Dilantin)
  Primidone (Mysoline)
  Barbiturates (Amytal, Seconal, and Phenobarbital)
  Oral contraceptives
  Cycloserine
  Tetracycline
  Salicylates
  Phenylbutazone (Butazolidin)

Anticonvulsants, principally diphenylhydantoin (Dilantin), and to a lesser extent primidone (Mysoline), and barbiturates, interfere with the absorption of folate from the small intestine and can lead to megaloblastosis. Anemia improves when these drugs are discontinued. If stoppage of drugs is not clinically advisable, supplementary folate may be given. By this same mechanism of interference with folate absorption oral contraceptives may also produce megaloblastic anemia. Rare instances of megaloblastic anemia have been reported with the use of the antituberculous drug cycloserine, and one instance has been attributed to long-term tetracycline therapy[183] and one to phenylbutazone.[364]

Chronic ingestion of an analgesic containing aspirin, salicylamide, and caffeine has been reported to result in megaloblastic anemia, presumably as a result of interference with folate metabolism.[369] Nitrofurantoin (Furadantin) has been reported to lead to megaloblastic anemia, but this may have been secondary to hemolysis caused by G-6-PD deficiency and increased folate demand.[225]

Absorption of vitamin B_{12} in the distal ileum can be impaired by colchicine, neomycin, and para-aminosalicylic acid.[73,360] Colchicine appears to induce reversible vitamin B_{12} malabsorption by altering mucosal function.[362] Frank megaloblastic anemia, however, has not been recorded from use of these drugs.

Other Drug-Induced Anemias

IRON DEFICIENCY ANEMIA. Drug-induced gastrointestinal bleeding can lead to iron deficiency anemia. Apart from obvious massive bleeding, slow oozing may ultimately cause anemia. Aspirin is by far the commonest offending drug, especially when used chronically in large doses. Aspirin-induced gastrointestinal blood loss varies among individuals, but appears to be consistent for a given patient at a given dose.[221] Such blood loss may contribute to anemia in illnesses such as rheumatoid arthritis in which protracted aspirin therapy is often used.

When iron deficiency anemia is treated with oral iron preparations, tetracycline, antacids, and milk can chelate iron and diminish its absorption, thus reducing its clinical effectiveness.

Administration of isoniazid may also produce anemia which is responsive to pyridoxine therapy.

PURE RED BLOOD CELL APLASIA. Pure red blood cell aplasia, an unusual form of anemia most often associated with thymomas, can also be produced by drugs. Chloramphenicol has caused most reported cases. Other implicated drugs include diphenylhydantoin (Dilantin), sulfathiazole, arsphenamine, penicillin, phenobarbital, chenopodium, isoniazid, tolbutamide (Orinase), chlorpropamide (Diabinese), and isoniazid and para-aminosalicylic acid used con-

CLINICAL MANIFESTATIONS

TABLE 4-16. Drugs Known to Cause Methemoglobinemia

Phenacetin
Acetanilid
Nitrites
Nitroglycerine
Nitrates
Sulfonamides
Sulfones
Chlorates
Aniline dyes
Chloroquine
Primaquine
Diaminodiphenylsulfone
Benzene derivatives (especially nitro compounds)
---

currently. Most patients have recovered when the offending drug was discontinued.[290] Diphenylhydantoin has been found to specifically inhibit DNA, but not RNA, synthesis in erythrocyte precursors, and this may be the mechanism by which this drug induces pure red blood cell aplasia.[378]

Methemoglobinemia and Sulfhemoglobinemia

When the iron in hemoglobin is converted from the ferrous to the ferric form, methemoglobin is produced. Methemoglobin is not capable of releasing oxygen and therefore limits tissue oxygenation. When methemoglobin levels reach 1.5 gm per 100 ml, cyanosis develops. Headache, weakness, malaise, and dyspnea appear in rare cases when half the hemoglobin is converted to methemoglobin. A variety of oxidizing drugs can cause methemoglobinemia (Table 4-16).[252,364] Prophylactic administration of chloroquine, primaquine, and diaminodiphenylsulfone in Vietnam to fight malaria has also resulted in methemoglobinemia with cyanosis.[67] In most instances, discontinuing the offending drug will reverse the abnormality.

When present in a concentration of 0.5 gm per 100 ml sulfhemoglobin produces cyanosis, although methemoglobin also is usually present. Chronic ingestion of acetanilid or phenacetin, found in a variety of proprietary analgesics, and ingestion of sulfides may lead to sulfhemoglobinemia.[252,364]

DRUG-INDUCED WHITE BLOOD CELL DISEASES

Agranulocytosis

A marked decrease or total absence of granulocytes caused by drugs may occur with aplastic anemia or as an isolated abnormality.

CLINICAL MANIFESTATIONS

The total white blood cell count is also decreased in agranulocytosis. Fever, malaise, and sore throat with mucosal ulcerations usually occur abruptly. These initial symptoms are not related to infection, but infection is the great danger in this condition and a common cause of death.

Aminopyrine and dipyrone probably induce agranulocytosis by an immunologic mechanism. In the presence of both serum and drug, granulocytes are lysed. Challenge with small doses of these drugs in susceptible individuals results in disappearance of neutrophils in 6 to 10 hours.

Most instances of agranulocytosis, however, are probably not a result of an immunologic mechanism. Up to 20 days after drug therapy has been started, a sharp decrease in the number of circulating granulocytes and a decrease in bone marrow production of these cells occurs. Chlorpromazine (Thorazine), one of the drugs more frequently implicated in this type of agranulocytosis, has been found to impair DNA synthesis in white blood cells.

If agranulocytosis is diagnosed early, and the causative drug is stopped, the patient's recovery is hastened. In the immunologic type, granulocytes may return rapidly, while in the type produced by chlorpromazine, recovery may take a week or more. The mortality rate is about 20 per cent, and death is usually caused by infection. Prophylactic antibiotics do not prevent infection, but are associated with infection attributable to resistant organisms. If infection does occur, it should be treated promptly.

Drugs which may cause agranulocytosis are listed in Table 4–17.[56,78,86,148,207,223,282,287,292,298,340,364]

Antineoplastic drugs can produce dose-related agranulocytosis as part of their bone marrow suppressant effects. Chloramphenicol can depress the white blood cell count as part of the clinical picture of aplastic anemia, or in a separate reaction. Other antibiotics, including penicillin, ampicillin, carbenicillin, methicillin, and cephalothin,[148,292] occasionally produce granulocytopenia, or rarely, agranulocytosis. Sulfonamides, as well as phenothiazines and propylthiouracil, are among the drugs that cause agranulocytosis more frequently.[340] Other drugs have been reported sporadically as inciting agents.

Other White Blood Cell Changes

ACTH and corticosteroids often elevate the white blood cell count, a symptom which may lead to the mistaken impression that there is a bacterial infection. Other drugs that may cause leukocytosis are listed in Table 4–18.

PSEUDOLEUKEMIC HEMATOLOGIC FINDINGS. Pseudoleukemic or leukemoid hematologic findings in the peripheral blood and bone marrow, suggesting acute myelocytic leukemia, have been

TABLE 4-17. *Drugs Known to Cause Agranulocytosis**

Antineoplastic drugs:	Hypoglycemics:
Busulfan	<u>Carbutamide</u>
Vincristine	Tolbutamide (Orinase)
Nitrogen mustard	Chlorpropamide (Diabinese)
Triethylenemelamine	Diuretics:
6-Mercaptopurine	Thiazides
Analgesics:	Chlorthalidone (Hygroton)
<u>Aminopyrine</u>	Acetazolamide (Diamox)
<u>Dipyrone</u>	Ethacrynic acid (Edecrin)
Phenylbutazone (Butazolidin)	Mercurial diuretics
Oxyphenbutazone (Tandearil)	Anticonvulsants:
Aspirin	Diphenylhydantoin (Dilantin)
Phenacetin	Trimethadione (Tridione)
Acetanilid	Ethosuximide (Zarontin)
Antibacterial:	Antihistamines:
<u>Chloramphenicol</u>	Tripelennamine (Pyribenzamine)
Penicillin	Methaphenilene (Diatrin)
Methicillin	Thenalidine
Ampicillin	Others:
Carbenicillin	<u>Phenindione</u> (Danilone, Dindevan, Hedulin)
Cephalothin	Dapsone
Thiosemicarbazone (Tibione)	Meprobamate
Ristocetin	Imipramine (Tofranil)
Novobiocin	Desipramine (Pertofrane)
<u>Sulfonamides</u>	Procainamide
Dapsone	Hydroxychloroquine (Plaquenil)
Organic arsenicals	Pamaquine (Plasmochin)
Phenothiazines:	Penicillamine
<u>Chlorpromazine</u> (Thorazine)	Metronidazole (Flagyl)
<u>Promazine</u> (Sparine)	Barbiturates
<u>Mepazine</u>	Pyrithyldione (Presidon)
Prochlorperazine (Compazine)	Quinine
Promethazine (Phenergan)	Neostibophen (antimony compound)
Thioridazine (Mellaril)	Gold compounds
Antithyroid drugs:	Organic arsenicals
<u>Propylthiouracil</u>	Dinitrophenol
Methimazole (Tapazole)	

* Underlined drugs indicate frequent cause of reaction.

TABLE 4-18. *Drugs Known to Cause Leukocytosis*

Adrenocorticotropic hormone (ACTH)
Corticosteroids
Phenacetin
Para-aminosalicylic acid
Belladonna alkaloids
Chlordiazepoxide (Librium)
Phenothiazines
Diphenylhydantoin (Dilantin)
Penicillin
Phenindione (Danilone, Dindevan, Hedulin)
Iodides
Iron dextran
Sympathomimetic amines

noted in a patient recovering from dapsone-induced agranulocytosis.[223] Both phenylbutazone[98] and oxyphenbutazone[333] have been reported to produce leukemoid reactions.

PSEUDO PELGER-HUËT ANOMALY. Sulfisoxazole (Gantrisin) has been known to induce a pseudo Pelger-Huët anomaly in which all granulocytes have a bilobed, dumbbell-shaped nucleus. This abnormality reverted to normal when the drug was discontinued. An increase in such bilobed granulocytes has also been noted in patients treated with busulfan and 6-azauracil for acute and chronic myelocytic leukemia.[186]

BLEEDING DISORDERS

Thrombocytopenia

Decreased platelet counts are so frequently drug-induced that in any case of thrombocytopenia drugs should always be considered as possible causative agents. Drug-induced thrombocytopenia is frequently produced by immunologic mechanisms. In such cases, when a drug is administered to a previously sensitized patient, the platelet count may fall minutes or hours later. If thrombocytopenia continues for more than two weeks after a drug is stopped, it is probably not drug-induced.[252]

An immunologic mechanism in drug-induced thrombocytopenia was first demonstrated with apronalide (Sedormid), a previously popular sedative which was removed from the market because of this effect. Sedormid was found to form an antigenic complex with platelets which incited antibody formation. The drug-platelet-antibody complex resulted in complement fixation and platelet lysis. Many other drugs that produce thrombocytopenia probably do so in a similar fashion.[252]

When thrombocytopenia is felt to be drug-induced, all suspect drugs should be stopped. If necessary, chemically unrelated compounds with similar pharmacologic effects should be substituted. In severe cases in which bleeding is threatened or occurs, corticosteroid therapy may prove helpful.

A list of the many and varied drugs known or suspected to cause thrombocytopenia by immunologic mechanisms is given in Table 4–19.[18,86,157,252,364] Some principles of immunologically-induced thrombocytopenia are exemplified by the action of these drugs. Minute quantities of a drug, often taken in disguised form, can induce thrombocytopenia and purpura; for example, the quinine in tonic water has produced thrombocytopenia in susceptible persons.[19] The drug itself may not always be the offending agent, but one of its metabolites may incite the immunologic response. Such a response

TABLE 4–19. *Drugs that Produce Thrombocytopenia by Known or Suspected Immune Mechanisms*

Analgesics:	Hypoglycemic agents:
Phenacetin°	Insulin
Antipyrine°	Tolbutamide° (Orinase)
Aspirin	Chlorpropamide° (Diabinese)
Sodium salicylate	Carbutamide
Acetaminophen	Anticonvulsants:
Phenylbutazone (Butazolidin)	Diphenylhydantoin° (Dilantin)
Oxyphenbutazone (Tandearil)	Mephenytoin°
Codeine	Trimethadione°
Meperidine (Demerol)	Paramethadione
Cinchona alkaloids:	Antihistamines:
Quinine°	Chlorpheniramine°
Quinidine°	Diphenhydramine°
Antimicrobial agents:	Heavy metals:
Sulfonamides°	Gold compounds
Penicillin	Silver
Cephalothin°	Bismuth
Chloramphenicol	Copper
Erythromycin	Other agents:
Novobiocin°	Dextroamphetamine°
Rifampicin°	Reserpine
Streptomycin	Digitoxin°
Tetracyclines	Vitamin K°
Isoniazid	Thiouracil
Para-aminosalicylic acid	Colchicine
Pyrazinamide	Carbamazepine (Tegretol)
Organic arsenicals	Heparin
Stibophen° (Fuadin)	Nitroglycerin
Sedatives and tranquilizers:	Prednisone
Apronalide (Sedormid)°	Estrogens
Barbiturates°	Methyldopa°
Meprobamate	Potassium iodide
Prochlorperazine	Chloroquine°
Promethazine	Hydroxychloroquine°
Methylparafynol°	Chlorophenothane
Desipramine°	Procaine
Diuretics:	Thalidomide
Thiazides°	Ergot
Acetazolamide° (Diamox)	Dinitrophenol
Diazoxide	
Mercurial diuretics	

° Definite immunologic mechanism.

has been found to occur with para-aminosalicylic acid, in which cases a glycine-conjugated metabolite was found to be responsible for causing the thrombocytopenia.[111] The immunologic response may be so specific that compounds that are closely related structurally are not necessarily able to produce thrombocytopenia. Digitoxin-induced thrombocytopenia is specific. However, platelets are not decreased when digoxin, ouabain, lanatoside C (Cedilanid), or digitoxigenin are administered. Quinine and quinidine are optical isomers, but they do not cross-react in producing thrombocytopenia. Also, chlorothiazide has been used without untoward effect in a patient who had hydrochlorothiazide-induced purpura.[377]

Drug-induced thrombocytopenia can also result from suppression of platelet formation in the bone marrow, as occurs in aplastic anemia. It may also occur as a dose-dependent phenomenon with many antineoplastic compounds: cyclophosphamide (Cytoxan), busulfan, nitrogen mustard, 6-mercaptopurine, azathioprine (Imuran), vincristine (Oncovin), 5-fluorouracil, cytosine arabinoside, and others.

Ristocetin, an antimicrobial agent, has been reported to cause a dose-related direct toxic effect on circulating platelets.[129] Platelet production can also be suppressed by thiazide diuretics, estrogens, and ethanol.[18,227]

Nonthrombocytopenic drug-induced purpura can occur as a result of capillary changes. This happens most often with the use of corticosteroids and ACTH. Other drugs that have caused nonthrombocytopenic purpura include anticoagulants, atropine, iodides, quinine, penicillin, phenacetin, salicylates, thiazide diuretics, chloral hydrate, bismuth, and mercury.[364]

Anaphylactoid (allergic or Henoch-Schönlein) purpura is discussed in the section on multisystem diseases.

Coagulation Defects

Treatment with heparin, or any of the oral anticoagulants, can lead to various hemorrhagic complications. Bleeding involving separate organ systems will be discussed in the appropriate sections. Heparin acts on blood by inhibiting many factors in the coagulation cascade, while the oral anticoagulants inhibit the hepatic synthesis of vitamin K-dependent clotting factors (prothrombin, factors VII, IX, and X). With the use of oral anticoagulants, hemorrhage occurs not only when the prothrombin time is excessively prolonged, but also when it is in the acceptable therapeutic range.

The oral anticoagulants interact with many drugs that may either prolong or diminish the prothrombin time. Anticoagulants can be displaced from their serum albumin binding sites, leading to an increased pharmacologically active blood level of these drugs, and a resultant prolonged prothrombin time. Drugs that are known to displace anticoagulants from their binding sites include phenylbutazone (Butazolidin), and salicylates.[3,86,104,252]

Diphenylhydantoin (Dilantin), disulfiram (Antabuse), and phenyramidol (Analexin), a muscle relaxant, increase the effect of oral anticoagulants by inhibiting their metabolic degradation in the liver.[55,252,270]

Quinidine, quinine, thyroxine, anabolic steroids, and monamine oxidase inhibitors may prolong the prothrombin time by mechanisms that are not clearly understood.[133,204,252]

The prothrombin time also may be prolonged by malabsorption of vitamin K if cholestyramine (Questran), a bile acid sequestrant in the gut, is used, or if bowel sterilization is undertaken with a variety of antibiotics.[252]

The effect of oral anticoagulants can be diminished by drugs that increase the activity of drug-metabolizing enzymes in the liver cell microsomes. This, in turn, requires an increased dose of the anticoagulant to keep the prothrombin time in the therapeutic range. Danger of bleeding arises if the microsomal enzyme-inducing drug is discontinued without an appropriate decrease in the anticoagulant dose. The following drugs are known to increase the catabolism of anticoagulants: barbiturates (amobarbital [Amytal], secobarbital [Seconal], phenobarbital), chloral hydrate, glutethamide (Doriden), meprobamate, haloperidol (Haldol), ethchlorvynol (Placidyl), and griseofulvin.[104,145,252]

There is an enhanced anticoagulant effect in hyperthyroidism (a similar effect occurs with the use of thyroxine), and a reverse phenomenon in hypothyroidism for reasons that are not yet known.[351]

Drugs and illnesses known to increase or decrease the prothrombin time in combination with the use of oral anticoagulants are shown in Table 4–20.

Another category of drug-induced bleeding disorders is that of the so-called "anticoagulant malingerers" or "Dicumarol eaters."[38] These individuals, many of whom have a paramedical background, secretly take oral anticoagulants to induce hemorrhagic phenomena. They are found to have a prolonged prothrombin time, and the anticoagulant can be identified in their blood. Bleeding may occur at various sites, but the abnormality is quickly corrected by the use of vitamin K.

TABLE 4–20. Drugs and Illnesses that Change Prothrombin Time by Interacting with Anticoagulants

Increase prothrombin time:	Monamine oxidase inhibitors
Phenylbutazone (Butazolidin)	Cholestyramine (Questran)
Oxyphenbutazone (Tandearil)	Bowel sterilization
Clofibrate (Atromid-S)	Hyperthyroidism
Indomethacin (Indocin)	Decrease prothrombin time:
Salicylates	Barbiturates
Diphenylhydantoin (Dilantin)	Chloral hydrate
Phenyramidol (Analexin)	Glutethamide (Doriden)
Disulfiram (Antabuse)	Meprobamate
Quinidine	Haloperidol (Haldol)
Quinine	Ethchlorvynol (Placidyl)
Thyroxine	Griseofulvin
Anabolic steroids	Hypothyroidism

OTHER DRUG-INDUCED BLOOD AND LYMPH DISORDERS

Lymphoid Tissue Changes

Long-term therapy with anticonvulsants, notably diphenylhydantoin (Dilantin), and less often with mephenytoin (Mesantoin), phensuximide (Milontin), ethotoin (Peganone), and primidone (Mysoline), can produce a *pseudolymphoma syndrome* that mimics Hodgkin's disease or lymphosarcoma, both clinically and histologically. Lymph node enlargement may be local or generalized. In some patients splenomegaly and hepatomegaly occur, as well as rash, fever, and eosinophilia. These abnormalities subside when the drug is discontinued. In one recorded case, a fatal malignant lymphoma developed after these abnormalities had disappeared following the cessation of diphenylhydantoin.[128]

Phenylbutazone (Butazolidin) has produced a similar clinical picture, with tender lymphadenopathy, splenomegaly, and peripheral atypical lymphocytes resembling those seen in infectious mononucleosis.[275,284] Para-aminosalicylic acid, iron dextran, and meprobamate also have been reported to cause lymph node enlargement.[128] Lymphadenopathy also occurs in serum sickness and drug-induced systemic lupus erythematosus. Drugs known to bring about this syndrome are enumerated in Table 4–21.[128,275,284]

Sarcoid-like granulomas in the liver, and at times in lymph nodes, have been caused by sulfonylureas, phenylbutazone, and diphenylhydantoin.[202]

Leukemia and Lymphoma

Some instances of chloramphenicol-induced aplastic anemia have been followed by acute myeloblastic leukemia.[39,68] Phenylbutazone therapy, without intervening aplastic anemia, has been statistically associated with an increased incidence of acute myeloblastic and acute lymphoblastic leukemia.[98] Acute leukemia has also been reported to follow oxyphenbutazone therapy.[333] Radioactive thorium dioxide (Thorotrast), previously used as a radiological con-

TABLE 4–21. Drugs Known to Cause Pseudolymphoma Syndrome or Lymph Node Enlargement

Pseudolymphoma syndrome:	Lymph node enlargement:
Diphenylhydantoin (Dilantin)	Phenylbutazone (Butazolidin)
Mephenytoin (Mesantoin)	Para-aminosalicylic acid
Phensuximide (Milontin)	Iron dextran
Ethotoin (Peganone)	Meprobamate
Primidone (Mysoline)	

trast medium, has been associated with the late development of acute myelocytic, acute monocytic, and chronic myelocytic leukemias.[87]

Long-term azathioprine (Imuran) and prednisone therapy in renal transplant patients is associated with an increased incidence of malignancies, principally histiocytic lymphomas, which are most often located intracranially.[94,302] A case of a fatal lymphoma following the diphenylhydantoin-induced pseudolymphoma syndrome mentioned earlier has been reported, but the causal relationship is unclear.[128]

3. CARDIOVASCULAR MANIFESTATIONS

Adverse drug reactions involving the cardiovascular system are mostly due to digitalis intoxication and to the effects of antihypertensive agents. Many other drugs, however, can produce multiple effects on the heart and circulation. In this section, reactions will be considered from both their anatomic and physiologic aspects. Drugs affecting the heart valves, myocardium (including coronary arteries), and pericardium will be dealt with first, followed by those that may induce congestive heart failure. Cardiac disorders produced by digitalis intoxication will be considered next, followed by a discussion of rhythm disturbances. Circulatory changes involving arterial pressure, venous thromboses, and pulmonary embolism will be discussed last.

Drugs Affecting the Heart Valves

The heart valves are rarely affected by drugs. Methysergide (Sansert), used in the prevention of migraine headaches, can produce retroperitoneal fibrosis. In a minority of patients thus affected, the coronary arteries and heart valves may be involved. Aortic insufficiency is produced by fibrosis of the aortic valve leaflets. The resultant murmur may regress wholly or partially after the drug is discontinued.[149]

Drug addicts develop bacterial endocarditis, caused by unusual and virulent organisms from the intravenous use of various contaminated drugs.

Drugs Affecting the Myocardium

Angina pectoris and acute myocardial infarction can be induced by drugs that decrease myocardial perfusion by constricting coronary arteries or by diminishing arterial blood pressure. Vasopressin (Pitressin), oxytocin (Pitocin), and ergot preparations produce coronary artery vasoconstriction that can precipitate angina pectoris and myocardial infarction. Vasopressin, which is used intravenously as a splanchnic vasoconstrictor to stop bleeding from esophageal varices, can produce myocardial ischemia and damage.[20] Ergotamine tartrate, used in the treatment of migraine headaches, has caused angina and acute myocardial infarction when given intramuscularly in therapeutic doses.[140] Methysergide (Sansert) can produce fibrosis at the root of the aorta, with narrowing of the coronary artery ostia. Instances of angina pectoris and acute myocardial infarction have been associated with the use of this drug. Angina has improved after discontinuance of the drug.[149,172]

Antihypertensive agents may produce a marked fall in blood

pressure, with consequent decrease in myocardial perfusion, which may precipitate angina pectoris and myocardial infarction. Hydralazine (Apresoline) may aggravate or precipitate angina pectoris by decreasing cardiac output despite an increased pulse rate. Marked hypotensive episodes as a complication of phentolamine (Regitine), when used as a test to diagnose pheochromocytoma, have led to acute myocardial infarction.[142] We have personally seen an instance of insulin-induced hypoglycemia result in a myocardial infarction. In hypertrophic subaortic stenosis, the use of digitalis and nitroglycerine may increase the number and severity of anginal attacks.

Emetine, used to treat amebic liver abscess, is potentially cardiotoxic, and may cause a myocardiopathy with tachycardia, T wave inversion, deformity of the ST segment and QRS complex, and prolonged P-R and Q-T intervals. Premature ventricular contractions, atrial tachycardia, and pericarditis have also been observed with the use of this drug.[86]

Other drugs that have produced myocardial damage, usually as part of a generalized allergic reaction with eosinophilia and skin lesions, include sulfonamides, aspirin, para-aminosalicylic acid, phenylbutazone (Butazolidin), methimazole (Tapazole), and benzathine penicillin G (Bicillin).[86]

Freons, used as propellants in aerosols, are rapidly acting, potent cardiotoxins. Inhaling these propellants for their euphoric effect has led to acute heart failure, hypotension, bradyarrhythmias, ventricular tachyarrhythmias, and asphyxia.[162]

Drugs Affecting the Pericardium

As mentioned above, emetine can produce pericarditis as part of its cardiotoxic effect.[186] The syndrome of drug-induced systemic lupus erythematosus (SLE) may be associated with pericarditis. Hydralazine (Apresoline)-induced SLE has resulted in pericarditis and pericardial tamponade. This disorder has responded dramatically to prednisone therapy and disappeared after cessation of the offending drug.[52]

The use of anticoagulants in patients with acute myocardial infarction has caused hemopericardium, tamponade, and death.[305] Anticoagulants have been used in patients with acute benign pericarditis because of the mistaken impression that chest pain was due to an acute myocardial infarction. Subsequent pericardial bleeding, with tamponade and death, has occurred. Anticoagulants are contraindicated in acute benign pericarditis because of the hazard of bleeding from an inflamed pericardium.[367] Hemopericardium with tamponade has also occurred in anticoagulated patients without previous evidence of heart disease.[119] Constrictive pericarditis has rarely followed anticoagulant-induced hemopericardium.[217]

Congestive Heart Failure

Propranolol (Inderal) may precipitate or worsen congestive heart failure in susceptible individuals by decreasing the strength of myocardial contraction and thus reducing the cardiac output.[115,176]

Intravenous fluids containing sodium, large amounts of orally ingested sodium in medicines (e.g., sodium bicarbonate), corticosteroid therapy, and intravenous mannitol infusions can increase intravascular volume and lead to congestive heart failure. By increasing the load on the heart, drug-induced hypertension and decreased cardiac output brought about by drug-induced myocarditis or arrhythmias, are capable of precipitating or worsening heart failure. Intravenous opiates, when used for therapeutic purposes or by narcotic addicts, can lead to pulmonary edema that responds well to narcotic antagonists but poorly to the usual measures.

Cardiac Manifestations of Digitalis Intoxication

Digitalis intoxication is a frequently encountered adverse drug effect. In hospital studies, up to 20 per cent of patients receiving digitalis glycosides develop toxicity. Digitalis compounds increase the force of myocardial contraction, enhance myocardial irritability, depress the refractory period of conduction tissue, and increase vagal activity on the heart.[86] These effects result in a variety of cardiac manifestations of digitalis intoxication. Digitalis compounds also produce gastrointestinal reactions, visual disturbances, gynecomastia, and rare allergic reactions which are discussed elsewhere.

ECG CHANGES. Digitalis produces electrocardiographic (ECG) changes that are not indicative of the adequacy of digitalization: pronounced ECG changes may follow small doses and minor changes may occur with large doses. The typical ECG effects of digitalis are flattening or inversion of T waves, sagging of the S-T segment below the baseline, prolongation of the P-R interval, and shortening of the Q-T interval.

The arrhythmias produced by digitalis can be viewed as exaggerations of the pharmacologic effects of the drug. Increased myocardial excitability can lead to premature ventricular contractions and various arrhythmias. Complete heart block results from both increased vagal tone and depressed refractory period of conduction tissue.

PREDISPOSING FACTORS. Certain factors predispose to digitalis intoxication. Depleted body potassium, which is not always manifested by hypokalemia, is the most frequent factor associated with digitalis toxicity. Potassium may be lost from diuretic therapy, mostly after administration of thiazides, ethacrynic acid (Edecrin), and furosemide (Lasix), and from corticosteroid treatment, hyperaldosteronism, potassium-losing nephropathy, hemodialysis, and gastrointestinal losses from vomiting and diarrhea. Intravenous glucose infusions and insulin both promote the shift of potassium from the extracellular into the intracellular compartment, which may precipitate digitalis intoxication. Intravenous calcium infusions, aminophylline, reserpine, guanethidine (Ismelin), and sympathomimetic amines used in conjunction with digitalis can produce arrhythmias. Increased myocardial sensitivity to digitalis occurs with acute myocardial infarction, myocardiopathies, severe heart disease of any type, marked congestive failure, and cor pulmonale with hypoxia. Older patients are more prone to develop toxicity from digitalis because of their decreased body size and reduced renal function.[96,189]

About 75 to 85 per cent of oral digitalis is absorbed, little is metabolized, and most is excreted in the urine. Propantheline (Pro-Banthine) decreases gastrointestinal motility and allows for increased absorption. Metoclopramide decreases digitalis absorption by enhancing gastrointestinal motility.[246] Digitalis absorption is also hindered in sprue, and by oral neomycin therapy.[96] Hyperthyroidism produces digitalis resistance by increasing the metabolism of the drug, while hypothyroidism may lead to digitalis intoxication with conventional doses of the drug because of impaired metabolism.[96] Impaired renal function rarely leads to digitalis intoxication, probably because of the associated potassium retention.

Individuals who undergo electrical cardioversion show an increased sensitivity to digitalis which may lead to serious arrhythmias after cardioversion. It is recommended that digitalis be discontinued for a day or so before anticipated cardioversion, but there is no risk in reinstituting or beginning digitalis immediately after cardioversion.[96]

DIGITALIS-INDUCED CARDIAC ARRHYTHMIAS. A cardiac arrhythmia in any patient taking a digitalis compound should always be suspected of being induced by the drug. The toxic effects of different digitalis preparations are essentially similar, but the purer glycosides, e.g., digoxin, produce fewer extracardiac effects. Digitalis intoxication can produce nearly all known cardiac arrhythmias, especially complex arrhythmias. An electrocardiogram is essential for proper diagnosis of these arrhythmias.

The most common and characteristic digitalis-induced arrhythmia is premature ventricular contractions. These may be isolated, multiple, multifocal or bigeminal. Premature ventricular contractions also occur in individuals who are not taking digitalis. The origin of these contractions sometimes alternates between the left and right ventricles. This arrhythymia may progress to ventricular tachycardia or ventricular fibrillation, especially if digitalis is continued.[174]

The vagal effects of digitalis toxicity can retard impulse formation at the sinoatrial node, with resultant sinus bradycardia, sinus arrhythmia, sinus arrest (intermittent failure of atrial impulse formation), sinoatrial block (lack of transmission of sinus impulse), and wandering atrial pacemaker.

At the atrioventricular node, prolongation of the P-R interval (first-degree heart block) is diagnosed by the ECG and is probably the second most common digitalis-induced arrhythmia. The Wenckebach phenomenon—progressive lengthening of the P-R interval until the atrial beat is completely blocked, with a consequently absent ventricular beat followed by recurrence of this cycle—is frequently digitalis-induced. Complete heart block is manifested by a regular, slow rhythm (usually less than 45 beats per minute) originating in the ventricles, while atrial impulses are blocked at the atrioventricular node. The atrial rhythm may arise in the sinus node or be atrial fibrillation.

In atrioventricular dissociation, the atria and ventricles beat independently. There is no bradycardia, and the ventricular rate is more rapid than the atrial rate. An atrial complex is occasionally transmitted through the atrioventricular node and results in a ventricular complex, termed a captured beat.[174]

The most frequent digitalis-induced ectopic tachycardia is atrial tachycardia with block. The atrioventricular block is usually 2 to 1, but may often be of the Wenckebach type. Although this arrhythmia is typical of digitalis intoxication, it may be due to other causes. It is uncommon for atrial fibrillation and rare for atrial flutter to be digitalis-induced.[174]

Nodal rhythm, nodal tachycardia, and nodal premature beats are relatively common arrhythmias of digitalis toxicity. Paroxysmal ventricular tachycardia may be digitalis-induced, as may ventricular fibrillation. Occasionally, electrical alternans with pulsus alternans may be caused by digitalis.[174]

Digitalis intoxication in the presence of atrial fibrillation produces certain recognizable ECG changes. Among the first that occur are atrioventricular junctional escape beats, which are usually slightly different in contour from other QRS complexes, and may occur as isolated beats or in regular runs. This change may progress to a regular nodal rhythm at a rate of about 70 beats per minute. Junctional tachycardia with exit block produces groups of progressively shortening intervals separated by pauses. The pause is less than twice the length of any two consecutive short intervals, and the interval before the pause is shorter than the interval after the pause. Lastly, bidirectional tachycardia is due to conduction down alternate bundle branches to the ventricles.[189]

SPURIOUS HEART DISEASE. Spurious heart disease has been induced by a reducing pill containing digitalis, a diuretic, thyroid extract, amphetamine, and a cathartic. Sagging ST segments suggesting ischemia, first- and second-degree heart block with associated hypokalemia, and a false positive response to Master's "2-step" test were produced by this curious combination-medicine.[190]

Treatment of digitalis intoxication includes discontinuing digitalis and all drugs that might contribute to potassium loss. Supplementary potassium should be given even if the serum potassium level is not depressed, since potassium losses are not always mirrored by hypokalemia. Antiarrhythmic drugs such as propranolol (Inderal), lidocaine (Xylocaine), diphenylhydantoin (Dilantin), procainamide, and quinidine are useful under certain circumstances. Cardiac pacing and cardioversion also have their place in treatment of some arrhythmias.[174]

Drug-Induced Arrhythmias

Sinus tachycardia (heart rate greater than 100 beats per minute) can be produced by the vagolytic effect of atropine. This effect is markedly exaggerated in patients with Down's syndrome (mongolism).[163] Other drugs that induce sinus tachycardia include sympathomimetic amines, especially epinephrine, ephedrine, and isoproterenol (Isuprel), amyl nitrite, thyroid extract, and phenothiazines.

Sinus bradycardia (heart rate slower than 60 beats per minute) is often produced by digitalis, especially in combination with reserpine. The vagotonia and bradycardia induced by reserpine are exaggerated by the concomitant use of barbiturates, monamine oxidase inhibitors, or phenothiazines.[86] Both propranolol (Inderal) and diphenylhydantoin (Dilantin), which are used to treat cardiac arrhythmias, can lead to sinus bradycardia.[71,258a] Pressor amines, opiates, and cyclopropane can also cause sinus bradycardia.

Sinoatrial block can be induced by digitalis, quinidine, atropine, and salicylates.[174]

Digitalis can produce premature atrial contraction as well as atrial tachycardia, usually with 2 to 1 block. Methylphenidate (Ritalin), administered intravenously, and emetine, may also precipitate atrial tachycardia.[59,86] Infrequently, atrial flutter may be caused by digitalis or quinidine.[86] Atrial fibrillation is an uncommon digitalis-induced arrhythmia, and also has occurred with intravenously administered methylphenidate (Ritalin).[59]

Digitalis and quinidine can produce a nodal rhythm. Atrioventricular dissociation can result from administration of digitalis, quinidine, procainamide, atropine, and salicylates.[174]

First-degree atrioventricular block occurs as an electrocardiographic finding with the use of digitalis, quinidine, and procainamide. Quinidine and procainamide also can lead to second-degree heart block, while digitalis can induce the Wenckebach phenomenon, as mentioned earlier. Complete heart block may result from digitalis intoxication, propranolol (Inderal), guanethidine (Ismelin), and cyclopropane anesthesia.[86,115,116,174]

Premature ventricular contractions are often the result of digitalis toxicity. Sympathomimetic amines (epinephrine, ephedrine, isoproterenol, amphetamines, etc.), even when used in nose drops or nasal sprays, may lead to premature ventricular contractions. This effect is enhanced by the concomitant administration of a monamine oxidase inhibitor. Quinidine, procainamide, cyclopropane, and emetine can also produce premature ventricular contractions.[86,116,174]

Ventricular tachycardia may be induced by digitalis, quinidine, procainamide, sympathomimetic amines, papaverine, potassium, intravenous mercurials, chloroform, cyclopropane, and thioridazine (Mellaril).[116,174,311]

Digitalis, procainamide, and quinidine can produce ventricular fibrillation.[269] Drug-induced arrhythmias are classified in Table 4–22.

TABLE 4–22. Drug-Induced Arrhythmias

Sinus tachycardia:
  Atropine
  Sympathomimetic amines
  Amyl nitrite
  Thyroid extract
  Phenothiazines
Sinus bradycardia:
  Digitalis
  Reserpine
  Propranolol (Inderal)
  Diphenylhydantoin (Dilantin)
  Pressor amines
  Opiates
  Cyclopropane
Sinoatrial block:
  Digitalis
  Quinidine
  Atropine
  Salicylates
Premature atrial contractions:
  Digitalis
Atrial tachycardia:
  Digitalis
  Methylphenidate (Ritalin)
  Emetine
Atrial flutter:
  Digitalis
  Quinidine
Atrial fibrillation:
  Digitalis
  Methylphenidate (Ritalin)
Nodal rhythm:
  Digitalis
  Quinidine
Atrioventricular dissociation:
  Digitalis
  Quinidine
  Procainamide
  Atropine
  Salicylates

First-degree atrioventricular block:
  Digitalis
  Quinidine
  Procainamide
Second-degree atrioventricular block:
  Digitalis (also Wenckebach phenomenon)
  Quinidine
  Procainamide
Complete heart block:
  Digitalis
  Propranolol (Inderal)
  Guanethidine (Ismelin)
  Cyclopropane
Premature ventricular contractions:
  Digitalis
  Sympathomimetic amines
  Quinidine
  Procainamide
  Cyclopropane
  Emetine
Ventricular tachycardia:
  Digitalis
  Quinidine
  Procainamide
  Sympathomimetic amines
  Papaverine
  Potassium
  Mercurials
  Chloroform
  Cyclopropane
  Thioridazine (Mellaril)
Ventricular fibrillation:
  Digitalis
  Quinidine
  Procainamide

Hypertension

On occasion, corticosteroid therapy may produce or aggravate hypertension. Infrequently, oral contraceptives may intensify existing hypertension or produce hypertension in normotensive women. However, hypertensive women have been placed on oral contraceptives without an increase occurring in blood-pressure levels. Oral contraceptives have been implicated in producing malignant hypertension with papilledema and left ventricular hypertrophy, which all reverted to normal after discontinuance of the drug. Increased concentration of renin substrate has been found in many but not all hypertensive women taking oral contraceptives, but the significance of this finding in relation to the cause of hypertension is unknown.[161,307,375]

Women taking oral contraceptives have been found to develop loud, high-pitched systolic bruits over the abdominal aorta, which at times radiate into either flank in the absence of hypertension or abdominal aneurysms. The significance of this finding is unknown. The bruits diminish in loudness when oral contraceptives are discontinued.[43]

Sympathomimetic amines may induce hypertension as part of their pharmacologic effect. Marked hypertension, with a positive reaction to the phentolamine (Regitine) test, has resulted from ingestion of phenylpropanolamine in Ornade.[102] The combination of sympathomimetic amines and certain antihypertensive drugs that deplete peripheral stores of norepinephrine, such as methyldopa (Aldomet), guanethidine (Ismelin), and reserpine, can lead to marked hypertension.[86]

Infrequently, parenteral guanethidine, reserpine, and methyldopa may produce paradoxical hypertension.[224] Vasopressin (Pitressin) and oxytocin are vasoconstrictors and can induce hypertension. Pentazocine (Talwin) regularly produces mild elevations of blood pressure, not necessarily into the hypertensive range, and in rare

TABLE 4-23. *Drugs Known to Cause Hypertension*

Corticosteroids
Oral contraceptives
Sympathomimetic amines
Vasopressin (Pitressin)
Oxytocin
Pentazocine (Talwin)

Paradoxical effect:
   Guanethidine (Ismelin)
   Reserpine
   Methyldopa (Aldomet)

cases can lead to marked hypertension.[95] Drugs known to cause hypertension are listed in Table 4-23.

Monamine oxidase inhibitors, in combination with other monamine oxidase inhibitors, sympathomimetic amines, foods containing tyramine, and other drugs can lead to a hypertensive crisis with headache, central excitation, seizures, intracerebral hemorrhage, fever, diaphoresis, and cardiac arrhythmias. Intracerebral hemorrhage has led to death.[86] Hypertension should be treated by discontinuing the responsible drugs and by administering intravenous phentolamine (Regitine). Reserpine should not be used because it produces heightened CNS excitement. Drugs which lead to hypertensive crisis when used with monamine oxidase inhibitors are listed in Table 4-24.

Hypotension

Postural hypotension is a frequent effect of the treatment of hypertension with antihypertensive drugs. Thiazides, when used alone (e.g., hydrochlorothiazide [Hydrodiuril]), rarely produce postural hypotension, but their use in combination with other antihypertensive drugs often leads to a postural fall in blood-pressure levels. Thiazides, given in combination with monamine oxidase inhibitors, can lead to profound hypotension.[86]

Postural hypotension often follows the use of reserpine parenterally, but rarely occurs with oral administration. Risk of hypotension

TABLE 4-24. *Drugs and Foods Known to Produce Hypertensive Crisis When Taken with Monamine Oxidase Inhibitors*

Other monamine oxidase inhibitors:	Amphetamines
Isocarboxazid (Marplan)	Dopamine
Nialamide (Niamid)	Levodopa (Dopar, Larodopa)
Phenelzine (Nardil)	Methyldopa (Aldomet)
Tranylcypromine (Parnate)	Tryptophan
Pargyline (Eutonyl)	Other drugs:
Furazolidone (Furoxone)	Phenothiazines
Tricyclic antidepressants:	Narcotics
Imipramine (Tofranil)	Foods with large amount of tyramine:
Amitriptyline (Elavil)	Strong and aged cheeses
Desipramine (Norpramin, Pertofrane)	Sour cream
Nortriptyline (Aventyl)	Pickled herring
Protriptyline (Vivactl)	Aged meats
Doxepin (Sinequan)	Yeast extract
Sympathomimetic amines (often found	Wines (especially chianti)
in proprietary cold and hay fever	Beer
remedies and reducing pills):	Chicken livers
Epinephrine	Canned figs
Norepinephrine (Levophed)	Raisins
Metaraminol (Aramine)	Broad beans
Ephedrine	Soy sauce
Phenylephrine	Excessive caffeine
Methylphenidate (Ritalin)	Excessive chocolate

is increased when reserpine, which produces peripheral norepinephrine depletion, is used concomitantly with phenothiazines or before general anesthesia.[86]

Other antihypertensive agents such as hydralazine (Apresoline), methyldopa (Aldomet), guanethidine (Ismelin), and ganglionic blocking agents frequently produce postural hypotension. Their effects are additive and are potentiated by thiazides. Use of these drugs may lead to pronounced hypotension in patients with either severe cardiovascular disease or a sympathectomy, or in those receiving phenothiazines, barbiturates, or undergoing general anesthesia.[86]

The intravenous use of the antiarrhythmic drugs procainamide, diphenylhydantoin (Dilantin),[71] and propranolol (Inderal)[176] may lead to hypotension.

Alpha-adrenergic blocking agents such as phentolamine (Regitine) and phenoxybenzamine (Dibenzyline) produce hypotension as a result of vasodilatation. Nitroglycerine occasionally produces a fall in blood pressure. The combination of nitroglycerine and alcohol has led to cardiovascular collapse with marked hypotension.[321]

Phenothiazines, notably chlorpromazine (Thorazine), can cause orthostatic hypotension, usually after parenteral administration. When patients receiving chlorpromazine or haloperidol (Haldol), which have an alpha-adrenergic blocking effect, are given epinephrine concomitantly, paradoxical hypotension may result.[86]

Narcotics administered intravenously, especially morphine, may cause hypotension. This effect is exaggerated by the attendant use of a monamine oxidase inhibitor.[86] Imipramine (Tofranil) and amitriptyline (Elavil) may produce hypotension rarely, as may emetine because of its cardiotoxic effects.[86] Both furosemide (Lasix) and ethacrynic acid (Edecrin) can cause hypotension by producing a massive diuresis and a contracted intravascular volume. Ethacrynic acid, however, has produced hypotension without a significant diuresis or electrolyte changes.[170]

Tetracycline treatment of patients with louse-borne relapsing fever has led to a Herxheimer type of reaction with fever and a brief elevation of blood pressure, followed by a fall in central venous pressure and arterial pressure. Although hypotension is usually not severe or prolonged, there have been cases in which patients have died early in the course of therapy, possibly as a result of marked hypotension and shock.[274]

Newborn babies, especially premature infants, when given more than 25 mg/kg of chloramphenicol as prophylaxis against infection, have developed the "gray syndrome." Within two to nine days after chloramphenicol has been instituted, abdominal distention with or without vomiting appears followed by hypothermia, ashen gray cyanosis, irregular respiration, and vasomotor collapse. This syn-

TABLE 4-25. Drugs Known to Cause Hypotension

Antihypertensive therapy:
Thiazide diuretics
Reserpine
Hydralazine (Apresoline)
Methyldopa (Aldomet)
Guanethidine (Ismelin)
Ganglionic blockers
Antiarrhythmic drugs:
Procainamide
Diphenylhydantoin (Dilantin)
Propranolol (Inderal)
Alpha-adrenergic blockers:
Phentolamine (Regitine)
Phenoxybenzamine (Dibenzyline)
Nitroglycerine
Phenothiazines
Narcotics
Imipramine (Tofranil)
Amitriptyline (Elavil)
Emetine
Ethacrynic acid (Edecrin)
Furosemide (Lasix)
Tetracyclines (in treatment of louse-borne relapsing fever)
Chloramphenicol (Gray syndrome)

drome is caused by the accumulation of toxic levels of chloramphenicol because of the inability of the immature liver to conjugate the drug with glucuronide.[363] Drugs known to cause hypotension are listed in Table 4-25.

Intravascular Clotting and Pulmonary Embolism

Long-term therapy with ACTH and corticosteroids may predispose to intravascular thrombosis and thrombophlebitis. When used in women or in men to treat prostatic carcinoma, estrogens can lead to thromboembolic disease. Oral contraceptives are associated with a significant incidence of deep vein thrombosis and pulmonary embolism. The mechanism by which oral contraceptives predispose to thromboembolic complications is not known.

There is no change in risk between brief or prolonged use of oral contraceptives, but sequential preparations are more hazardous than combined preparations.[86] Oral contraceptives are best avoided by women with a history of thrombophlebitis or pulmonary embolism. If these complications occur, oral contraceptives should be discontinued and the usual forms of therapy for thrombophlebitis or pulmonary embolism should be instituted.

4. GASTROINTESTINAL MANIFESTATIONS

Adverse drug reactions frequently involve the gastrointestinal tract. Nausea, vomiting, gastrointestinal bleeding, and diarrhea are the most common symptoms of drug-induced digestive disorders. This section will deal with drug-induced disease of the gastrointestinal tract exclusive of those involving the liver.

Drugs Affecting the Mouth

DRY MOUTH. Dry mouth is a frequent accompaniment of treatment with anticholinergic drugs (atropine and its congeners) and drugs with anticholinergic side effects (reserpine and tricyclic antidepressants such as amitriptyline [Elavil]). Monilial stomatitis may accompany the use of broad-spectrum antibiotics. The buccal mucosa may be involved in drug-induced cutaneous reactions, especially in erythema multiforme, and rarely in contact dermatitis of the mouth caused by denture cleaning powders, mouthwash, and toothpaste.[13]

SWOLLEN OR HAIRY TONGUE. The tongue may swell as part of the syndrome of angioneurotic edema. A hairy tongue produced by elongation of the filiform papillae of the anterior two-thirds of the tongue, which may range in color from yellowish to black, is usually the result of broad-spectrum antibiotic treatment, especially with tetracyclines. Occasionally, oral corticosteroids, throat lozenges, or mouthwashes may be the cause. These agents probably act by altering the normal mouth flora and allowing an overgrowth of new organisms, mostly fungi. Discontinuing the causative drug produces a reversal of this condition.[122]

ENAMEL HYPOPLASIA AND DISCOLORATION. The tetracyclines are deposited in growing teeth and can result in permanent enamel hypoplasia and discoloration which is related to the total dose of the drug. Tetracyclines cross the placenta and also can affect developing teeth in utero. During the early stages of their development, between two months and two years of age, permanent teeth also are affected. Susceptibility to dental damage from tetracyclines, however, probably exists up to age seven.[363]

GINGIVAL HYPERTROPHY. Diphenylhydantoin (Dilantin) may produce gingival hypertrophy, especially in individuals with poor dental hygiene. Bismuth compounds and mercury poisoning may result in blue-gray discoloration of the gums at the base of the teeth.[122]

Drugs Affecting the Salivary Glands

Phenylbutazone (Butazolidin) and oxyphenbutazone (Tandearil) have produced *parotitis* with fever and dry mouth, which clears when these drugs are discontinued, but recurs with drug readministration.[155] Guanethidine (Ismelin) and Bretylium (an antihypertensive drug similar to guanethidine used in Europe) have produced parotid swelling and pain.[86] Asymptomatic parotid swelling has been caused by isoproterenol (Isuprel), and parotid pain while eating has resulted from treatment with vincristine (Oncovin) and vinblastine (Velban).[86,295]

Drugs Affecting the Esophagus

Atropine and other anticholinergic drugs can worsen the symptoms of peptic esophagitis by increasing gastric reflux as a result of decreased resting tone of the lower esophageal sphincter.

A rare instance of dysphagia, produced by a retroesophageal hematoma resulting from coumarin anticoagulation, has been reported.[291]

Drugs Causing Nausea and Vomiting

Nausea and vomiting are among the most frequently occurring drug-induced symptoms, and have been observed more often in women. Almost any orally administered drug can produce nausea or vomiting by a direct irritant effect on the gastric or small-bowel mucosa (e.g., ferrous sulfate), or by central stimulation of the chemoreceptor zones and vomiting center in the medulla (e.g., digitalis compounds).[342] Only a few drugs that often produce nausea or vomiting will be discussed.

Digitalis toxicity is frequently ushered in by anorexia, followed in a day or two by nausea and vomiting. In some instances there may be abdominal discomfort accompanying these symptoms, and less often diarrhea occurs.[174] Levodopa (Larodopa, Dopar) commonly produces nausea and vomiting, probably via a central mechanism.[342]

Other drugs that are frequently associated with nausea and vomiting include salicylates, narcotic analgesics, colchicine, potassium chloride, ferrous sulfate, indomethacin (Indocin), phenylbutazone (Butazolidin), aminophylline, tetracycline, erythromycin, and para-aminosalicylic acid.

Drug-Induced Peptic Ulceration and Gastrointestinal Hemorrhage

Drug-induced peptic ulceration may be complicated by hemorrhage or perforation. Aspirin and other salicylates are the commonest cause of gastroduodenal injury. Gastrointestinal blood loss occurs in about 70 per cent of aspirin users, with a mean daily loss of less than 5 cc. In a minority of patients, severe bleeding with hematemesis and melena may occur. Diffuse hemorrhagic gastritis, peptic erosion, or ulceration also may occur. A previous peptic ulcer may be reactivated, but this is not a great risk.[105]

Reserpine increases gastric acid secretion which has led to peptic ulcer, and in a few cases to ulcer perforation.[86]

The antiarthritic compounds phenylbutazone (Butazolidin), oxyphenbutazone (Tandearil), and indomethacin (Indocin) can produce peptic ulcer and bleeding. Other drugs that may induce gastrointestinal bleeding include ethacrynic acid (Edecrin), mefenamic acid (Ponstel), colchicine, tolbutamide (Orinase), histamine, and alcohol.[86]

ACTH and corticosteroids induce peptic ulceration that may develop rapidly, and increases in frequency with larger doses and prolonged therapy. About 60 per cent of such ulcers are found in the stomach. There is an inconsistent increase in gastric acid secretion and a decreased mucosal resistance. Symptoms are often absent until hemorrhage or perforation make known the presence of the ulcer. Ulcers may heal slowly when treated with antacids and multiple feedings, even though corticosteroids are continued. Corticosteroid-induced peptic ulceration is more common in patients with rheumatoid arthritis and systemic lupus erythematosus, and less common in patients with asthma, pemphigus, or ulcerative colitis.[86] The combination of corticosteroids and azathioprine (Imuran), used in treating patients with renal transplants, often leads to the formation of gastric ulcers.[253]

Gastrointestinal bleeding from anticoagulant therapy may occur from the stomach or the small intestine. There is an increased hazard of bleeding in patients who are receiving concomitant ulcerogenic drugs, or if a peptic ulcer is already present.[305] Drugs known to cause peptic ulceration and gastrointestinal bleeding are shown in Table 4-26.

Drugs Causing Small Bowel Lesions

Digitalis has been associated with the production of acute hemorrhage and necrosis of the small and large bowel in aged, arteriosclerotic patients. Increased splanchnic venous pressure at the level of the liver has been felt to be the cause of this syndrome.[132]

TABLE 4-26. Drugs Known to Cause Peptic Ulceration and Gastrointestinal Bleeding

Aspirin	Mefenamic acid (Ponstel)
Corticosteroids	Colchicine
Reserpine	Tolbutamide (Orinase)
Phenylbutazone (Butazolidin)	Histamine
Oxyphenbutazone (Tandearil)	Alcohol
Indomethacin (Indocin)	Anticoagulants
Ethacrynic acid (Edecrin)	

Patients with chronic congestive heart failure, especially if accompanied by hypotension or arrhythmias, have developed abdominal pain, hematemesis, melena, distension, and adynamic ileus associated with the administration of digitalis or norepinephrine. Diffuse, patchy, mucosal and submucosal hemorrhagic lesions in the absence of vascular obstruction have been found from the stomach to the small bowel. Perforation has occurred. The pathogenesis is unknown, but is probably due to bowel ischemia and to decreased cardiac output.[29]

Superior mesenteric artery thrombosis with infarction of the midgut has been associated with the use of oral contraceptives.[42]

Enteric-coated potassium chloride tablets and combined potassium chloride and thiazide diuretic tablets dissolve in the small bowel and lead to local high concentrations of potassium which can cause ulceration that may heal with stenosis.

Anticoagulants may produce hemorrhage within the bowel wall which can lead to ileus. Paralytic ileus brought on by ganglionic blocking drugs (hexamthionium, pentolinium, and mecamylamine) may persist after cessation of the drug and have a fatal outcome.[86] Large doses of parenteral anticholinergic drugs (e.g., atropine) can lead to ileus, which is reversible when the drug is stopped.

Diarrhea Caused by Drugs

Diarrhea, exclusive of steatorrhea, is a frequent drug-induced problem. Laxatives and antacid combinations of aluminum and magnesium hydroxide are common causes. Use of eye drops containing echothiophate (phospholine iodide), a potent cholinesterase, can result in enough systemic absorption of this drug to lead to diarrhea.[134] Other drugs that often cause diarrhea include colchicine, quinidine, reserpine, guanethidine, broad-spectrum antibiotics (e.g., tetracyclines, ampicillin), alkylating agents, and digitalis.[342]

Malabsorption Caused by Drugs

Aluminum hydroxide chelates iron and prevents its absorption. Neomycin and colchicine can cause steatorrhea. Para-aminosalicylic acid can decrease fat and cholesterol absorption and produce steatorrhea without diarrhea.[86] Megaloblastic anemia from selective folate malabsorption can be caused by diphenylhydantoin (Dilantin), primidone (Mysoline), barbiturates, oral contraceptives, cycloserine, tetracyclines, salicylates, and phenylbutazone (Butazolidin).[183,360,364,369] Vitamin B_{12} malabsorption, of a degree not severe enough to cause megaloblastic anemia, has been produced by cholchicine and neomycin. Para-aminosalicylic acid has produced subacute combined degeneration as a result of vitamin B_{12} malabsorption, which responded to parenteral vitamin B_{12} treatment.[159]

Choléstyramine (Questran), a bile salt binder, can lead to steator-

TABLE 4-27. Drugs Known to Cause Pancreatitis

Corticosteroids
Thiazide diuretics
Chlorthalidone (Hygroton)
Salicylazosulfapyridine (Azulfidine)
Azothiaprine (Imuran)
Oral contraceptives (secondary to hyperlipidemia)
Tetracyclines (only those which result in hepatic damage)

rhea and to malabsorption of fat-soluble vitamins. Children treated with corticosteroids have developed pancreatic necrosis with secondary malabsorption.[86]

Constipation Caused by Drugs

Narcotic analgesics often are associated with the occurrence of constipation. Anticholinergic drugs, ganglionic blockers, aluminum hydroxide, and vincristine (Oncovin) are other drugs which bring on constipation. Cholestyramine (Questran) has resulted in obstipation caused by colonic impaction that required surgical removal.[66]

Other Drug-Induced Bowel Disorders

Patients with ulcerative colitis may develop toxic megacolon as a result of the constipating effects of anticholinergic drugs and opiates. Broad-spectrum antibiotics, especially tetracyclines, have led to ulcerative proctitis. Oral contraceptives have been associated with reversible vascular damage to the colon, manifested by abdominal pain and bloody stools.[196] Pruritus ani and perianal moniliasis also may result from the use of broad-spectrum antibiotics.

Drug-Induced Pancreatitis

Acute pancreatitis is rarely drug-induced. Corticosteroids, especially when given in high doses and to children, can induce acute pancreatitis that may progress to pancreatic insufficiency. This may occur after the drug has been discontinued or the dose is being decreased. Other drugs that have caused pancreatitis are thiazide diuretics (chlorothiazide and hydrochlorothiazide), chlorthalidone (Hygroton), salicylazosulfapyridine (Azulfidine), and azathioprine (Imuran).[191]

Oral contraceptives have produced massive hyperlipidemia with associated pancreatitis that did not recur after discontinuance of the drug.[88] Pancreatitis has occasionally been a concomitant of hepatic damage caused by tetracyclines.[199] Drugs known to cause pancreatitis are presented in Table 4-27.

Narcotic analgesics, oral anticoagulants, heparin, chlorothiazide (Diuril), and pentobarbital (Nembutal) may produce elevations in serum amylase levels without causing pancreatitis.

5. LIVER MANIFESTATIONS

The liver plays an important role in the detoxification and metabolism of many drugs. It acts as a gateway between intestinal absorption and systemic distribution of orally administered drugs. The liver is especially vulnerable to drug-induced damage, which is most often detected clinically as jaundice. Because of the great functional reserve of the liver, however, injury may be manifested only as abnormalities in liver-function studies with no clinical symptoms. There is no specific way of differentiating drug-induced liver disease from that produced by other causes. The clinical history remains the cornerstone of proper diagnosis.

The liver can be injured by drugs in various ways. Jaundice can be simulated by quinacrine (Atabrine) and picrates, which produce a yellowish discoloration of the skin. Drug-induced hemolysis can lead to jaundice. Hepatic damage, however, is usually manifested as obstructive, hepatocellular, or mixed types of jaundice, or as alterations in tests of liver function. Cirrhosis and granulomas can occasionally be drug-induced. Certain drug effects can precipitate hepatic encephalopathy or worsen the detrimental effects of neonatal jaundice and produce kernicterus. Infrequently, the Budd-Chiari syndrome, peliosis hepatitis, and hepatic tumors follow drug use.

Drugs that can produce liver disease must be differentiated from hepatotoxins such as carbon tetrachloride and phosphorus. The former produce sporadic instances of hepatic damage, while the latter are substances that cause liver injury in man and in animals that is predictable, dose-related, and has a short latent period (e.g., carbon tetrachloride and phosphorus). Substances with significant hepatotoxic effects are not used as drugs, but some that are relatively nontoxic in normal adult doses may still be used to some extent (e.g., chloroform).

Drug-induced jaundice can usually be classified as cholestatic or hepatocellular. In most instances, there is both morphologic and chemical evidence of one of these mechanisms predominating almost to the exclusion of the other. However, sharp distinctions cannot always be drawn. In some instances, there is a mixed type of hepatic damage. Certain drugs characteristically produce one or the other type of liver injury.

Cholestatic Jaundice Caused by Drugs

Drug-induced cholestatic jaundice occurs in only a small fraction of individuals exposed to implicated drugs. The reaction is not dose-related, and has a variable latent period. In some patients there are systemic signs of allergy (eosinophilia, fever, rash, and arthralgias) that precede jaundice. Usually, there is hepatomegaly and occasionally, splenomegaly. The urine becomes dark, stools become acholic, and itching may be a troublesome symptom. Levels of serum bilirubin are elevated, bilirubin is mostly direct-reacting, and alkaline phosphatase levels may be markedly elevated. Increased values of serum cholesterol also occur often, and if this becomes chronic, xanthomatoses may develop. There is usually a variable, but not marked, rise in transaminase levels. Histologic examination of the liver shows bile stasis, an inflammatory reaction in the portal triads, and little hepatocellular damage.

These changes usually disappear within a few weeks after the inciting drug is stopped. In some instances cholestasis may be prolonged, and may progress rarely to biliary cirrhosis.

Therapy consists of discontinuing the implicated drug, and general supportive measures. Corticosteroids are of little value, but may produce beneficial effects in some patients early in the course of jaundice. In cases of protracted cholestasis, cholestyramine (Questran) may help relieve itching. Fat malabsorption may develop, with resultant decreased vitamin D and calcium absorption requiring dietary supplements.[199]

Methyltestosterone (Metandren), anabolic steroids, and other C-17 alpha-alkyl-substituted steroids produce a different form of cholestasis. There are no signs of allergy, and clinical and chemical signs of obstruction are typical except that cholesterol is not elevated. Liver biopsy shows cholestasis but no inflammation. These drugs probably produce cholestasis by inhibiting bile excretion in the liver. Recovery usually occurs within three months after the drug is discontinued.[199]

Those drugs that can produce cholestatic jaundice are listed in Table 4–28.[199,202] Comments will be confined here to drugs that produce common or troublesome reactions.

Among the phenothiazines, chlorpromazine (Thorazine) produces cholestatic jaundice most often. This reaction is not dose-related. About 1 to 2 per cent of patients taking this drug become icteric, but anicteric reactions occur in from 20 to 50 per cent. Symptoms usually begin one to four weeks after onset of drug treatment, but reactions have occurred after only one dose of the drug or as long as 18 days after stopping the drug. Readministration usually produces a recrudescence of symptoms, but not always. On occasion, jaundice may disappear even though the drug is continued.

Jaundice is usually preceded by fever, nausea, vomiting, epigastric distress, skin rash, or arthralgias. The urine becomes dark, stools become pale, and itching appears. The liver is enlarged and often tender. Occasionally, there is splenomegaly and lymph node enlargement. Eosinophilia may occur early in the course of illness. Most of the bilirubin is direct-reacting. Levels of alkaline phosphatase and cholesterol levels are elevated. There are variable increases

TABLE 4-28. Drugs Known to Cause Cholestatic Jaundice

Phenothiazines:	Oral contraceptives
Chlorpromazine (Thorazine)	Sulfonylureas:
Promazine (Sparine)	Tolbutamide (Orinase)
Trifluoperazine (Stelazine)	Chlorpropamide (Diabinese)
Thioridazine (Mellaril)	Acetohexamide (Dymelor)
Fluphenazine (Permitil, Prolixin)	Metahexamide (Euglycin)
Mepazine (Pacatal)	Antimicrobial agents:
Perphenazine (Trilafon)	Tetracyclines
Prochlorperazine (Compazine)	Erythromycin estolate (Ilosone)
Promethazine (Phenergan)	Oxacillin (Prostaphlin)
Trimeprazine (Temaril)	Nitrofurantoin (Furandantin)
Sedatives and tranquilizers:	Sulfonamides
Chlordiazepoxide (Librium)	Antithyroid drugs:
Meprobamate	Thiouracil
Ectylurea (Cytran)	Methimazole (Tapazole)
Tricyclic antidepressants:	Antineoplastic drugs:
Imipramine (Tofranil)	6-Mercaptopurine
Amitriptyline (Elavil)	Thioguanine
Desipramine (Norpramin)	Other drugs:
Nortriptyline (Aventyl)	Arsphenamine (and other organic arsenicals)
Androgens and anabolic steroids:	Chlorothiazide (Diuril)
Methyltestosterone (Metandren)	Indomethacin (Indocin)
Norethandrolone (Nilevar)	Griseofulvin
Ethylestrenol (Maxibolin)	Carbamazepine (Tegretol)
Fluoxymesterone (Halotestin)	Phenindione (Danilone, Dindevan, Hedulin)
Oxandrolone (Anavar)	Tripelennamine (Pyribenzamine)
Oxymetholone (Anadrol)	Nicotinic acid (Niacin)
Methandrostenolone (Dianabol)	Carbarsone (Amebarsone)
	Dinitrophenol

in transaminase levels. Liver biopsy shows dilated canaliculi, portal inflammation, and little or no hepatic cell necrosis. Jaundice clears in about two to four months after chlorpromazine is discontinued. In a minority of cases, corticosteroids have a beneficial effect. Prolonged jaundice lasting from four months to five years after the drug is discontinued occurs rarely, and may lead to portal fibrosis or biliary cirrhosis with xanthomatoses.[199]

Other phenothiazines, including those used as antiemetics, such as prochlorperazine and promethazine (Compazine and Phenergan), and antipruritics such as trimeprazine (Temaril), have infrequently produced cholestatic jaundice.

Cross-sensitivity in producing cholestasis has been noted between chlorpromazine (Thorazine) and promazine (Sparine), and between thioridazine (Mellaril) and trifluoperazine (Stelazine).[199]

Chlordiazepoxide (Librium) may cause elevations of transaminase levels and rare instances of cholestatic jaundice.[1]

Infrequently, the tricyclic antidepressants may produce transient cholestatic jaundice, which responds to drug withdrawal.[199,202]

As mentioned before, androgens and anabolic steroids, notably methyltestosterone (Metandren) and norethandrolone (Nilevar), produce cholestasis by inhibiting bile secretion, with no accompanying signs of inflammation or allergy. Jaundice slowly abates when these drugs are discontinued.[199]

Naturally occurring estrogens may increase bromsulphalein (BSP) retention and produce increases in concentration of alkaline phosphatase, but do not alter liver structure. Hepatic changes are not produced by natural progestins. Synthetic estrogens combined with progestins in oral contraceptives probably act synergistically to produce jaundice.[199] These synthetic hormones are C-17 alpha-alkyl-substituted steroids structurally similar to those mentioned as causes of cholestasis.

Between 20 and 40 per cent of women taking oral contraceptives show some degree of BSP retention. Occasionally, there are mild elevations of either alkaline phosphatase or transaminase levels. Rarely, a syndrome of cholestatic jaundice with hepatocellular damage is produced. Jaundice usually appears within the first three cycles of drug administration. It is preceded by malaise, anorexia, nausea, pruritus, and dark urine. Serum bilirubin is mostly direct-reacting. There may be moderately elevated transaminase values, and levels of alkaline phosphatase are variably elevated. Liver biopsy shows bile stasis, a minimal or absent inflammatory reaction, and mild hepatocellular damage. Cessation of the drug results in complete recovery in a few weeks or months. However, almost half of the women who have developed this syndrome while taking oral contraceptives have had recurrent jaundice or severe pruritus in the third trimester of pregnancy. Women with such a history should not be placed on oral contraceptives.[268]

The sulfonylurea antidiabetic drugs are a rare cause of cholestasis that clears rapidly when the drug is withdrawn. Chlorpropamide (Diabinese)-induced cholestasis does not appear when tolbutamide (Orinase) is given. Consequently, when necessary the latter drug can be substituted for the former.[199]

Erythromycin estolate (Ilosone), the lauryl sulfate salt of the propionyl ester of erythromycin, is the only form of erythromycin that produces cholestasis. Erythromycin ethylsuccinate (Erythrocin) does not produce liver damage.[199]

The tetracyclines—tetracycline (Achromycin), chlortetracyline (Aureomycin), and oxytetracycline (Terramycin)—when administered orally, can produce fatty changes in the liver. Intravenous therapy with large doses (2.4 to 3.5 gm daily) of these drugs for pyelonephritis in the third trimester of pregnancy, postpartum, and occasionally in nonpregnant women may result in severe hepatic damage with fatality rates of up to 80 per cent. A few days after treatment is begun nausea, vomiting, and abdominal pain occur; these are rapidly followed by jaundice, azotemia, and acidosis. Acute pancreatitis may supervene. During pregnancy, the liver appears to be more susceptible to those

CLINICAL MANIFESTATIONS

tetracyclines that depress protein anabolism. Autopsy findings typically show a fatty liver with necrosis.[199,210]

Sulfonamides can also cause jaundice that shows features of cholestasis. There is associated fever and rash, suggesting allergy as the causative mechanism.[241]

Antineoplastic drugs, particularly 6-mercaptopurine, can produce cholestasis with typical changes in the liver microstructure as well as some hepatocellular damage.[329]

The other drugs listed in Table 4-28 cause cholestasis more infrequently, except for the organic arsenicals that are no longer used clinically.

Hepatocellular Jaundice Caused by Drugs

Drugs can produce hepatocellular damage ranging from scattered foci of necrosis to massive necrosis. With severe necrosis there is a high mortality rate. Survivors may develop postnecrotic cirrhosis. In some instances, e.g., with iproniazid (Marsilid) and cinchophen (both drugs are no longer in use), the clinical course and histologic appearance of lesions are indistinguishable from those of lesions in viral hepatitis. In fact, it has been argued that in such cases hepatocellular damage is caused by viral hepatitis rather than by the drug, or that the drug in some way facilitates the appearance of or aggravates viral hepatitis.[12]

Jaundice may be preceded by symptoms suggesting allergy: fever, chills, rash, and eosinophilia. Early in the course of the disease there may be obstructive symptoms such as dark urine, light stools, and pruritus. The clinical picture, however, rapidly changes to one of hepatocellular damage. Right upper quadrant distress and an enlarged tender liver occur frequently. Occasionally, the spleen may be palpable. As in viral hepatitis, transaminase levels are usually markedly elevated, but higher levels of alkaline phosphatase are more common in hepatocellular jaundice than in viral hepatitis.

Therapy consists of discontinuing the inciting drug. Jaundice may abate in a few days or in two or three weeks. In instances of severe hepatocellular necrosis, corticosteroids may provide some benefit if the patient has not progressed to a comatose state. Patients suffering from drug-induced acute hepatic failure have been reported to have improved after exchange blood transfusions.[218]

The many drugs implicated in producing hepatocellular jaundice are listed in Table 4-29.[199,202]

All halogenated anesthetic agents are potentially hepatotoxic. However, halothane (Fluothane) and methoxyflurane (Penthrane) cause hepatitis, often with hepatic necrosis, by allergic mechanisms. In halothane hepatitis, unexplained postoperative fever is one of the

TABLE 4-29. *Drugs Known to Cause Hepatocellular Jaundice*

Anesthetics:	Anticonvulsants:
Halothane (Fluothane)	Phenacemide (Phenurone)
Methoxyfluorane (Penthrane)	Diphenylhydantoin (Dilantin)
Vinyl ether	Mephenytoin (Mesantoin)
Ethyl chloride	Ethotoin (Peganone)
Chloroform	Trimethadione (Tridione)
Monamine oxidase inhibitors:	Phenobarbital
Iproniazid (Marsilid)	Other drugs:
Isocarboxazid (Marplan)	Zoxazolamine (Flexin)
Nialamide (Niamid)	Griseofulvin
Phenelzine (Nardil)	Thiouracil
Antituberculous agents:	Propylthiouracil
Isoniazid	Methimazole (Tapazole)
Pyrazinamide (Aldinamide)	Quinacrine (Atabrine)
Ethionamide (Trecator)	Carbutamide
Para-aminosalicylic acid	Acetohexamide (Dymelor)
Antimicrobial agents:	Metahexamide (Euglycin)
Sulfonamides	Chlordiazepoxide (Librium)
Penicillin	Nicotinamide (vitamin B_3)
Novobiocin	Vitamin A
Triacetyloleandomycin (TAO)	Methyldopa (Aldomet)
Antirheumatic drugs:	Dapsone
Cinchophen	Phenolphthalein
Phenylbutazone (Butazolidin)	Iodochlorhydroxyquin (Carbasone,
Oxyphenbutazone (Tandearil)	Entero-Vioform)
Indomethacin (Indocin)	Melarsopol (antitrypanosomal)
Probenecid (Benemid)	Stibophen (Fuadin)
Allopurinol (Zyloprim)	Antimony potassium tartrate
Gold compounds	Phenindione (Dindevan, Danilone, Hedulin)
Aspirin	Trimethobenzamide (Tigan)
Antineoplastic drugs:	Carbamazepine (Tegretol)
Cyclophosphamide (Cytoxan)	Aminocaproic acid (Amicar)
6-Mercaptopurine	Methoxsalen (Meloxine)
Mithramycin (Mithracin)	Cholecystographic dyes:
Chlorambucil (Leukeran)	Bunamiodyl (Orabilex)
Urethane	Iopanoic acid (Telepaque)
Azathioprine (Imuran)	Iodipamide (Cholografin)

features most indicative of liver damage. The incidence is about 1 in 10,000 patients exposed to the drug. Between one-third to one-half of all cases may terminate fatally, mostly in obese individuals who have received halothane once or twice in the previous month. Frequently there is an abrupt onset with chills and fever. Occasionally a rash, arthralgias, and eosinophilia are present. Jaundice appears three to four days after the onset of fever. In many patients this is followed by liver failure with hepatic precoma and coma. The liver is usually slightly enlarged and tender. Levels of serum bilirubin are elevated, with variable elevation of alkaline phosphatase levels. Prothrombin time may be prolonged. Hypoglycemia may occur in instances of severe liver damage. Histologically, the hepatic lesions are identical to those of viral hepatitis.

Methoxyflurane (Penthrane) has produced similar reactions, with cross-sensitivity to halothane being reported in some cases.

Treatment consists of supportive measures. Corticosteroids may be of benefit if administered before coma supervenes. Exchange blood transfusions have been used in extreme circumstances.[199,278]

In support of the theory of an allergic basis for halothane hepatitis, a case has been reported of an anesthetist who experienced recurrent acute hepatitis as a result of exposure to halothane at work; this eventuated in cirrhosis.[200]

Iproniazid (Marsilid), a hydrazine derivative, was the prototype of the monamine oxidase inhibitors. Because of its severe hepatotoxic effects, resembling those of viral hepatitis, it was withdrawn from use. Other hydrazine derivatives (isocarboxazid, nialamide, and phenelzine) have a much lower incidence of hepatic damage. Tranylcypromine (Parnate), which is not a hydrazine derivative, does not produce hepatitis.[199]

The antituberculous drug isoniazid is structurally related to iproniazid (Marsilid), and also can produce hepatitis. Recurrence of hepatitis has occurred with readministration of the drug.[242] Pyrazinamide (Aldinamide) can produce fulminant hepatic necrosis. Instances of hepatitis also have been recorded with use of ethionamide (Trecator) and para-aminosalicylic acid.[199]

Sulfonamides may produce hepatic damage that is mainly hepatocellular, but which usually has a cholestatic component. Cross-sensitivity between sulfonamide drugs (sulfamethoxazole and sulfisoxazole) has been demonstrated.[124] The probable allergic basis of this reaction is suggested by the reappearance of hepatitis when the drug is readministered.[101]

Penicillin may produce hepatitis, but only as part of a systemic allergic reaction usually associated with exfoliative dermatitis.[199] Novobiocin and triacetyloleandomycin cause hepatitis rarely.

Cinchophen, an antiarthritic drug that is no longer used, produced hepatocellular damage that was fatal in about one-half of the cases. Other antiarthritic drugs have produced infrequent cases of hepatocellular damage.[199] Aspirin has recently been implicated in producing hepatocellular damage, notably in patients with systemic lupus erythematosus. The hepatic changes are reproduced when the drug is readministered.[371]

In rare instances, antineoplastic drugs (see Table 4-29) may produce hepatocellular damage serious enough to lead to death.[199,202]

Phenacemide (Phenurone) often produces severe hepatitis that may be fatal. Diphenylhydantoin (Dilantin)-induced hepatitis is usually associated with other signs of allergy. All instances of hepatitis due to phenobarbital have been accompanied by cutaneous reactions.[199]

Hepatocellular damage produced by zoxazolamine (Flexin) has

*TABLE 4–30. Other Drugs
Known to Cause Jaundice*

Streptomycin
Chloramphenicol
Organic antimony compounds
Potassium p-aminobenzoate (Potaba)
Quinethazone (Hydromox)

been severe and often fatal.[199] Quinacrine (Atabrine) can produce a yellowish discoloration of the skin, but frank hepatocellular injury occurs infrequently.[199]

Acetohexamide (Dymelor) and metahexamide (Euglycin) may produce parenchymal liver disease, which in rare cases may progress to postnecrotic cirrhosis.[141,199]

Chlordiazepoxide (Librium) has produced hepatic reactions resembling cholestasis. An instance of acute hepatic necrosis, confirmed by liver biopsy, has also been reported to have been produced by the drug.[281]

Nicotinamide (vitamin B_3), given in large doses for the treatment of schizophrenia, has caused hepatic injury which recurred at the time of drug readministration. Vitamin A, used in the treatment of acne and occasionally as a means of preventing colds, can lead to hepatocellular damage that may progress to portal cirrhosis.[259]

Many other drugs have produced sporadic cases of hepatocellular damage. Some cholecystographic dyes, which are listed in Table 4–29, can also injure hepatic cells.[199]

On rare occasion, jaundice has been reported to have been caused by other drugs (see Table 4–30). In these instances, either the data given were inadequate to determine the mechanism of hepatic injury, or a mixed hepatocellular-cholestatic type of reaction occurred.[89,127,199]

Other Drugs that Affect Liver Function

Drugs can alter liver-function tests without producing jaundice. In most instances, either transaminase levels or alkaline phosphatase levels are elevated. Azathioprine (Imuran) and methyldopa (Aldomet) can produce elevated levels of both of these enzymes.[199,202]

Erythromycin estolate (Ilosone) produces elevations of serum glutamic oxaloacetic transaminase (SGOT), which are spurious and not due to true elevations of enzyme levels. An unidentified substance produced in relation to the administration of the antibiotic interferes with the colorimetric method used to measure SGOT.[308]

Triacetyloleandomycin (TAO) and oxacillin (Prostaphlin) can produce elevations in SGOT levels. Ampicillin (Polycillin), nafcillin

(Unipen), and cephalothin (Keflin) also may result in rises in SGOT levels, more commonly in children.[202]

Coumarin derivatives—warfarin (Coumadin) and bishydroxycoumarin (Dicumarol)—occasionally produce elevations in SGOT levels. This effect can create difficulty in diagnosing a recent or suspected myocardial infarction. These anticoagulants should not be used in patients with severe liver disease because of the increased risk of hemorrhage.[202]

Mithramycin (Mithracin) and levodopa (Dopar, Larodopa) may also lead to elevations in SGOT levels.[202]

Corticosteroids may produce an enlarged liver, secondary to fatty infiltration.[199,202]

Use of oral contraceptives is associated with an increased incidence of venous thrombosis, mostly in the lower legs. Thrombosis of the hepatic vein also has occurred in patients receiving oral contraceptives, resulting in the Budd-Chiari syndrome.[199]

Drug-Induced Fibrosis and Granulomas

Fibrosis or cirrhosis of the liver can be produced by drugs (see Table 4-31). Postnecrotic cirrhosis has followed severe hepatocellular damage induced by cinchophen, halothane (Fluothane), iproniazid (Marsilid), metahexamide (Euglycin), and acetohexamide (Dymelor).[141,199] Biliary cirrhosis has occurred after prolonged cholestasis produced by organic arsenicals, chlorpromazine (Thorazine), tolbutamide (Orinase), and metahexamide (Euglycin).[199] Hepatic fibrosis has eventuated from liver damage caused by vitamin A toxicity.[259]

Long-term methotrexate therapy for psoriasis can produce hepatic fibrosis with portal inflammation. This reaction is dose-related and

TABLE 4-31. Drugs Known to Cause Cirrhosis

Postnecrotic cirrhosis:
  Cinchophen
  Halothane (Fluothane)
  Iproniazid (Marsilid)
  Metahexamide (Euglycin)
  Acetohexamide (Dymelor)
Biliary cirrhosis:
  Organic arsenicals
  Chlorpromazine (Thorazine)
  Tolbutamide (Orinase)
  Metahexamide (Euglycin)
Hepatic fibrosis:
  Hypervitaminosis A
  Methotrexate
  Chlorambucil (Leukeran)
  Thorium dioxide (Thorotrast)

is not preceded by drug-induced hepatitis. The degree of fibrosis does not correlate with liver-function studies, so that a liver biopsy must be given in order to detect or determine the degree of fibrosis.[347] Similar fibrosis has been produced by chlorambucil (Leukeran).[199] Hepatic fibrosis can occur many years after the use of thorium dioxide (Thorotrast), a radioactive radiological contrast medium.[179]

Granulomas resembling those seen in Hodgkin's disease or sarcoidosis may occur in the liver and in the lymph nodes during treatment with sulfonylureas (e.g., carbutamide), phenylbutazone (Butazolidin), oxyphenbutazone (Tandearil), hydantoins (e.g., Dilantin), and allopurinol (Zyloprim).[202]

Drug-Induced Kernicterus

The blood-brain barrier is not fully developed in the neonate. Unconjugated (indirect-reacting) bilirubin is bound to serum albumin, but once the binding capacity of the serum albumin is exceeded, unconjugated bilirubin diffuses into the central nervous system producing spasticity, muscle twitching, and convulsions. Infants that survive develop kernicterus, with mental retardation and spastic paraplegia with athetosis. Hemolysis increases unconjugated bilirubin levels (e.g., as in erythroblastosis fetalis), and drug-induced hemolysis has the same effect. Sulfonamides and salicylates displace bilirubin from its serum albumin binding site. Although the total amount of unconjugated bilirubin remains unchanged, increased amounts of unbound bilirubin are available for passage into the central nervous system. Kernicterus can also result from the administration of vitamin K analogues that produce hemolysis, and from the use of novobiocin, which increases levels of serum bilirubin by interfering with hepatic conjugation of bilirubin, especially in the neonate.[199]

Drug-Induced Hepatic Encephalopathy

Hepatic encephalopathy can be precipitated by severe liver necrosis induced by many of the drugs listed in Table 4–29. In severe liver disease, regardless of the cause, ammonium chloride increases the level of blood ammonia and often results in hepatic encephalopathy. Diuretic-induced electrolyte disturbances, principally hypokalemia, correlate with the induction of hepatic coma. While the thiazide diuretics and acetazolamide (Diamox) often produce hypokalemia, ethacrynic acid (Edecrin) and furosemide (Lasix) are more potent diuretics and have a much higher incidence of associated hypokalemia and hepatic decompensation.[327]

Drug-Induced Peliosis Hepatis and Hepatic Tumors

Estrogenic and androgenic steroids can produce varied changes in the liver, including neoplastic transformation. Peliosis hepatis, a rare hepatic lesion, consists of islands of dilated portal sinusoids lined by endothelial or hepatic parenchymal cells that are scattered throughout the liver. Fatal bleeding may occur. Both oral contraceptives and anabolic steroids have been implicated as causative drugs.[107]

Oral contraceptives have produced benign hepatic adenomas. The initial sign may be a right upper quadrant mass or an intraperitoneal hemorrhage that may be fatal.[16] Long-term androgenic and anabolic steroid therapy (longer than 10 months) for aplastic anemia has been associated with the development of hepatocellular carcinoma. No metastases have been noted. In one case the tumor decreased in size when androgen therapy was discontinued, suggesting a mechanism of hormone dependence. Oxymetholone (Anadrol), methyltestosterone (Metandren), and methandrostenolone (Dianabol) were the drugs implicated. Their use by athletes who believe that they increase strength and stamina may lead to potentially deleterious effects.[181] On the basis of the above findings, it has been suggested that estrogens induce benign liver tumors, while androgens produce malignant liver tumors.[16]

Thorotrast (thorium dioxide) was used between 1930 and 1953 as a radioactive radiological contrast material. Thorium has a biologic half-life of about 400 years. The material is deposited in the reticuloendothelial system. About 100 cases of malignant liver tumors have been reported in patients who received Thorotrast. About half of these tumors have been hemangioendotheliomas, which are almost specific for thorium dioxide, and the rest have been hepatomas or cholangiocarcinomas.[179] Because of a 20-year or more latent period before these tumors appear, they are still being encountered even though Thorotrast is no longer used.

6. RESPIRATORY MANIFESTATIONS

Drug reactions affecting the respiratory system are infrequent, but can mimic most known pulmonary diseases. Besides disorders affecting the lungs, drugs may produce nasal symptoms (nasal congestion from reserpine, abuse from vasoconstricting nose drugs, and epistaxis from anticoagulants), and infrequently corticosteroids may induce episternal fat accumulation in individuals with other cushingoid features.[235]

Bronchoconstriction and Asthma

Bronchoconstriction and asthma are the commonest drug-induced pulmonary reactions (Table 4–32). Bronchoconstriction and wheezing occur frequently as a part of anaphylactic reactions.

Aspirin can induce wheezing in 2 to 10 per cent of asthmatic patients. Characteristically, these patients have a low incidence of atopy, but often have rhinorrhea, nasal polyps, and asthma which usually precede the onset of aspirin sensitivity. Within a few minutes to two hours after these patients ingest aspirin, bronchospasm develops which is usually severe and protracted and may be fatal. The usual bronchodilator drugs tend to be ineffective in treating these attacks, and corticosteroid treatment is usually required. Most of these patients have perennial asthma, negative reactions to skin tests, normal IgE levels, and also wheeze when aspirin is not given. Although the mechanism of aspirin-induced bronchospasm is not known, it is not immunologic. There appears to be an autosomal recessive type of inheritance of this disorder. The sensitivity is specific for aspirin. Asthma is not induced by other salicylates. These patients must be warned not only against taking aspirin, but must avoid the myriad of proprietary medicines that contain aspirin.[86,231]

Patients with aspirin-induced asthma also have been found to be sensitive to other structurally dissimilar drugs that produce the same clinical syndrome: indomethacin (Indocin), aminopyrine, mefenamic acid (Ponstel), and the yellow food coloring tartrazine.[231,352]

TABLE 4–32. *Drugs Known to Cause Asthma or Wheezing*

Aspirin	Methylcholine
Indomethacin (Indocin)	Pituitary snuff
Aminopyrine	Aerosols:
Mefenamic acid (Ponstel)	Isoproterenol (Isuprel)
Tartrazine (yellow food dye)	Cromolyn (Intal, Aarane)
Propranolol (Inderal)	Acetylcysteine (Mucomyst)
	Polymyxin B

CLINICAL MANIFESTATIONS 143

Propranolol (Inderal), the beta-adrenergic blocker, can produce bronchoconstriction, especially in asthmatics and patients with pulmonary insufficiency. This is probably caused by the unopposed bronchoconstrictor activity of the parasympathetic nervous system. Propranolol-induced asthma responds well to aminophylline, but not to corticosteroids.[115,299]

Methylcholine, an acetylcholine-like drug, can precipitate asthma attacks.[86] Paradoxically, isoproterenol (Isuprel) aerosols used to treat asthma can incite or worsen bronchospasm about 30 to 60 minutes after use. This effect is not produced by parenterally administered isoproterenol. The mechanism is unknown, but it is conjectured that drug metabolites may have weak beta-adrenergic blocking properties.[192,299] Aerosols of the newly introduced drug cromolyn (Intal, Aarane), which is used to prevent asthma attacks, occasionally produce mild bronchospasm. Pituitary snuff, aerosolized acetylcysteine (Mucomyst), and aerosolized polymyxin B have caused bronchospasm.[299]

Pulmonary Infiltrates and Fibrosis

NITROFURANTOIN REACTION. Many unrelated drugs can lead to the production of pulmonary infiltrates and fibrosis (Table 4–33). Nitrofurantoin (Furadantin) can cause two types of pulmonary reactions: (1) an acute infiltrative form, and (2) a chronic fibrotic process.

(1) The more common acute form is characterized by chills, fever, dyspnea, orthopnea, cough with or without frothy sputum, and occasionally cyanosis. These symptoms begin abruptly from two hours to ten days after patients receive the drug. Basilar rales are present, although the chest x-ray film may show no abnormalities or diffuse alveolar infiltrates, and occasionally a pleural effusion occurs. The white blood cell count is elevated, often with concurrent eosinophilia. There may be hypoxia with mild hypercapnia. When nitrofurantoin is discontinued, there is clinical and radiographic clearing within two days. With readministration of the drug, this syndrome recurs, suggesting that it is caused by an allergic mechanism. This disorder may be mistaken for pulmonary edema, pulmonary embolus, pneumonia, or bronchitis.[262,267] A similar clinical picture also can be produced by para-aminosalicylic acid, sulfonamides, penicillin, chlorpropamide (Diabinese), imipramine (Tofranil), and mephenesin.[299] Hydrochlorothiazide (Hydrodiuril) has produced a similar acute reaction in patients within 45 minutes of their taking an initial oral dose of 50 mg. Fever and eosinophilia are absent, but dyspnea, orthopnea, cough, rales, and wheezes, with diffuse pulmonary infiltrates showing on chest x-ray film, are typical. This reaction is not due to underlying heart disease and is probably idiosyncratic in nature.[338]

(2) The chronic nitrofurantoin reaction appears insidiously after

TABLE 4-33. *Drugs Known to Cause Pulmonary Infiltrates and Fibrosis*

Nitrofurantoin (Furadantin)
Hydrochlorothiazide (Hydrodiuril)
Busulfan (Myleran)
Cyclophosphamide (Cytoxan)
Methotrexate
Methysergide (Sansert)
Ganglionic blockers:
   hexamethonium
   mecamylamine
   pentolinium
Pituitary snuff
Oxygen
Oil aspiration

---

the patient has been taking the drug for six months to six years. Dyspnea, orthopnea, cough, and cyanosis develop over a period of weeks or months. Fever, pleural effusion, and eosinophilia are absent. The chest x-ray film shows bilateral diffuse basilar interstitial infiltrates. Pulmonary function studies show restrictive disease and decreased carbon monoxide diffusion. On a lung biopsy, there is either chronic interstitial pneumonitis, fibrosis, or an admixture of these. The process is partially reversible when the drug is discontinued. Recovery is hastened by corticosteroid treatment.[300,337]

BUSULFAN. Busulfan (Myleran) therapy administered to patients for three or four years can lead to the insidious onset of dyspnea, cough, and fever with pulmonary fibrosis. The chest x-ray film shows diffuse intra-alveolar and interstitial infiltrates. This process is usually irreversible, but corticosteroids may produce some clearing. Cyclophosphamide (Cytoxan) can lead to similar changes. Bleomycin (Blenoxane), a new chemotherapeutic agent used in the treatment of epidermoid carcinoma, lymphoma, and other neoplasms, can lead to pulmonary fibrosis that may be fatal.[299]

METHOTREXATE. Methotrexate may cause an acute or subacute pulmonary reaction with cough and dyspnea, which occurs in patients after 10 days to 4 months of therapy. The chest x-ray film shows bilateral, diffuse, patchy infiltrates. The histologic changes are similar to those produced by busulfan or may resemble granulomas. The prognosis is better than that for busulfan lung.[299]

METHYSERGIDE. Fibrosis due to methysergide (Sansert) usually involves the retroperitoneal space, but pulmonary and pleural fibrosis occur also. After six months to several years of treatment with the drug, there is a gradual onset of cough and dyspnea. Chest pain, fever, chronic pleural effusion, and a friction rub may appear. Although a lung biopsy shows fibrosis around the terminal bronchioles and vessels, this regresses slowly when the drug is discontinued. Symptoms recur as the drug is readministered.[149]

GANGLIONIC BLOCKING AGENTS. The ganglionic blocking agents, hexamethonium, mecamylamine, and pentolinium, which are rarely used now, may produce intra-alveolar and interstitial fibrosis after a few months to a year of therapy. Cough and dyspnea may begin acutely or gradually. Dyspnea is often relieved in patients by lying down.[299]

PITUITARY SNUFF. Pituitary snuff (porcine or bovine posterior pituitary extract) can produce an allergic alveolitis with dyspnea, cough, and rales. Widespread micronodular infiltrates which can progress to interstitial fibrosis are found on chest x-ray film. Pituitary snuff more commonly induces acute asthmatic attacks.[299]

OXYGEN THERAPY. High-concentration oxygen therapy can lead to increased respiratory distress and patchy or confluent infiltrates detected by chest x-ray. Typically, these patients are treated with artificial ventilation. A decrease in vital capacity and pulmonary compliance develops, with consequent hypoxia and difficulty in weaning the patient from the ventilator. As pulmonary compliance decreases, a greater ventilatory pressure and a higher partial pressure of alveolar oxygen are needed to maintain the same inspiratory volume and arterial oxygenation. This process may occur in patients with no previous history of cardiorespiratory disease. Some patients may die of progressive pulmonary insufficiency. An initial exudative phase with intra-alveolar fibrin exudate, hyaline membranes, and interstitial edema is followed by a proliferative phase with interstitial edema, fibroblastic proliferation, fibrosis, and hyperplasia of the alveolar lining cells. At autopsy, the lungs are heavy. The use of 90 to 100 per cent oxygen in patients for more than 10 days is associated with the worst findings.[266]

Newborns, especially premature infants, when treated with oxygen at any level can develop pulmonary hemorrhage.[324]

OTHER FACTORS. Drug-induced systemic lupus erythematosus can produce pulmonary complications such as interstitial pneumonitis, areas of atelectasis, and pleurisy with or without effusion, Drug-induced vasculitis and polyarteritis can cause pulmonary infiltrates.[86]

Aspiration of mineral oil, other neutral oils, or petrolatum jelly can lead to acute or chronic pneumonitis (lipoid pneumonia) which may be localized or diffuse, or may produce a granuloma.[299] Lymphangiography produces oil embolism in about half of patients and decreased carbon monoxide diffusion in all patients following exposure. This can lead to respiratory insufficiency in patients with preexisting lung disease or in those with large amounts of oil embolism.[299]

Other Pulmonary Disorders

Oral contraceptives are associated with an increased incidence of thromboembolic disease. Embolization of particulate matter such as glass, rubber, and plastic can occur from the use of intravenous fluids and indwelling venous catheters. These inert materials can cause granulomas or pulmonary hypertension.[299]

Bleeding into the lungs, mediastinum, and pleural space can occur from anticoagulant therapy, even when the clotting or prothrombin times are within the therapeutic range. Pulmonary hemorrhage can produce dyspnea, bloody sputum, rales, and infiltrates on the chest x-ray film.[291]

Pulmonary edema can follow intravenous infusions of salt containing fluids and blood. As previously mentioned, acute reactions to nitrofurantoin and other drugs can produce a clinical picture resembling acute pulmonary edema. Opiates in large doses also can lead to frank pulmonary edema. The most common cause of such drug-induced pulmonary edema is the illicit use of heroin. The edema develops several hours after recovery from the stuporous state. The causative mechanism is unclear, but does not involve heart failure. Treatment consists of assisted ventilation, oxygen, and narcotic antagonists. After recovery from heroin-induced pulmonary edema, asymptomatic functional lung changes persist which cause a decrease in vital capacity and hinder carbon monoxide diffusion. Pulmonary edema may also occur with overdoses of methadone and propoxyphene (Darvon), and uncommonly with barbiturate intoxication.[299]

Calcification of the lung has been noted in vitamin D intoxication, in high-dose therapy with calcium or inorganic phosphate, and in the milk-alkali syndrome.[299]

Aminorex, an appetite suppressant used in Europe that is structurally similar to amphetamine and epinephrine, has been associated with the production of pulmonary hypertension after about nine months of treatment. This occurs mostly in women. It is thought that the drug acts as a vasoconstrictor of the small pulmonary arteries by stimulating alpha-adrenergic receptors.[299]

Hypoventilation and Apnea

Morphine and other opiates, as well as pentazocine (Talwin),[265] produce respiratory depression as part of their pharmacologic effects. This can lead to hypoventilation, and even apnea, especially in patients with chronic ventilatory insufficiency, hypoadrenalism, hypopituitarism, or severe liver disease.

The aminoglycoside and polymyxin group of antibiotics have a neuromuscular blocking action which can lead to respiratory muscle paralysis and apnea more often than is generally thought (Table 4–

TABLE 4–34. Drugs Known to Produce Neuromuscular Blockade

Aminoglycoside antibiotics:
  Streptomycin
  Neomycin
  Kanamycin (Kantrex)
  Gentamicin (Garamycin)
  Viomycin
Polymyxin antibiotics:
  Polymyxin B
  Colistin (Coly-Mycin)

---

34). Respiratory muscle paralysis is more likely to occur under certain circumstances: high blood levels of these drugs secondary to renal insufficiency; intravenous, intraperitoneal, or intrapleural administration; accidental overdose; the simultaneous use of muscle relaxants with these drugs during surgery, such as succinylcholine (Anectin, Sucostrin) and d-tubocurarine; and the presence of neuromuscular disease (e.g., myasthenia gravis).[299]

Respiratory muscle fatigability produces dyspnea and restlessness which can progress to apnea in from 1 to 26 hours. Neuromuscular blockade may also lead to blurred vision, diplopia, slurred speech, difficulty in swallowing, generalized weakness, and generalized areflexia.[228]

Competitive neuromuscular blockade can be produced by neomycin, kanamycin (Kantrex), and streptomycin. This can be reversed by the use of neostigmine. Noncompetitive blockade is caused by polymyxin B, colistin (Coly-Mycin), and possibly kanamycin. Noncompetitive blockade may be worsened by neostigmine, but may be ameliorated in its early stages by intravenously administered calcium gluconate. The cornerstone of therapy for muscular paralysis is endotracheal intubation and mechanically assisted ventilation, until the neuromuscular blockade wears off.[228] Paromomycin, tetracyclines, and sulfonamides may also produce neuromuscular blockade, but clinical respiratory paralysis has not been reported with these drugs.[228]

Prolonged and occasionally fatal apnea may result in patients given succinylcholine as a muscle relaxant during surgery. Individuals so affected have a hereditary lack of pseudocholinesterase, an enzyme necessary for the inactivation of succinylcholine. Systemic absorption of an anticholinesterase (phospholine iodide) in eye drops used to treat glaucoma has resulted in prolonged apnea when patients using these eye drops received succinylcholine during anesthesia.[134]

Drug interactions that can enhance or prolong neuromuscular blockade are listed in Table 4–35.[86,228]

*TABLE 4–35. Drug Interactions that Enhance or
Prolong Neuromuscular Blockade*

Drug	Agent Interacting with
Streptomycin Neomycin Kanamycin Gentamicin Viomycin Polymyxin B Colistin	Succinylcholine d-Tubocurarine
Succinylcholine d-Tubocurarine	Quinidine Monamine oxidase inhibitors Anticholinesterases
Succinylcholine	Lidocaine (Xylocaine) Promazine (Sparine)
d-Tubocurarine	Hypokalemia

The intramuscular, but especially the intravenous, use of diazepam (Valium) for sedation before cardioversion, endoscopies, and surgical procedures may lead to respiratory depression, cyanosis, and apnea.[49] Regardless of the cause of respiratory depression or apnea, aspiration pneumonia is a frequent complication.

Pulmonary Infection

The use of corticosteroids, immunosuppressive drugs, and antineoplastic agents often leads to pulmonary infection with opportunistic pathogens. Corticosteroids are associated with bacterial pneumonia and the reactivation of tuberculosis. Antineoplastic agents and immunosuppressive drugs, often in combination with corticosteroids, may be associated with infections due to fungi (e.g., aspergillosis, actinomycosis), *Pneumocystis carinii*, and cytomegalovirus.

Lung Tumors

Arsenic therapy has been associated with the development of bronchogenic carcinoma many years after its use.[86] Rare cases of bronchiolar cell carcinoma have occurred in patients with busulfan-induced pulmonary fibrosis.[299]

Pleural Involvement

Pleurisy and pleuritic chest pain occur in association with the respiratory syndromes produced by methysergide, methotrexate, and drug-induced SLE. Methysergide can produce pleural fibrosis.

Acute pleural effusions may occur in the acute pulmonary reaction caused by nitrofurantoin and in drug-induced SLE. Chronic pleural effusions may occur in methotrexate-induced pleuropneumonic fibrosis.[299]

Mediastinal Involvement

Patients treated with corticosteroids who become clinically cushingoid may also be found to have mediastinal widening on chest x-ray, as a result of mediastinal fat accumulation. Often, the epicardial fat pad is also more prominent in these patients.[34]

Diphenylhydantoin (Dilantin) can produce generalized lymph node enlargement, which infrequently leads to mediastinal lymphadenopathy that regresses when the drug is stopped. Methotrexate has also produced enlarged mediastinal lymph nodes.[299]

7. ENDOCRINE MANIFESTATIONS

Drugs can affect the functioning of endocrine organs or can produce endocrine effects by their pharmacologic actions. In addition to the usual endocrine dysfunctions, breast changes and impaired ovarian and testicular function will be discussed.

Drug-Induced Posterior Pituitary Disorders

INAPPROPRIATE ANTIDIURETIC HORMONE SECRETION. Drugs can cause the syndrome of inappropriate antidiuretic hormone secretion characterized by hyponatremia, hypotonic plasma, and simultaneous hyperosmolar urine in the absence of dehydration or hypovolemia (see Table 4-36). Edema is absent, and the concentration of blood urea nitrogen is usually low. In order for a drug to induce this syndrome, there must be excess water intake with drug usage. Large doses of vasopressin can produce these symptoms as part of the drug's normal pharmacologic effect. Oxytocin, used in deliveries and gynecologic procedures, has an antidiuretic effect and has produced this disorder.

The syndrome has also been caused by drugs that do not have a direct endocrine effect: vincristine (Oncovin), cyclophosphamide (Cytoxan), chlorpropamide (Diabinese), and thiazide diuretics. Clofibrate (Atromid-S) and carbamazepine (Tegretol) can produce increased urine osmolality regardless of levels of serum osmolality, but these drugs have not been reported to produce the full symptom complex, with hyponatremia and serum hypotonicity.[15,91]

Treatment consists of discontinuing the causative drug and of restricting water intake until the blood and urine abnormalities revert to normal.

NEPHROGENIC DIABETES INSIPIDUS. Nephrogenic diabetes insipidus caused by impaired renal concentrating ability, and ac-

TABLE 4-36. Drugs Known to Cause the Syndrome of Inappropriate Antidiuretic Hormone Secretion

Vasopressin
Oxytocin
Vincristine (Oncovin)
Cyclophosphamide (Cytoxan)
Chlorpropamide (Diabinese)
Thiazide diuretics

companied by polyuria, polydipsia, and weakness, has been produced by lithium carbonate[248] and demeclocycline (Declomycin).[331] These effects are reversible when the drug is discontinued.

Diabetes Mellitus

Drugs can worsen diabetes mellitus, even to the extent of inducing ketoacidosis, and can produce glucose intolerance in individuals who have latent diabetes, and in pregnant women (Table 4-37). It is problematic whether drug-induced glucose intolerance can be produced in normal individuals without latent diabetes. Certain drugs, such as corticosteroids and thiazide diuretics, although frequently diabetogenic, neither exacerbate diabetes in all diabetic patients nor induce glucose intolerance in all those with latent diabetes.

ACTH and corticosteroids, nevertheless, frequently worsen diabetes or produce glucose intolerance. The exact mechanism of the corticosteroid diabetogenic effect is not known, but decreased peripheral insulin sensitivity is present.[24] In some instances, there is increased glucagon secretion.[247] Ketonuria without glycosuria may occur, and, rarely, ketoacidosis can be precipitated.[31] Adjustment of the dosage of insulin or of the oral hypoglycemic agent will usually provide adequate control.

Oral contraceptives can worsen existing diabetes and produce glucose intolerance during the third trimester of pregnancy in women with a family history of diabetes or a history of an abnormal glucose tolerance test.[86]

Thiazide diuretics, chlorthalidone (Hygroton), furosemide (Lasix), and probably ethacrynic acid (Edecrin) can be diabetogenic.[41,86,263] Thiazide diuretics lead to decreased levels of serum insulin.[41] Diazoxide, a thiazide derivative with potent hypotensive effects, regularly causes hyperglycemia and is, therefore, used to treat hypoglycemic states. Diazoxide, administered intravenously, used to treat severe hypertension in a patient with moderate renal insufficiency but without previous evidence of diabetes, has resulted in acute diabetic ketoacidosis.[349]

Diabetic patients who receive excessive doses of insulin may develop hypoglycemia that is often asymptomatic. Rebound hyperglycemia occurs in response to the hypoglycemia. This sequence of events leads to a clinical picture simulating inadequately controlled diabetes, because the hyperglycemic phase is usually detected by the occurrence of marked glycosuria. This diagnosis may result in the mistaken impression that the patient needs insulin, because the hyperglycemia is not recognized as a reaction to antecedent hypoglycemia. The sequence of excessive insulin dosage, given in response to essentially asymptomatic hypoglycemia, followed by hyperglycemia, is termed the *Somogyi effect*. Posthypoglycemic hyperglycemia should be suspected if the following conditions are present: periods in which the urine is negative for glucose and ketones are followed by marked glycosuria and ketonuria as early as four hours later; wide fluctuations in blood glucose occur in a period of several hours, and are unrelated to meals; glycosuria fluctuates between negative and 4+ without intermediate gradations; and marked glycosuria occurs during the day, with sweating at night and morning hypothermia or headache, suggesting hypoglycemia. Treatment consists of gradually reducing insulin dosage; too rapid a reduction will result in persistent hyperglycemia and ketonuria.[33]

Other drugs that have produced hyperglycemia or diabetic glucose tolerance tests are listed in Table 4–37 and include epinephrine, cyclophosphamide (Cytoxan), diphenylhydantoin (Dilantin), isoniazid, nicotinic acid, lithium carbonate, and excessive amounts of thyroxine.[86,248,285]

Hypoglycemia

Hypoglycemia is caused either by excessive doses of insulin, or may be related to delay or omission of a meal or unexpected exercise in a diabetic receiving a usual insulin dose. If insulin is incorporated into intravenous fluids, up to 20 per cent may be absorbed by the bottle and tubing. If the same system is used again, insulin will no longer be bound, and the same dose may produce hypoglycemia.

The mixing of regular insulin and protamine zinc insulin (PZI) in the same syringe results in variable combinations of protamine with regular insulin. The amount of available regular insulin is reduced

TABLE 4–37. Drugs Known to Cause Hyperglycemia

Corticosteroids
Oral contraceptives
Thiazide diuretics
Diazoxide
Chlorthalidone (Hygroton)
Furosemide (Lasix)
Ethacrynic acid (Edecrin)
Insulin (Somogyi effect)
Epinephrine
Cyclophosphamide (Cytoxan)
Diphenylhydantoin (Dilantin)
Isoniazid
Nicotinic acid
Lithium carbonate
Thyroxine

and the effect of PZI is exaggerated, with resultant delayed hypoglycemia.

Oral hypoglycemic agents also may produce symptomatic hypoglycemia. Acetohexamide (Dymelor) poses a particular problem in patients with impaired renal function because its active metabolite, hydroxyhexamide, requires renal excretion for its elimination.[213] Other drugs given in combination with sulfonylureas, tolbutamide (Orinase), chlorpropamide (Diabinese), acetohexamide (Dymelor), and tolazamide (Tolinase), often enhance the hypoglycemic effect of these drugs. Sulfonamides, phenylbutazone (Butazolidin), oxyphenbutazone (Tandearil), and salicylates displace sulfonylureas from their serum protein binding sites, making them more pharmacologically active.[86] Phenylbutazone also interferes with the renal excretion of hydroxyhexamide, the active metabolite of acetohexamide, and can lead to prolonged hypoglycemia.[120] Thiazide diuretics, monamine oxidase inhibitors, coumarol anticoagulants, propranolol, and alcohol increase the hypoglycemia effects of sulfonylureas.[86,332]

An enhanced insulin effect and hypoglycemia may occur when other drugs are used concomitantly with insulin: monamine oxidase inhibitors, propranolol, and sulfonylureas.[86]

Propranolol alone, but usually in patients receiving insulin or oral hypoglycemics, can induce hypoglycemia. By virtue of its beta-adrenergic blocking effect, the drug opposes catecholamine action and can abolish the usual symptoms of hypoglycemia.[115] Phenformin produces hypoglycemia rarely.[88] Decreased glucose release from the liver induced by norethandrolone (Nilevar) can lead to hypoglycemia. Alcohol, in the absence of liver disease, can depress blood glucose levels.[92]

Patients who surreptitiously took insulin or chlorpropamide to feign illness have been reported. Symptoms often have led to the suspicion that insulinoma was present.[26]

TABLE 4–38. Drugs Known to Cause Hypoglycemia

Insulin:	Phenylbutazone (Butazolidin)
Enhanced effect with:	Oxyphenbutazone (Tandearil)
Monamine oxidase inhibitors	Salicylates
Propranolol (Inderal)	Thiazide diuretics
Sulfonylureas	Monamine oxidase inhibitors
Sulfonylureas:	Coumarol anticoagulants
Tolbutamide (Orinase)	Propranolol (Inderal)
Chlorpropamide (Diabinese)	Alcohol
Acetohexamide (Dymelor)	Phenformin
Enhanced effect with:	Propranolol (Inderal)
Insulin	Norethandrolone (Nilevar)
Sulfonamides	Alcohol

Drugs which are known to cause hypoglycemia are indicated in Table 4-38.

Drug-Induced Thyroid Gland Disorders

HYPERTHYROIDISM. Hyperthyroidism can be produced by excessive doses of exogenous thyroid hormone preparations. Withdrawal of iodide therapy for hyperthyroidism may result in a rebound hyperthyroid state.[47] Radioiodine treatment of hyperthyroidism has eventuated in release of stored thyroid hormone and resultant hyperthyroidism and thyroid storm.[62]

Drugs can affect thyroid function studies in such a way that hyperthyroidism is suggested. Long-term perphenazine (Trilafon) therapy can elevate the protein-bound iodide (PBI) without altering thyroid function.[79] Oral contraceptives do not alter thyroid function but increase the amount of thyroid-binding globulin, leading to elevated PBI levels. Iodinated radiographic dyes increase the PBI level and depress radioiodine uptake by the thyroid gland. Conversely, the antihistamine parabromdylamine maleate (Dimetane) can suppress thyroid radioiodine uptake in both hyperthyroid and euthyroid individuals.[325] Phenindione (Dindevan) has been found to lead to reversible depression of radioiodine uptake.[368]

HYPOTHYROIDISM. Chronic ingestion of large amounts of iodide or iodide-generating organic compounds can lead to goiter and varying degrees of hypothyroidism, with or without goiter formation. The excess thyroidal inorganic iodide inhibits synthesis of thyroid hormone. When iodide ingestion is discontinued, the individual usually becomes euthyroid.[261,373]

Hypothyroidism is a well-recognized and not unusual complication of ^{131}I therapy for hyperthyroidism. However, years may pass before it appears.

Hypothyroidism occurs significantly more often in diabetics treated with either tolbutamide (Orinase) or chlorpropamide (Diabinese) than in those treated with insulin.[173] Rare instances of hypothyroidism have resulted from therapy with para-aminosalicylic acid and, in the past, from long-term thalidomide ingestion.[86] Nontoxic goiter has been produced by combined therapy with phenylbutazone (Butazolidin) and vitamin A.[22]

Long-term use of lithium carbonate can produce a diffuse goiter. Patients are usually euthyroid, but hypothyroidism may occur.[106]

Hypothermic myxedema coma has been induced in hypothyroid patients who were receiving either chlorpromazine (Thorazine) or imipramine (Tofranil).[238]

A few instances of *hypoparathyroidism* have followed administration of ^{131}I therapy for hyperthyroidism. Symptoms appeared after 10 weeks to 13 months. Usual doses of ^{131}I were used. Myxedema was not present when tetany occurred. The pathogenesis of this unusual complication is not known.[109]

Drug-Induced Adrenal Gland Disorders

The typical features of Cushing's disease can be induced by exogenous ACTH and corticosteroids. Although individual differences in susceptibility exist, both total corticosteroid dose and duration of therapy are important contributing factors. Cushingoid side effects can be mitigated if a single morning dose or alternate day therapy is feasible.

Corticosteroid therapy, except when given only for short periods, induces adrenal atrophy and hypofunction by suppressing pituitary ACTH secretion. Since under these circumstances the adrenal glands are unable to respond to stresses, such as infection, trauma, surgery, or anesthesia, when corticosteroid output is increased, a hypoadrenal state can ensue with accompanying hypotension and shock. The same dangers exist when corticosteroids are suddenly discontinued or the dose is rapidly decreased after prolonged administration. There is wide individual variation in the duration of suppressed adrenal response to stress after corticosteroids have been withdrawn. Some degree of suppression may last for two years.

Corticosteroids cross the placenta and have produced adrenal crisis and shock in the newborn.[86]

The antileukemic agent busulfan (Myleran) may induce a syndrome characterized by hyperpigmentation, fatigue, muscle weakness, and weight loss that simulates adrenal insufficiency, but in which adrenal cortical function is normal.[212]

Busulfan-induced adrenal insufficiency, however, may occur as a result of decreased pituitary ACTH reserve. The syndrome improves when the drug is discontinued, but added corticosteroids may be needed during stressful periods.[353]

Acute adrenal insufficiency as a result of bilateral adrenal hemorrhage secondary to anticoagulation with the use of heparin or dicoumarol has led to death.[60]

Hyperaldosteronism with hypokalemia has resulted from chronic abuse of various laxatives. The laxative-induced watery diarrhea resulted in sodium depletion (and enhanced potassium losses), which led to elevated blood renin and aldosterone levels.[123]

Drug-Induced Breast Changes

GYNECOMASTIA. *Gynecomastia* occurs with the use of many drugs (Table 4-39). This is probably caused by the estrogen or progesterone peripheral effects of these drugs. Breast enlargement in men tends to disappear when these drugs are discontinued.[86,353]

TABLE 4-39. *Drugs Known to Cause Gynecomastia*

Estrogens (diethylstilbestrol)	Isoniazid
Androgens (methyltestosterone)	Ethionamide
Desoxycorticosterone	Methyldopa (Aldomet)
Spironolactone (Aldactone)	Griseofulvin
Digitalis compounds	Busulfan (Myleran)
Phenothiazines	Phenaglycodol (Ultran)
Reserpine	

Besides estrogens, spironolactone (Aldactone), because of its molecular structure, is associated with a high incidence of gynecomastia.

GALACTORRHEA. Drug-induced mammary hypertrophy and *galactorrhea* in women is often associated with amenorrhea. Breast enlargement often occurs with the use of oral contraceptives, and may be accompanied by galactorrhea.[153] About 10 to 15 per cent of women treated with phenothiazines, most often with trifluoperazine (Stelazine), develop breast engorgement and galactorrhea. In many instances, increased levels of lactogenic hormone have been found. This is felt to be the result of drug action on the hypothalamic-pituitary axis. Those drugs that can produce galactorrhea are listed in Table 4-40.

Drug-Induced Gonadal Changes

MENSTRUAL CYCLE CHANGES. Oral contraceptives may produce changes in the *menstrual cycle*. Breakthrough bleeding, spotting, and alterations in the amount of menstrual flow, as well as amenorrhea, may be encountered. Long-term treatment has led to amenorrhea for up to 18 months after oral contraceptives were discontinued. There is an increased incidence of anovulatory cycles. Ovaries have shown fibrosis which regresses after cessation of treatment.[86]

Cyclophosphamide (Cytoxan) frequently leads to amenorrhea, which lasts up to a year after the cessation of therapy in one-half of women who receive the drug. The main ovarian changes are a lack of follicular maturation with absent ova, or only a few follicles in an

TABLE 4-40. *Drugs Known to Cause Galactorrhea*

Oral contraceptives	Haloperidol (Haldol)
Phenothiazines:	Reserpine
Trifluoperazine (Stelazine)	Chlordiazepoxide (Librium)
Thioridazine (Mellaril)	Imipramine (Tofranil)
Others	Amitriptyline (Elavil)
Chlorprothixene (Taractan)	Methyldopa (Aldomet)

inactive state.[359] Busulfan (Myleran) therapy also may lead to amenorrhea and ovarian atrophy.[353]

VIRILIZING EFFECTS AND SPERMATOGENESIS. Androgens and anabolic steroids produce *virilizing effects* in women, with resultant diminished menses, clitoral hypertrophy, and increased libido.

Many antineoplastic agents suppress *spermatogenesis* in men: cyclophosphamide (Cytoxan), vincristine (Oncovin), procarbazine (Matulane), and nitrogen mustards. Cyclophosphamide has been the most intensively studied. During drug therapy, sertoli and Leydig cells remain intact and libido and potentia are unaffected, but spermatogenesis is absent in the majority of men. Spermatogenesis may return after cessation of therapy.[326,353]

Anabolic steroids may also suppress spermatogenesis, and in prepubertal males may lead to precocious sexual development.[86]

8. URINARY TRACT MANIFESTATIONS

The kidneys are often the site of adverse drug reactions because many drugs are excreted through the kidneys, and because of the inherent nephrotoxicity of some drugs. Drugs may lead to decreased renal function, acute tubular necrosis, the nephrotic syndrome, crystallization within the kidney, renal calculi, hematuria, bladder involvement, and tumors.

Decreased Renal Function Caused by Drugs

Many drugs can impair renal function, even to the point of causing acute renal failure (Table 4–41). Heavy metals, both as inorganic and organic preparations, are potent nephrotoxins. Inorganic mercury produces acute tubular necrosis. Organic mercurial diuretics can lead to renal failure and acute tubular necrosis, possibly as the result of the conversion of organic mercury to inorganic mercury which binds sulfhydryl groups in renal enzymes. Bismuth compounds, previously used in the treatment of syphilis, have an effect similar to that of mercury poisoning. Gold salts used in the treatment of rheumatoid arthritis have produced fatal anuric nephritis. Transient renal failure has occurred from the use of antimony compounds in the treatment of kala-azar.[312]

Chronic analgesic abuse can lead to nephropathy. The incriminated drug is phenacetin, usually in combination with aspirin or caffeine. The earliest histologic lesion occurs as a result of an increase in interstitial collagen, with scarring in the medulla. Renal papillary necrosis occurs often, even without the presence of pyelonephritis, which, however, is a frequent complication. Secondary cortical atrophy then occurs which may be fatal.[131,197] The initial functional derangement is an impaired ability to concentrate urine. Progressive azotemia follows, often with renal papillary necrosis and nonobstructive pyelonephritis. If phenacetin is discontinued, the renal lesions are partially reversible and renal function stabilizes or improves.

Acute renal failure has followed salicylate overdose. Even in the normal adult dose, salicylates are renal irritants which lead to the appearance of cells, casts, and small amounts of albumin in the urine. These effects are dose-related and clear within a week if the drug is discontinued. No renal damage is produced.[86,312]

Aminopyrine, an analgesic related to phenacetin, may cause renal damage.[86] Phenazone has produced acute tubular necrosis as a result of an allergic mechanism.[271] Phenylbutazone (Butazolidin) has led to acute renal failure by producing either tubular necrosis or cortical necrosis.[312]

TABLE 4-41. Drugs Known to Be Nephrotoxic

Heavy metals:	Penicillin
Mercurials	Methicillin (Staphcillin)
Bismuth	Oxacillin (Prostaphlin)
Gold	Ampicillin
Antimony	Cephaloridine (Loridine)
Arsenic	Cephalothin (Keflin)
Iron	Vancomycin
Uranium	Ristocetin
Lead	Amphotericin B
Silver	Radiographic contrast media:
Cadmium	Bunamiodyl (Orabilex)
Copper	Intravenous and intra-arterial injection
Thallium	Other drugs:
Analgesics:	Para-aminosalicylic acid
Phenacetin	Phenindione (Dindevan, Danilone, Hedulin)
Salicylates	Pentamidine
Aminopyrine	d-Penicillamine
Phenazone	Methoxyflurane (Penthrane)
Phenylbutazone (Butazolidin)	Epsilon-amino caproic acid (Amicar)
Antimicrobial agents:	Dextran (low molecular weight)
Sulfonamides	Sucrose
Streptomycin	Mannitol
Kanamycin (Kantrex)	Cyclophosphamide (Cytoxan)
Gentamicin (Garamycin)	Mithramycin (Mithracin)
Neomycin	Acetazolamide (Diamox)
Polymyxin B	Zoxazolamine (Flexin)
Colistin (Coly-Mycin)	Thiazide diuretics
Bacitracin	Erythromycin
Paromomycin (Humatin)	Quinine
Tetracyclines	

Antimicrobial agents can impair renal function by various mechanisms. Sulfonamides can crystallize in and obstruct the kidney. This occurs most often in concentrated urine of low pH, and leads to renal pain, hematuria, azotemia, oliguria, and anuria. Drug crystallization is less likely to occur with the presently used more soluble compounds. Treatment consists of giving fluids and alkalinizing the urine. Infrequently, sulfonamides produce renal damage by causing direct tubular necrosis, interstitial nephritis, and necrotizing angiitis.[312]

The combination of sulfamethoxazole and trimethoprim (Bactrim, Septra) may produce a decrease in renal function.[184]

The inherent nephrotoxicity of the aminoglycoside and polymyxin group of antibiotics is enhanced by increased blood levels of these drugs produced by large doses and subsequent decreased renal function. Renal damage is reversible with cessation of these drugs. Streptomycin infrequently causes mild proximal tubular damage. Kanamycin (Kantrex) and gentamicin (Garamycin) may produce severe renal damage secondary to tubular necrosis. Azotemia also occurs frequently with these antimicrobial agents. Only a small proportion of oral neomycin is absorbed, but toxic effects have occurred in patients with preexisting renal insufficiency. Polymyxin B and colistin (Coly-Mycin) often produce tubular damage and azotemia.[312]

Bacitracin is highly nephrotoxic and therefore is not used parenterally. Paromomycin (Humatin), used in the treatment of amebiasis, can produce tubular damage.[86]

The tetracyclines, notably oxytetracycline, can produce transient azotemia in patients being treated for a urinary tract infection, especially if the blood urea nitrogen level was moderately elevated before the onset of treatment. Tetracyclines administered intravenously can lead to jaundice, fatty liver, and uremia, usually in the setting of treating pregnant women for urinary tract infections.[86]

Interstitial nephritis and renal failure usually associated with fever, rash, and eosinophilia have been caused by penicillin, methicillin (Staphcillin), oxacillin (Prostaphlin), and ampicillin. There may be accompanying hematuria, proteinuria, and pyuria. The underlying mechanism is probably allergic.[14,48]

Cephaloridine (Loridine) produces a predictable, dose-related (more than 4 gm daily), reversible nephrotoxic effect. Associated proteinuria, cylindruria, and hematuria may be found, and, on occasion, fatal acute tubular necrosis has occurred.[187,245] Cephalothin (Keflin), particularly when given in very large doses (12 to 24 gm administered intravenously each day), has led to renal failure.[187]

Amphotericin B produces some renal damage in most patients. This is manifested by azotemia, plus renal tubular acidosis and deposit of calcium in the renal medulla. The urine may show casts, and not have significant proteinuria, red blood cells, and white blood cells. Mild renal impairment may persist for many years.[350]

Bunamiodyl (Orabilex), an oral radiographic contrast medium previously used for visualizing the gall bladder, was removed from the market because of its marked nephrotoxicity. Other oral contrast media rarely lead to renal functional impairment. High concentrations and rapid injection of other contrast media, given either intravenously for pyelography or intra-arterially for abdominal angiography, have led to renal impairment ranging from mild azotemia to acute renal failure.[312] When an intravenous pyelogram is given, preparatory dehydration in a patient with multiple myeloma can lead to the precipitation of proteinaceous material in the renal tubules. Dehydration in a patient with diabetic nephropathy in whom a drip-infusion pyelogram was performed with meglumine diatrizoate (Renografin 60) has led to oliguria.[25]

Para-aminosalicylic acid has caused fever, rash, hemolysis, and acute renal failure.[312] Rarely, the anticoagulant phenindione (Dindevan, Danilone, Hedulin) causes severe and often fatal tubular necrosis, which is often preceded by a rash.[86]

The treatment of *Pneumocystis carinii* pneumonia with pentami-

CLINICAL MANIFESTATIONS

dine has led to reversible oliguria and azotemia with proteinuria, granular and white blood cell casts in the urine, and glycosuria.[13] Although d-penicillamine usually produces the nephrotic syndrome, reversible nephropathy with decreased renal function has also occurred.[178] The anesthetic methoxyflurane (Penthrane) has induced a renal tubular disorder with azotemia, inability to concentrate urine, and resultant dehydration with hypernatremia. Mild renal dysfunction may persist for several months.[112]

Glomerular capillary thrombosis and acute renal failure have ensued after use of epsilon-aminocaproic acid (Amicar), an inhibitor of fibrinolysis.[57] Dextran, in preparations of low molecular weight, has adversely affected renal function by producing damage of large and small renal vessels.[243] Sucrose and mannitol infusions can cause tubular damage.[312]

Cyclophosphamide (Cytoxan) can lead to acute tubular damage and glomerular capillary thickening, with hematuria and proteinuria.[233] Another antineoplastic drug, mithramycin (Mithracin), can cause tubular damage and azotemia.[194]

Deposition of crystals in the tubules has resulted from treatment with acetazolamide (Diamox). Favorable responses to this condition have occurred after treatment of the patient with fluids, and after alkalinizing the urine.[272] Zoxazolamine (Flexin), a uricosuric agent, has produced renal damage possibly as a result of urate precipitation in the kidney.[312] Uric acid nephropathy may follow successful treatment of acute leukemia. Cell destruction leads to the release of purines that are catabolized to uric acid. Pretreatment with allopurinol (Zyloprim) often prevents this complication.[354]

Renal function can be markedly compromised by necrotizing renal vasculitis produced by thiazide diuretics, sulfonamides, phenylbutazone (Butazolidin), penicillin, tetracyclines, erythromycin, and quinine.[86]

Drug-induced systemic lupus erythematosus rarely produces renal involvement, but proteinuria may occur, which abates when the inciting drug is discontinued. Drug-induced serum sickness often causes mild renal damage.

Acute drug-induced hemolysis, as occurs in glucose-6-phosphate dehydrogenase deficiency, may on occasion produce severe enough hemoglobinuria to lead to renal dysfunction. Drug-induced hypercalcemia (e.g., vitamin D intoxication) produces nephrocalcinosis and impaired renal concentrating ability. Hypokalemic nephropathy can be caused by potassium loss due to therapy with diuretics.

Drug-Induced Nephrotic Syndrome

The nephrotic syndrome, with proteinuria, hypoalbuminuria, edema, and hypercholesterolemia, can be induced by many struc-

TABLE 4-42. *Drugs Known to Produce the Nephrotic Syndrome*

Mercurial diuretics
Gold salts
Bismuth compounds
Trimethadione (Tridione)
Paramethadione (Paradione)
d-Penicillamine
Phenindione (Danilone, Dindevan, Hedulin)
Probenecid (Benemid)
Tolbutamide (Orinase)
Gamma globulin

turally unrelated drugs. Discontinuing the causative drug usually results in prompt improvement. The anticonvulsants trimethadione (Triadone) and paramethadione (Paradione) are the most frequently implicated drugs in this effect. The nephrotic syndrome recurs with readministration of these drugs.[86] Other drugs that have brought about this renal abnormality are listed in Table 4-42.[86,312]

Drug-Induced Renal Tubular Acidosis

Outdated tetracyclines have caused reversible renal tubular dysfunction resembling Fanconi's syndrome, or cystinosis, with glycosuria, aminoaciduria, phosphaturia, and proteinuria. Renal tubular acidosis was a common feature, and nitrogen retention with hypokalemia was sometimes observed. This disorder was found to be due to tetracycline degradation products (anhydro-4-epitetracycline produced the syndrome in rats and dogs) which were produced by heat, moisture, and a low pH resulting from the presence of citric acid. Lactose has replaced citric acid in these drug preparations, with resultant greater stability of tetracyclines and no recent reports of this syndrome.[125]

Amphotericin B induces a renal tubular lesion which is manifested by impaired urine concentrating ability, excessive urinary potassium loss with hypokalemia, and renal tubular acidosis caused by a defect in acid secretion with a resultant alkaline urine. With cessation of the drug, tubular function slowly returns to normal.[45,99]

Drug-Induced Retroperitoneal Fibrosis

Methysergide (Sansert), a prophylactic drug against migraine headaches, induces retroperitoneal fibrosis in about one per cent of users. Symptoms have appeared after nine months to two years of therapy. The aorta, heart, and lungs may also be involved. Abdominal and flank pain may occur. The retroperitoneal fibrosis produces ureteral obstruction and hydronephrosis, which leads to renal infection and azotemia. Histologic examination of retroperitoneal tissue shows inflammation, followed by fibrosis. With cessation of the drug, there is regression of fibrosis, which may be enhanced by corticosteroid therapy. Hydronephrosis and azotemia also improve.[149]

Renal Calculi Produced by Drugs

Calcium phosphate stones have occurred after long-term therapy with acetazolamide (Diamox).[272] Vitamin D intoxication leads to hypercalciuria, which may result in stone formation. A rare instance of allopurinol (Zyloprim)-induced xanthine stones has been reported in treatment of the Lesch-Nyhan syndrome. This syndrome is characterized by mental retardation, self-mutilation, and hyperuricemia; the hyperuricemia is a result of excessive purine production. When allopurinol was used to block the conversion of hypoxanthine and xanthine to uric acid, the increased xanthinuria resulted in stone formation.[52]

Other Drug-Induced Urinary Tract Disorders

Anticoagulation caused by heparin or coumarin derivatives can lead to microscopic or gross hematuria.[305]

Lithium carbonate[248] and demeclocycline (Declomycin)[331] have produced reversible *nephrogenic diabetes insipidus*. Renal concentrating ability is impaired, with consequent polyuria and polydipsia, but without azotemia.

Cyclophosphamide (Cytoxan) has produced *hemorrhagic cystitis*, probably as a result of drug metabolites in the urine causing irritation to the bladder. Hemorrhagic cystitis is severe, and can be fatal. Forcing fluids is the recommended therapy. Nonhemorrhagic cystitis and fibrosis of the bladder have also been reported with the use of this drug.[256]

Urinary retention due to bladder atony, especially in elderly men with prostatic hypertrophy, is frequently induced by anticholinergic drugs such as atropine. Antihistamines, sedatives, and ganglionic blocking agents may have the same effect.[86]

Drug-Induced Tumors

Analgesic abuse with phenacetin has been associated with the development of transitional cell carcinomas of the renal pelvis and bladder. Treatment of Hodgkin's disease with high doses of chlornaphazine has produced bladder tumors. Renal carcinomas have occurred in individuals in whom thorium dioxide (Thorotrast) had been used as a radiographic contrast medium. Patients with arsenic-induced basal cell carcinomas of the skin tend to have associated bronchial and genitourinary tumors.[86]

9. GYNECOLOGIC ABNORMALITIES

Drugs can alter menses, damage the ovaries, induce virilization, increase susceptibility to vaginitis, and produce vaginal carcinomas.

Altered Menses Caused by Drugs

Changes in the menstrual cycle, such as breakthrough bleeding, spotting, and changes in menstrual flow, may occur with the use of oral contraceptives. Amenorrhea may appear after long-term treatment with these drugs, and may last for 18 months after cessation of treatment. Fibrosis of the ovaries with anovulatory cycles may occur, but this condition regresses when oral contraceptives are discontinued.[86] Already present uterine fibroids may enlarge under the hormonal effects of oral contraceptives.

About one-half of the women treated with cyclophosphamide (Cytoxan) develop amenorrhea that may last for a year after therapy is discontinued. The ovaries show poor follicular maturation, with absent ova, or only a few follicles in an inactive state.[359] Ovarian atrophy and amenorrhea have followed busulfan (Mylleran) therapy.[353]

As mentioned in the section of endocrine manifestations, amenorrhea is often associated with drug-induced breast hypertrophy and galactorrhea. Phenothiazines, especially trifluoperazine (Stelazine), reserpine, chlorprothixene (Taractan), haloperidol (Haldol), imipramine (Tofranil), amitriptyline (Elavil), chlordiazepoxide (Librium), and methyldopa (Aldomet) can bring about this syndrome. These effects have been attributed to drug-induced depletion of hypothalamic catecholamines and the resultant removal of the hypothalamic inhibiting effects on the secretion of prolactin.[51,348]

Drug-Induced Virilization

The virilizing effects of androgens and anabolic steroids can lead to scanty menses and clitoral hypertrophy in women, as well as to increased libido, deepening of the voice, and hirsutism.

Drug-Induced Candida Vaginitis

Oral contraceptives, probably by inducing a state of pseudopregnancy, can lead to intractable *Candida vaginitis* which is resistant to local treatment until oral contraceptives are discontinued.[376] Broad-spectrum antibiotics and corticosteroids, and potentially immunosuppressive agents and antineoplastic drugs, can precipitate *Candida vaginitis*.[318]

Drug-Induced Vaginal Adenocarcinoma

It has recently been discovered that female infants born of mothers who were treated with diethyl stilbestrol during pregnancy may develop vaginal adenocarcinoma during adolescence and early adulthood. Malignancies of other portions of the urogenital tract have not been found in these offspring.[167]

10. FETAL AND NEONATAL MANIFESTATIONS

During the early period of fetal development, drugs can produce fetal death, abortion, or congenital anomalies. Malformations are most likely to occur during the first trimester of pregnancy, at the time of organ formation. Drugs can also cause growth defects, physiologic derangements, and postnatal abnormalities, which may be detectable soon after birth or not until many years later. A teratogenic drug may not always produce an abnormality. While some drugs tend to produce a specific effect, such as phocomelia induced by thalidomide, the same drug may also cause other abnormalities.

Drugs Which Produce Multiple Congenital Anomalies

Antineoplastic drugs may cause abortion, multiple congenital anomalies, or no apparent ill effects. Aminopterin has been used as an abortifacient. In instances in which abortion did not follow the use of this drug, infants were born with multiple congenital anomalies. Methotrexate, mercaptopurine, chlorambucil (Leukeran), and busulfan (Myleran) can produce various congenital anomalies.[325a] Chlorambucil has resulted in absence of the fetal kidney and ureter, an effect which was reproducible in rats.[344a] A few successful pregnancies have occurred in women treated with either mercaptopurine, cyclophosphamide (Cytoxan), azathioprine (Imuran), or nitrogen mustard, with the delivery of apparently normal infants.[56a,325a] Absence of or a reduced number of toes in the fetus has been attributed to the effects of cyclophosphamide.[325a]

Congenital anomalies have been attributed to the use of certain drugs during pregnancy with varying degrees of certainty. Thalidomide is a prototype of a known teratogenic drug. It was withdrawn from use because of frequently induced phocomelia (absence of the proximal portions of the limbs, hands, or feet). Abnormalities of the ears, eyes, heart, gastrointestinal tract, and urogenital system also were caused by this drug.[344a,380]

A high incidence of all types of congenital abnormalities has been attributed to the use of diphenylhydantoin (Dilantin) during pregnancy, but this occurrence has not always been found to be statistically significant.[258] Diphenylhydantoin has also been implicated in producing skeletal abnormalities consisting of hypoplasia or irregular ossification of the distal phalanges, with resultant short, narrow, misshapen ends of both fingers and toes.[234] The antiepileptic drug trimethadione (Tridione) is also possibly teratogenic.[325a]

Drugs Implicated in Prenatal Abnormalities

Dextroamphetamine, used as an appetite suppressant, when taken during pregnancy increases the risk of congenital heart disease and possibly of biliary atresia.[325a]

Coumarin derivatives cross the placenta and have caused fatal bleeding in the fetus when the mother's prothrombin time was in the therapeutic range.[56a,344a] Heparin does not cross the placenta. Thus when an anticoagulant is needed, women approaching term should be treated with heparin in order to prevent fetal hemorrhage during delivery.[352a]

The use of isoniazid for the treatment of tuberculosis during pregnancy has resulted in the birth of infants with psychomotor retardation, convulsions, and myoclonus felt to be caused by the interference of isoniazid with pyridoxine metabolism.[363] Methyl mercury contamination of fish in Japan has been implicated in causing fetal cerebral palsy and microcephaly.[325a]

The antihistamine-antiemetics meclizine (Antivert, Bonine), cyclizine (Marezine), and chlorcyclizine (found in Fedrazil) have been found to be teratogenic in rats, but there is no conclusive evidence of their induction of congenital anomalies in humans.[56a,344a,376a]

Tetracycline, given early in pregnancy or during lactation, may cause cataracts, but a clear-cut relationship has not been established.[344a] Also, tetracycline is deposited in bone and can retard skeletal growth, which rapidly returns to normal after short-term drug exposure.[68a,363] Streptomycin therapy during pregnancy has caused hearing loss in the fetus without impaired vestibular function.[363] Chloroquine (Aralen) has been reported to have been the cause of deafness in three children born to the same woman.[344a] Quinine possibly may produce nerve deafness in the fetus.[344a] There is some evidence that treatment with corticosteroids may produce a small risk of inducing cleft palate.[325a]

Radioactive iodine should not be used for either diagnostic or therapeutic purposes during pregnancy because it accumulates in the fetal thyroid gland, with resultant destruction and hypothyroidism. Neonatal goiter can be caused by iodine-containing drugs and antithyroid compounds such as propylthiouracil and methimazole (Tapazole). Goiters may subside, but they can also cause respiratory distress because of their size. Hypothyroidism may occur rarely,[56a] and rebound hyperthyroidism may follow cessation of drug exposure after delivery of the infant.[344a]

In the children of one woman, the use of phenmetrazine (Preludin), an appetite suppressant, has been suspected of causing absence of a leaf of the diaphragm, with herniation of the abdominal contents into the chest, but the association is probably coincidental.[325a]

There appears to be an increased risk of congenital heart disease and of other congenital abnormalities when oral contraceptives are taken during pregnancy.[56a]

The use of synthetic progestins, which have androgenic effects, and of androgenic steroids between the eighth and thirteenth weeks of pregnancy have resulted in the masculinization of the female fetus. Natural progesterone does not possess androgenic activity.[325a]

Infants of mothers who smoke weigh less at any given stage of gestation than those of nonsmoking mothers. Decreased birth weight correlates with the number of cigarettes smoked and the socioeconomic status of the mother. The incidence of prematurity is doubled when the mother smokes, and is again related to the number of cigarettes smoked. A slight increase in the number of abortions among smokers has been observed, but this has not been found to be statistically significant. No greater incidence of stillbirths, congenital anomalies, or maternal complications has been noted.[348a] It has been conjectured that these effects are related to carbon monoxide inhalation from smoking.[344a] Alcoholism also leads to decreased birth weight of infants, and has been correlated with mental retardation, and craniofacial, limb, and cardiac malformations in the neonate.[56a]

Drugs Implicated in Postnatal Abnormalities

Drugs taken during pregnancy can produce physiologic changes in the neonate at the time of birth or shortly thereafter. Depressant drugs such as narcotic analgesics and diazepam (Valium) given during labor can lead to a lethargic, hypotonic infant.[56a] The prolonged use of magnesium sulfate to treat pre-eclampsia can result in a hypotonic infant and may lead to paralysis and respiratory failure.[56a] Mepivacaine (Carbocaine), a local anesthetic used in obstetrical practice, can cause fetal intoxication by crossing the placenta after maternal absorption. The anesthetic is poorly detoxified by the fetus. Accidental direct injection of mepivacaine into the fetus has also occurred.[121,296,330] Reserpine, used to treat hypertension during pregnancy, may cause nasal stuffiness in the neonate and lead to upper airway obstruction that on rare occasion has caused death.[344a]

Hexamethonium, a ganglionic blocking agent previously used to treat hypertension, has caused paralytic ileus and death in neonates.[344a]

Coumarin derivatives, as mentioned, cross the placenta and can cause neonatal bleeding. Women with thromboembolic disorders requiring anticoagulants at the time of labor should be given heparin, which does not appreciably cross the placenta. Heparin should be substituted for one of the coumarin group of drugs about two weeks before delivery.[352a] Bleeding has also been caused by thrombocytopenia induced in both the mother and infant by quinine,[104a] and in the infant but not the mother by thiazides.[104a]

Insulin, which does not cross the placenta, is usually required to treat pregnant diabetic women. Women receiving oral hypoglycemic agents at term have given birth to infants who have evidenced prolonged hypoglycemia.[56a] Prednisone is rapidly metabolized to prednisolone, which does not cross the placenta. A few instances of hypoglycemia in the neonate have been reported in mothers receiving prednisone. In such instances, enough corticosteroid probably crossed the placenta to suppress the fetal pituitary-adrenal axis.[56a]

Phenothiazines cross the placenta and have led to rare instances of extrapyramidal signs in neonates.[56a]

Narcotics[344a] and long-term use of barbiturates[56a] have led to addiction in the neonate followed by a withdrawal syndrome which can be fatal. Symptoms are similar to those observed in adults: restlessness, yawning, stretching, poor feeding, vomiting, diarrhea, pallor, dyspnea, cyanosis, and rarely, convulsions.

Kernicterus results from unconjugated bilirubin entering the central nervous system across an immature neonatal blood-brain barrier. Unconjugated bilirubin is bound to serum albumin. When serum levels exceed the binding capacity of albumin, unconjugated bilirubin becomes available for diffusion into the central nervous system. One source of excessive unconjugated bilirubin is hemolysis from excessive doses of synthetic vitamin K, given either to the mother during labor or to the infant after delivery.[344a] Sulfonamides, especially the long-acting varieties, and salicylates bind to serum albumin in preference to unconjugated bilirubin, which increases the amount of unconjugated bilirubin available for diffusion into the central nervous system. For this reason sulfonamides should not be administered to newborns. Novobiocin interferes with the conjugation of bilirubin in the liver, more markedly so in the neonate, and may lead to kernicterus.[199]

Chloramphenicol given to the neonate, especially to premature infants, in doses greater than 25 mg/kg of body weight, has resulted in the "gray syndrome." In two to nine days after the drug is begun, abdominal distension, occasionally vomiting, hypothermia, a gray ashen cyanosis, respiratory difficulty, and vascular collapse appear. Because of the inability of the neonate's liver to conjugate chloramphenicol, toxic blood levels of the drug develop which lead to the syndrome.[363]

Delayed Drug-Induced Changes

Drugs administered during pregnancy can produce changes that are delayed in appearance. Tetracyclines are deposited in growing teeth, and if sufficient amounts are taken during pregnancy, there may be permanent enamel hypoplasia and a yellow to brown discoloration of the young child's teeth.[363]

Female infants born of mothers treated with diethyl stilbestrol during pregnancy may develop adenocarcinoma of the vagina during adolescence or early adulthood. Other malignancies of the reproductive tract have not been found.[167]

Drugs administered during pregnancy pose a potential risk to both the mother and the fetus. Drugs with a known ability to affect the unborn child adversely should be sedulously avoided. All drugs should be administered reluctantly to the pregnant women, especially new drugs whose teratogenic potential is unknown. Special care must be taken during the first trimester of pregnancy, when severe malformations and fetal death are more likely to occur. Drugs should be used during pregnancy only for definite medical reasons, and the pregnant woman should be strongly advised not to take any nonprescribed drug, including over-the-counter preparations, without previous consultation with her physician.

11. METABOLIC MANIFESTATIONS

Drug-induced metabolic disorders, including electrolyte imbalance, disordered acid-base balance, shifts in fluid volume, altered serum calcium levels, elevated serum lipids, hyperuricemia and gout, hemochromatosis, and porphyria are discussed in this section. Some of these disorders, such as alterations in electrolyte, acid-base, and fluid balance, and elevated levels of serum uric acid, are frequently drug-induced; the others are less frequently caused by drugs.

ELECTROLYTE IMBALANCE

Drug-Induced Hypernatremia

The infusion of excessive amounts of hypertonic saline, especially in patients with compromised renal function, can lead to hypernatremia. The treatment of hypercalcemia with sodium sulfate infusion, as a means of increasing urinary excretion of calcium, often leads to marked hypernatremia. Concomitant hypercalcemic impairment of renal function increases the likelihood of hypernatremia.[165] Prolonged intravenous administration of mannitol as an osmotic diuretic in treatment of cirrhotic patients with renal failure has led to hypernatremia, as a result of renal water excretion with relatively little sodium loss.[137] Drugs which lead to hypernatremia are listed in Table 4–43.

Drug-Induced Hyponatremia

One of the hazards of diuretic therapy with mercurial diuretics, thiazides, ethacrynic acid (Edecrin), or furosemide (Lasix) is chronic sodium depletion, manifested by hyponatremia, hypochloremia, and slight elevations of the blood urea nitrogen (BUN) levels and hematocrit values.[103] These changes are reversed by judiciously increasing salt intake.

Excessive water intake or infusions of salt-poor fluids can depress serum sodium values, particularly in patients who are unable to excrete water easily, such as those with renal disease, severe heart failure, or cirrhosis. The treatment for this condition is water restriction.

TABLE 4–43. Drugs Known to Cause Hypernatremia

Hypertonic saline infusion
Sodium sulfate infusion
Mannitol (prolonged intravenous use)

TABLE 4-44. *Drugs, Drug-Induced Syndromes, and Fluids that Cause Hyponatremia*

Diuretics
Excessive water intake
Salt-poor parenteral fluids
Drug-induced inappropriate secretion of antidiuretic hormone:
    Vasopressin
    Oxytocin
    Chlorpropamide (Diabinese)
    Vincristine (Oncovin)
    Cyclophosphamide (Cytoxan)
    Thiazide diuretics
Corticosteroid withdrawal (adrenal crisis)
Enemas
Hypertonic mannitol

Inappropriate secretion of antidiuretic hormone induced by drugs is characterized by hyponatremia, hypotonicity of serum, and urine hyperosmolarity without edema. Chlorpropamide (Diabinese), thiazide diuretics, vincristine (Oncovin), and cyclophosphamide (Cytoxan) have produced this syndrome.[15]

Stress during corticosteroid therapy, or rapid withdrawal of corticosteroid treatment, can lead to acute adrenal insufficiency with hyponatremia as one of its manifestations.

Repeated enemas can cause colonic sodium loss and water absorption leading to hyponatremia.

Hypertonic mannitol, given intravenously during the early phase of acute renal failure, may not be excreted by the kidneys. Hyperosmolality with resultant hyponatremia may occur from vascular overfill.[9]

Drugs, drug-induced syndromes, and fluids that may cause hyponatremia are indicated in Table 4-44.

Drug-Induced Hyperkalemia

Oral or intravenous administration of potassium chloride can lead to hyperkalemia from excessive dosage or impaired renal function. The potassium salt of penicillin, which is the form used for intravenous treatment, contains 1.5 mEq of potassium per million units. Increased serum potassium levels can occur if renal function is compromised.[363] Any form of drug-induced renal insufficiency also can be accompanied by hyperkalemia.

Spironolactone (Aldactone) and triamterene (Dyrenium) are weak diuretics that inhibit sodium reabsorption and potassium secretion in the distal tubule. Used by themselves, or with a thiazide diuretic, they can lead to hyperkalemia which can be fatal.[64,201]

TABLE 4-45. Drugs and Drug-Induced Conditions Known to Cause Hyperkalemia

Potassium salts
Drug-induced renal insufficiency
Spironolactone (Aldactone)
Triamterene (Dyrenium)
Corticosteroid withdrawal (adrenal crisis)
Antineoplastic drugs (tumor lysis)

Elevated serum potassium levels occur in adrenal insufficiency, secondary to rapid corticosteroid withdrawal or to stress during corticosteroid therapy. Acute drug-induced hemolysis, as occurs in glucose-6-phosphate dehydrogenase deficiency, releases potassium from injured erythrocytes, with resultant hyperkalemia. Similarly, hyperkalemia has followed sudden lysis of a large volume of tumor cells in a patient receiving chemotherapy for Burkitt's lymphoma.[8]

Drugs and drug-induced conditions known to cause hyperkalemia are listed in Table 4-45.

Drug-Induced Hypokalemia

One of the more common causes of hypokalemia is diuretic therapy with the thiazide diuretics, or with the more potent compounds, ethacrynic acid and furosemide. Potassium loss is one of the most predictable results of effective diuresis. Potassium supplements are required to avoid the hazards of hypokalemia (metabolic alkalosis, weakness, depressed reflexes, nephropathy, ileus, and bladder atony), as well as of the enhanced potential that is created for digitalis intoxication.[103]

Drug-induced vomiting generally is not severe enough to lead to significant potassium depletion. Chronic laxative abuse resulting in watery stools has been reported to lead to secondary hyperaldosteronism; this is presumably caused by fecal sodium loss leading to activation of the renin-aldosterone axis. Marked hypokalemia has resulted from both hyperaldosteronism and diarrhea.[123]

Corticosteroids cause renal loss of potassium. Hypokalemia is especially likely to occur with the use of steroid preparations that have mineralocorticoid effects, such as desoxycorticosterone (Percorten) and fluorocortisone (Florinef).

Hypokalemia produced by renal potassium loss occurs in renal tubular acidosis that is induced by amphotericin B and outdated tetracyclines.[99,125] Renal potassium losses have induced hypokalemia in patients treated with sodium sulfate for hypercalcemia.[328]

TABLE 4-46. Causative Drugs and Predisposing Factors of Hypokalemia

Diuretics	Renal tubular acidosis:
Potassium-free fluids	Amphotericin B
Drug-induced vomiting	Outdated tetracyclines
Drug-induced diarrhea	Sodium sulfate infusions
Laxative abuse	Metabolic alkalosis (from absorbable alkali)
Enemas	Insulin
Corticosteroids	Glucose (intravenously)

Prolonged treatment with potassium-free intravenous fluids can lead to hypokalemia as a result of daily obligate renal potassium losses. Metabolic alkalosis, whether caused by potassium deficits or by ingestion of absorbable alkali (e.g., sodium bicarbonate), leads to enhanced renal potassium losses, and thus to a vicious cycle of potassium wasting.

In patients with borderline potassium deficiency, insulin or large amounts of intravenously administered glucose can lead to hypokalemia, caused by a shift of potassium from extracellular to intracellular fluid as glucose enters the cells.

Drugs which have been implicated in causing hypokalemia, and other predisposing factors of hypokalemia, are listed in Table 4-46.

ACID-BASE CHANGES

Drug-Induced Metabolic Alkalosis

Hypokalemia, regardless of its cause, leads to metabolic alkalosis. As the serum potassium level falls, intracellular potassium enters the extracellular fluid and is replaced in the cell by sodium and hydrogen ions, producing a relatively alkaline extracellular fluid. Chloride loss alone, but usually in association with diuretic-induced potassium loss, causes alkalosis. The electrolyte values in typical hypokalemic-hypochloremic alkalosis show low serum potassium and serum chloride levels and an elevated serum bicarbonate level. These abnormalities are corrected by the administration of potassium chloride.

The diuretics ethacrynic acid and furosemide lead to a loss of hydrogen ions and of potassium and chloride ions in the urine, thereby enhancing alkalosis.[216]

The ingestion of large amounts of absorbable alkali, notably bicarbonate and ions that are converted to bicarbonate (e.g., lactate and citrate), can lead to metabolic alkalosis with tetany. If this condition occurs concomitantly with dyspepsia, and large amounts of milk are ingested, the milk-alkali syndrome may result.

TABLE 4-47. Predisposing Factors of Metabolic Alkalosis

Drug-induced hypokalemia
Diuretic-induced hypochloremia
Absorbable alkali
Drug-induced vomiting

At times severe drug-induced vomiting, may lead to enough hydrogen and chloride ion loss from the stomach to produce alkalosis.

Predisposing factors of metabolic alkalosis are indicated in Table 4-47.

Drug-Induced Metabolic Acidosis

Chronic paraldehyde ingestion has led to severe metabolic acidosis from the accumulation of acetaldehyde, a paraldehyde metabolite.[158] Dialysis is necessary to correct acidosis.[156]

Lactic acidosis may result from phenformin (D.B.I., Meltrol) treatment of diabetes mellitus. Acidosis is severe, and the mortality rate is high because of the frequency of associated underlying disease. The mechanism of lactic acid production is poorly understood. Treatment consists of large doses of sodium bicarbonate and necessary supportive measures.[182]

Amphotericin B[99] and outdated tetracyclines[125] can cause renal tubular acidosis. A decrease in renal tubular acid secretion leads to an alkaline urine and metabolic acidosis.

The ingestion of ammonium chloride, which was used to enhance the effect of mercurial diuretics, has led to hyperchloremic acidosis. Acetazolamide (Diamox), presently used as an adjunct in the treatment of glaucoma rather than as a diuretic, can produce metabolic acidosis by increasing urinary bicarbonate loss. Typically, there is a depressed serum bicarbonate level and an elevated serum chloride level.

Causative drugs and predisposing factors of metabolic acidosis are included in Table 4-48.

TABLE 4-48. Causative Drugs and Predisposing Factors of Metabolic Acidosis

Paraldehyde
Lactic acidosis (resulting from phenformin)
Renal tubular acidosis:
  Amphotericin B
  Outdated tetracyclines
Ammonium chloride
Acetazolamide (Diamox)

FLUID BALANCE

Drug-Induced Hypovolemia

Loss of appreciable amounts of body fluid can occur with drug-induced vomiting or diarrhea. In the former, there may be loss of enough potassium or hydrogen ions to produce concomitant metabolic alkalosis. Diarrhea also may lead to potassium loss.

Acute fluid volume depletion is a common result of a brisk response to diuretic treatment. Even with hypovolemia, some residual edema may persist. Contraction of the blood volume leads to an increase in hematocrit value and a decreased renal perfusion, with resultant azotemia and a decrease in urine volume. Liberalized intake of salt and water corrects this disorder.[103]

Drug-Induced Fluid Retention and Edema

Retention of sodium, with consequent weight gain and edema, follows saline infusions, notably in patients with decreased renal function. Drugs may cause sodium retention and edema. This is a frequent effect of therapy with corticosteroids, especially mineralocorticoids, and with oral contraceptives. Rauwolfia alkaloids, phenylbutazone (Butazolidin), oxyphenbutazone (Tandearil), methyldopa (Aldomet), and diazoxide may produce edema. Diazoxide, a thiazide derivative with hypotensive effects when given parenterally, regularly causes salt and water retention with resultant edema.[356]

CHANGES IN SERUM CALCIUM LEVELS

Drug-Induced Hypercalcemia

The ingestion of large amounts of calcium in the form of milk and of absorbable alkali (principally sodium bicarbonate), usually for self-medication of a peptic ulcer, can lead to the milk-alkali syndrome,

TABLE 4–49.
Drugs and Drug-Induced Syndromes Known to Cause Hypercalcemia

Milk-alkali syndrome
Vitamin D
Thiazide diuretics

CLINICAL MANIFESTATIONS

TABLE 4-50. Drugs and Drug-Induced Conditions Known to Cause Hypocalcemia

Phosphate infusion
Sodium sulfate infusion
Mithramycin (Mithracin)
Drug-induced malabsorption
Drug-induced renal insufficiency

characterized by hypercalcemia and mild alkalosis. Renal function is often impaired, with associated azotemia, nephrocalcinosis, impaired concentrating ability, and polyuria and polydipsia. When milk and alkali are discontinued the hypercalcemia is reversed and renal function is improved.[239]

The use of vitamin D in large doses as ill-advised therapy for rheumatoid arthritis and osteoporosis, as a dietary supplement by food faddists, and in the treatment of hypoparathyroidism, usually leads to hypercalcemia with weakness, lethargy, nausea, and vomiting. Since vitamin D is stored in the body, calcium levels may remain elevated for prolonged periods after the drug is discontinued.[76]

Thiazide diuretics reduce urinary calcium excretion and can aggravate hypercalcemia in patients with actual or potential hypercalcemia.[273]

Drugs and drug-induced syndromes known to cause hypercalcemia are found in Table 4-49.

Drug-Induced Hypocalcemia

Hypocalcemia may occur during the treatment of hypercalcemia with intravenously administered phosphates or sodium sulfate. Phosphate treatment has caused prolonged hypocalcemia with hypotension.[320] The antineoplastic drug mithramycin (Mithracin) produces dose-related hypocalcemia.[194]

Serum calcium levels can be depressed secondary to malabsorption of vitamin D in drug-induced biliary cirrhosis. Hypocalcemia occurs as part of the uremic syndrome in severe drug-induced renal damage.

Drugs and drug-induced conditions known to cause hypocalcemia appear in Table 4-50.

OTHER METABOLIC DISORDERS

Gout and Changes in Serum Uric Acid Levels

Drug-induced hyperuricemia can precipitate gouty attacks in susceptible individuals. The thiazide diuretics, chlorthalidone

(Hygroton), ethacrynic acid, and furosemide decrease renal urate clearance and lead to hyperuricemia.[103,216]

Pyrazinamide therapy in tuberculosis regularly causes a rise in serum uric acid levels and a fall in urinary uric acid levels within two days of the onset of therapy. Resultant gouty attacks and tophus formation have occurred. Within two days after discontinuing the drug, there is increased uric acid output in the urine and serum uric acid levels return to pretreatment levels.[310]

Small doses of aspirin result in uric acid retention, while large doses are uricosuric. The combination of salicylates and phenylbutazone leads to urate retention. Also, the uricosuric action of probenecid (Benemid) is antagonized by salicylates.[86]

Initiating treatment with probenecid (Benemid) or allopurinol (Zyloprim) in gouty patients can lead to gouty attacks without an elevation of the serum uric acid level. This can be prevented by maintenance therapy with colchicine before these drugs are begun.

Treatment of lymphomas and acute leukemias with chemotherapy can cause acute hyperuricemia from the release of intracellular purines, which are metabolized to uric acid. In such cases uric acid nephropathy is the major danger, but gout may also be precipitated. However, hyperuricemia can be mitigated by pretreatment with allopurinol (Zyloprim), which inhibits the conversion of hypoxanthine and xanthine to uric acid.[354]

Drug-induced renal failure with uremia results in concomitant hyperuricemia that usually does not lead to gout.

Serum uric acid levels can be depressed by uricosuric drugs (e.g., probenecid) and by allopurinol. Drug-induced renal tubular acidosis leads to an increased uric acid clearance and to hypouricemia.[45]

Drugs and drug-induced conditions know to cause hyperuricemia are listed in Table 4–51.

Changes in Serum Cholesterol and Serum Lipid Levels

Oral contraceptives can increase plasma triglyceride levels.[164] Although hyperlipemia is usually not severe, a few patients with

TABLE 4–51. Drugs and Drug-Induced Conditions Known to Cause Hyperuricemia

Thiazide diuretics
Chlorthalidone (Hygroton)
Ethacrynic acid (Edecrin)
Furosemide (Lasix)
Pyrazinamide
Aspirin (small dose)
Chemotherapy for leukemia and lymphomas (cell lysis)
Drug-induced renal failure

massive hyperlipemia have been reported, some of whom developed acute pancreatitis.[88] Whether chronic hypertriglyceridemia caused by oral contraceptives will predispose the patient to atherosclerosis is not known.

Hypercholesterolemia may occur in drug-induced obstructive jaundice, biliary cirrhosis, hypothyroidism, and the nephrotic syndrome; and in diabetes mellitus that is poorly controlled because of hyperglycemia produced by drugs.

Drug-Induced Hemochromatosis

Fatal hemochromatosis, with bronzed skin, diabetes, hepatomegaly, and congestive heart failure, resulted from oral iron therapy of ten-years duration. It was estimated that during this period of time 1,000 gm of elemental iron were ingested.[180]

Drug-Induced Porphyria

Attacks of the various types of porphyria may be precipitated by drugs. Episodes of acute intermittent porphyria, an inherited disease transmitted by a dominant gene, are characterized by pain (usually abdominal), vomiting, constipation, peripheral neuropathy, psychic disturbances, fever, tachycardia, and transient hypertension, without photosensitivity. Drugs are an important factor in precipitating

TABLE 4–52. Drugs Known to Precipitate Attacks of Porphyria

Acute intermittent porphyria:
  Barbiturates
  Aminopyrine
  Chlordiazepoxide (Librium)
  Meprobamate
  Griseofulvin
  Sulfonamides
  Diphenylhydantoin (Dilantin)
  Sulfonmethane
  Chlorpropamide (Diabinese)
  Tolbutamide (Orinase)
  Androgens
  Estrogens
  Oral contraceptives
Porphyria cutanea tarda symptomatica:
  Barbiturates
  Chloroquine
  Tolbutamide (Orinase)
  Chlorpropamide (Diabinese)
  Androgens
  Estrogens
  Oral contraceptives
  Alcohol

attacks. Barbiturates are the most frequently implicated group of drugs, especially phenobarbital and thiopental (Pentothal). Other causative drugs include aminopyrine, chlordiazepoxide (Librium), meprobamate, griseofulvin, sulfonamides, diphenylhydantoin (Dilantin), sulfonmethane, chlorpropamide (Diabinese), tolbutamide (Orinase), androgens, estrogens, and oral contraceptives.[86,122] An attack may occur after a single dose of these drugs, but an attack may not necessarily be precipitated each time one of these drugs is taken.

Porphyria cutanea tarda symptomatica, which is associated with photosensitivity and superficial erosions, vesicles, and hyperpigmentation in light-exposed areas, can be exacerbated by barbiturates, chloroquine, tolbutamide, chlorpropamide, androgens, estrogens, oral contraceptives, and excessive alcohol intake.[86] South African mixed porphyria and hereditary coproporphyria, decidedly rare forms, may also be precipitated by barbiturates.[86]

Drugs known to precipitate attacks of porphyria are found in Table 4-52.

12. MUSCULOSKELETAL MANIFESTATIONS

The muscles, bones, and joints are not frequent sites of adverse drug reactions. Relatively few drugs are involved and they produce a small number of reactions, but the effects are notable because of the serious degree of incapacity that often occurs.

Drug-Induced Muscle Weakness

A modest degree of muscle weakness is common in patients who are treated with corticosteroids, but severe myopathy is an infrequent effect. Muscle weakness and atrophy occur symmetrically, with the pelvic and shoulder girdles most markedly affected. There is no muscle pain. Deep tendon reflexes are diminished as a result of muscle weakness rather than of neurologic involvement. Severity of the effect is not related to the duration of therapy. Myopathy can occur with any corticosteroid, but is encountered most frequently with fluorinated compounds such as dexamethasone (Decadron) and triamcinolone (Aristocort, Kenacort). Concomitant corticosteroid-induced hypokalemia can aggravate muscle weakness. Substitution of another glucocorticoid may result in improvement. After corticosteroid treatment is discontinued, complete recovery may not occur for several months.[86]

Drug-induced hypokalemia (see the section on metabolic manifestations) can cause severe myopathy with diffuse, severe weakness that responds rapidly to potassium replacement therapy. Muscle cramps, mostly in the calves, may accompany hypokalemia.

Prolonged chloroquine (Aralen) therapy infrequently induces a neuromyopathy, which principally affects the proximal limb muscles. Although there is evidence of neurologic involvement, sensory changes are absent.[86]

Emetine treatment of hepatic amebic abscesses may lead to cardiomyopathy and less often to skeletal muscle involvement with weakness.[86] Chronic colchicine toxicity has caused myopathy with weakness that slowly improved with decreased drug dosage.[206]

Drugs and drug-related conditions known to cause myopathy are presented in Table 4-53.

TABLE 4-53. Drugs and Drug-Induced Conditions Known to Cause Myopathy

Corticosteroids
Diuretic-induced hypokalemia
Chloroquine (Aralen)
Emetine
Colchicine

TABLE 4–54. *Drugs Known to Cause Myalgias*

Clofibrate (Atromid-S)
Thiabendazole (Mintezol)
Methysergide (Sansert)
Vitamin A intoxication

A small number of drugs infrequently may cause muscle syndromes which are characterized by myalgias (Table 4–54). Clofibrate (Atromid-S) can cause severe myalgias, muscle stiffness, and weakness. Levels of serum transaminase and of creatine phosphokinase are elevated in these patients and in some without muscular symptoms, suggesting subclinical myopathy. Discontinuing the drug produces prompt relief.[214] Thiabendazole (Mintezol) treatment of strongyloidiasis has led to muscle aches during exercise, some muscle tenderness, but no weakness. Serum aldolase levels were found to be elevated before and after exercise, but transaminase and creatine phosphokinase levels were normal.[83] Muscle pains and cramps have occurred with methysergide (Sansert) treatment of migraine.[172] Vitamin A intoxication may be associated with muscle stiffness which is exacerbated by exercise.[259]

Drug-Induced Bone Disorders

Tetracyclines are deposited in the skeleton of the human fetus, and can cause retarded bone growth. Measurement of fibulas in premature infants treated with these drugs has shown a 40 per cent depression of bone growth. This effect is reversible if time of drug exposure has been short.[363]

The use of prolonged corticosteroid therapy in children leads to retarded bone growth. When the drug dose is decreased or the drug is discontinued, a compensatory growth spurt may occur.[232]

Osteoporosis is a common effect of long-term corticosteroid treatment, and can be severe enough to cause vertebral compression fractures and pathologic fractures of long bones.[86] Large doses of heparin for six months or longer can also lead to osteoporosis, with resultant spontaneous vertebral and rib fractures.[154]

Drug-Induced Joint Disorders

Chronic corticosteroid therapy can result in aseptic necrosis of the femoral head which may be bilateral. Less often, aseptic necrosis of the humeral head may occur. These disorders produce pain, and decreased motion of the involved joint.[85] Intra-articular injection of

TABLE 4-55.
Drugs Known to Cause a Rheumatic Syndrome

Isoniazid
Pyrazinamide
Ethionamide

---

corticosteroids has led to septic arthritis by introducing microorganisms or by reactivating a smouldering infection.[147]

Three antituberculous drugs—isoniazid, pyrazinamide, and ethionamide—can produce a rheumatic syndrome (see Table 4–55). Isoniazid, most often in the fourth week of therapy, can lead to the sudden onset of joint pain, tenderness, and stiffness affecting the hands, especially the proximal interphalangeal joints, shoulders, elbows, wrists, knees, hips, and spine. Stiffness upon awakening from sleep may be striking. Swelling may appear, but joint effusions are unusual. Pain and contractures of the shoulders and hands are frequent sequelae.[144]

Pyrazinamide can cause joint pain in up to one-fifth of patients treated with the drug. The shoulders, elbows, and knees are most often affected. Joint pain may be severe enough to require stopping the therapy. Joint pains may appear in almost one-half of patients treated with both pyrazinamide and isoniazid.[310] Ethionamide has also produced joint pains.[144]

Arthralgias and arthritis also occur in drug-induced systemic lupus erythematosus, serum sickness, and other immunologically mediated drug reactions. Drugs that cause elevations of the serum uric acid level can precipitate attacks of gout (see section on metabolic manifestations).

13. NEUROLOGIC MANIFESTATIONS

Sedation is one of the most common drug-induced neurologic disorders. Other nonlocalizing neurologic symptoms, such as central excitation and coma, are encountered less often. Localizing signs can be produced by a direct drug effect on nervous tissue, or by an effect on the vascular supply to the central nervous system. Reactions will be divided into those that affect the peripheral nerves, the myoneural junction, and the brain and spinal cord. Drug-induced syndromes that predominantly produce mental changes will be discussed in the section on emotional disorders.

DRUG REACTIONS AFFECTING THE PERIPHERAL NERVES

Peripheral Neuropathies

Digitalis intoxication is a rare cause of toxic neuritis, with facial pain resembling that of trigeminal neuralgia.[297] Lesions of the optic nerve and of the eighth nerve will be considered in the sections on the eye and the ear, respectively.

Peripheral neuropathy is characterized by numbness, paresthesias, weakness, and distal (stocking and glove) loss of sensation. Many structurally related drugs can damage peripheral nerves. Heavy metals such as arsenic, especially as used in Fowler's solution, mercury, previously used in antisyphilitic therapy, gold salts, employed in treating rheumatoid arthritis, and lead, found in illegally distilled whiskey, can produce peripheral nerve damage.

The antituberculous drugs isoniazid and ethionamide, and the antihypertensive drug hydralazine (Apresoline), can cause peripheral neuritis that may be either prevented by or responds to pyridoxine therapy. Isoniazid polyneuritis is dose-related. The drug is inactivated in the liver by acetylation. About 60 per cent of all people have a genetically determined lack of hepatic acetylating enzymes which results in slow inactivation of isoniazid. Polyneuritis occurs more often in these slow inactivators.[363] Ethionamide also occasionally produces peripheral neuritis.[286] Hydralazine is structurally similar to isoniazid, and paresthesias occur in about 15 per cent of patients receiving this drug after low-dose, prolonged therapy (50 mg for seven days). Remission of symptoms follows pyridoxine treatment.[289]

Nitrofurantoin (Furadantin), furaltadone (Altafur), and nitrofurazone (Furacin) have caused peripheral neuropathy. Neurotoxicity resulting from these drugs is dose-related and is enhanced by decreased renal function.[249,304]

Certain antibiotics, notably colistin (Coly-Mycin), polymyxin B,

TABLE 4-56. Drugs Known to Cause Peripheral Neuropathy

Digitalis (trigeminal neuropathy)	Antibiotics:
Heavy metals:	Kanamycin (Kantrex)
Arsenic	Streptomycin
Mercury	Polymyxin B
Gold	Colistin (Coly-Mycin)
Lead	Vancomycin (Vancocin)
Pyridoxine responsive:	Chloramphenicol
Isoniazid	Antidepressants:
Ethionamide	Imipramine (Tofranil)
Hydralazine (Apresoline)	Amitriptyline (Elavil)
Nitrofurans:	Vinca alkaloids:
Nitrofurantoin (Furadantin)	Vincristine (Oncovin)
Nitrofurazone (Furacin)	Vinblastine (Velban)
Furaltadone (Altafur)	Other drugs:
	Chloroquine (Aralen)
	Emetine
	Thalidomide

and kanamycin, frequently produce variable degrees of peripheral nerve damage. Perioral paresthesias occur often. Neuropathy is enhanced by the presence of concomitant renal insufficiency.[86]

Imipramine (Tofranil) can produce a motor neuropathy with absent deep-tendon reflexes in the legs. Peroneal nerve palsy, with little recovery after cessation of drug therapy, has been reported.[86] Amitriptyline (Elavil) can cause polyneuritis.[86]

Vincristine (Oncovin) and vinblastine (Velban) therapy often produce paresthesias.

Long-term therapy with chloroquine (Aralen) infrequently causes neuromyopathy, which is manifested by proximal muscle weakness of the legs and later the arms. Weakness may progress to involve the trunk, neck, and face. Deep-tendon reflexes are depressed or absent, without sensory changes. Gradual improvement usually follows after the drug is discontinued.[86]

Emetine can cause muscle weakness and peripheral neuritis.[86] Thalidomide has produced neuropathy after six months or more of use.[86]

Drugs known to cause peripheral neuropathy appear in Table 4-56.

DRUG REACTIONS AFFECTING THE MYONEURAL JUNCTION

Myasthenia Gravis

Myasthenia gravis is a functional abnormality of synaptic transmission across the myoneural junction, characterized by weakness and easy fatigability. Weakness is most pronounced in the facial, oculomotor, pharyngeal, laryngeal, and respiratory muscles. Great danger arises from respiratory muscle weakness and consequent hypoventilation and apnea. When used to treat this condition, the anticholinesterase drugs neostigmine (Prostigmin) and pyridostigmine (Mestinon) improve strength. However, increasing doses of these drugs in an effort to produce optimal strength can lead to progressive weakness. More drug may erroneously be given, culminating in profound weakness termed a cholinergic crisis. Treatment consists of decreasing drug dosage.

Myasthenic weakness is aggravated by d-tubocurarine, quaternary ammonium compounds, quinine, quinidine, procainamide, chlorpromazine (Thorazine), aminoglycoside antibiotics (streptomycin, neomycin, kanamycin [Kantrex], viomycin), tetracyclines, polymyxin B, and colistin (Coly-Mycin).[228]

Colistin, at therapeutic blood levels, has led to reversible neuromuscular blockade that mimicked myasthenia gravis in a previously normal patient. Treatment with edrophonium produced increased strength.[139] Trimethadione (Tridione) has caused a similar edrophonium-responsive myasthenic syndrome after eight months of treatment with 1200 mg of the drug daily. Symptoms completely abated 4½ months after the drug was discontinued.[279]

Drugs that aggravate myasthenia gravis are found in Table 4–57. Neuromuscular blockade and respiratory paralysis caused by other drugs are discussed in the section on respiratory manifestations.

Extrapyramidal Syndromes

Extrapyramidal syndromes are frequent complications caused by drugs used to treat psychoses. These disorders indicate functional derangements of the basal ganglia. Extrapyramidal signs occur

TABLE 4–57. Drugs that Aggravate Myasthenia Gravis

Anticholinesterase drugs, excessive dose
d-Tubocurarine
Quaternary ammonium compounds
Quinine
Quinidine
Procainamide
Chlorpromazine (Thorazine)
Antibiotics:
  Streptomycin
  Neomycin
  Kanamycin (Kantrex)
  Viomycin
  Tetracyclines
  Polymyxin B
  Colistin (Coly-Mycin)

in about 40 per cent of patients treated with phenothiazines. These reactions have been attributed to almost all members of this group of drugs and are not dose-related. Haloperidol (Haldol), a non-phenothiazine drug used in the treatment of psychoses, produces extrapyramidal signs in up to 90 per cent of patients. The thioxanthenes—thiothixene (Navane) and chlorprothixene (Taractan)—another group of major tranquilizers, also cause extrapyramidal signs. Rauwolfia derivatives, no longer used as antipsychotic drugs, can produce dose-related extrapyramidal syndromes.[100]

ACUTE DYSTONIC REACTIONS. Acute dystonic reactions begin abruptly a day or two after the drug is started. There are bizarre muscle spasms, usually of the head and neck, but also of the arms, legs, and back. These may take the form of torticollis, retrocollis, facial distortions, dysarthria caused by involuntary movements of the tongue, scoliosis, lordosis, opisthotonus, and dystonic gait. In the oculogyric crisis that often accompanies this reaction, a momentary fixed stare occurs followed by upward or lateral rotation of the eyes. The patient, with his mouth open, tilts his head in order to see. This syndrome is more common with children under the age of 15 and in males. There is variable individual susceptibility.[86,100] Prochlorperazine (Compazine) often causes this syndrome, particularly in patients with hypoparathyroidism who are probably sensitized by hypocalcemia.[309] Prochlorperazine has also produced marked trismus and meningism without other extrapyramidal signs.[146] Antihistamines administered parenterally, barbiturates, and antiparkinsonian drugs bring dramatic relief.[100]

AKATHISIA. In akathisia, or motor restlessness, also produced by phenothiazines, there is an inability to sit or stand still. Patients walk or pace, tap their foot or shift their legs when sitting, rock back and forth or from side to side when standing, twist their fingers, roll their tongues, or perform chewing motions. Symptoms are alleviated by decreasing the drug dose or using antiparkinsonian drugs.[86,100]

PARKINSONISM. Parkinsonism occurs after varying intervals of drug therapy with phenothiazines or thioxanthenes, and may be dose-related or show individual susceptibility. There is typical rigidity, impaired motor activity, tremor, and cogwheeling. The syndrome is relieved by decreasing the dose or discontinuing the drug, or by treatment with antiparkinsonian drugs.

TARDIVE DYSKINESIA. Tardive dyskinesia, which may be irreversible, usually occurs after several years of phenothiazine therapy. Symptoms may also begin after several weeks or months of treatment, or shortly after cessation of drug therapy. The incidence of this condition is greater in the elderly, probably because of the existence of a more chronic condition requiring more prolonged drug therapy. Tardive dyskinesia is characterized by stereotyped, repetitive, involuntary movements of the mouth, lips, and tongue (sucking and smacking the lips, jaw movements, puffing the cheeks, thrusting the tongue), athetoid and choreiform movements, and axial hyperkinesis (to-and-fro movement of the spine). All involuntary movements disappear during sleep. Antiparkinsonian drugs are either not helpful or exaggerate symptoms. Reducing the dose or discontinuing the causative drug may relieve symptoms, but phenothiazines may have to be reinstituted because of worsening psychosis.[100] Since many of the symptoms of tardive dyskinesia are similar to those of catatonic schizophrenia, the drug reaction may be difficult to differentiate from the underlying disease.

Treatment of parkinsonism with levodopa (Dopar, Larodopa) can cause various involuntary movements: myoclonus, grimacing, jaw movements, intermittent choreiform movements of the legs, intermittent wavelike motion of the head, hemiballismus, rhythmic movements, and screams.[75] The effect of start-hesitation, produced by long-term levodopa therapy, consists of sudden episodes in which there is a sensation of extreme heaviness in both feet and an inability to walk; patients frequently fall and injure themselves. Once patients commence to walk, however, their gait is normal.[7] Decreasing the dose of levodopa ameliorates these symptoms.

DRUG REACTIONS AFFECTING THE CENTRAL NERVOUS SYSTEM

Central Nervous System Excitation

Central nervous system excitation can present as either restlessness, irritability, insomnia, aggressive behavior, or hallucinations. Marked excitation is manifested as delirium. Anticholinergic drugs such as atropine and scopolamine can produce these symptoms in association with other anticholinergic signs, such as flushed face, lack of sweating, and fever. Children can absorb enough atropine or homatropine from cycloplegic eye drops to produce this syndrome.[171]

Amphetamines can produce marked restlessness in some individuals. Sedatives, especially barbiturates, occasionally lead to paradoxical agitation and excitement in the very young or the elderly. Bromide intoxication can cause hyperactivity. Digitalis intoxication in elderly patients with arteriosclerosis and in patients with aortic valve lesions can produce delirium.[174]

Monamine oxidase inhibitors, in combination with certain drugs, often lead to central excitation. If sympathomimetic amines are administered concomitantly with these drugs, a hypertensive crisis associated with marked agitation ensues. When monamine oxidase inhibitors are combined with the tricyclic antidepressants imipramine (Tofranil) or amitriptyline (Elavil), delirium and seizures can occur.

CLINICAL MANIFESTATIONS

Monamine oxidase inhibitors and cocaine cause excitation. Narcotic analgesics given to patients receiving monamine oxidase inhibitors lead to a prolonged narcotic effect, but with associated excitation.[86]

Seizures

Certain drugs lower the seizure threshold and can produce convulsions in epileptic or normal individuals (see Table 4–58). These include analeptics (e.g., amphetamines), phenothiazines, rauwolfia alkaloids, chlorprothixene (Taractan), imipramine (Tofranil), amitriptyline (Elavil), and antihistamines.

Isoniazid, polymyxin B, and colistin (Coly-Mycin), all of which produce peripheral neuropathy, can also induce seizures, especially if there are high blood levels of these drugs, usually caused by impaired renal function.[61,86]

Penicillin, when administered in massive intravenous doses (20 to 80 million units daily), can cause convulsions. The presence of underlying brain disease and excessively high cerebrospinal fluid levels of penicillin caused by impaired renal function are important contributing factors.[363] In patients undergoing cardiopulmonary bypass for open heart surgery, penicillin given intravenously in doses of 50 million units a day can induce generalized convulsions. Experiments in dogs have shown that cardiopulmonary bypass makes the blood-brain barrier unduly permeable to penicillin, and results in the high cerebrospinal fluid concentrations of the drug necessary to precipitate seizures.[317]

TABLE 4–58. Drugs Known to Cause Seizures

Amphetamines
Phenothiazines
Rauwolfia alkaloids
Chlorprothixene (Taractan)
Imipramine (Tofranil)
Amitriptyline (Elavil)
Antihistamines
Isoniazid
Polymyxin B
Colistin (Coly-Mycin)
Penicillin (massive IV doses)
Lidocaine (Xylocaine)
Anticholinergics
Probenecid (Benemid)
Barbiturate withdrawal
Ethchlorvynol (Placidyl) withdrawal
Glutethimide (Doriden) withdrawal
Monamine oxidase inhibitors combined with either imipramine (Tofranil) or amitriptyline (Elavil)
Phenothiazines combined with piperazine (Antepar)

Lidocaine (Xylocaine), when given intravenously in excessive doses to combat cardiac arrhythmias, can cause focal or generalized convulsions.[135] Intoxication caused by anticholinergic drugs[171] and by probenecid (Benemid)[294] produces convulsions on rare occasions.

Abrupt withdrawal of treatment with barbiturates, ethchlorvynol (Placidyl), and glutethimide (Doriden) may produce anxiety, muscle twitches, tremor, and seizures which may be misdiagnosed as epilepsy.[130]

The combination of imipramine (Tofranil) or amitriptyline (Elavil) with a monamine oxidase inhibitor is apt to cause central excitation, delirium, and seizures. The concomitant use of a phenothiazine and piperazine (Antepar) used to treat pinworms in a child has led to seizures. Experiments in goats and dogs have supported the observation that this latter combination of drugs is epileptogenic.[37]

Drug-induced hyponatremia and hypoglycemia are conditions under which seizures can occur.

Central Nervous System Depression and Coma

Central nervous system depression ranging from lethargy and sleepiness to coma can be caused by many drugs, especially when they are taken in overdoses in suicide attempts. Drowsiness is produced by certain drugs as a frequent side effect, notably with sedatives, tranquilizers, antihistamines, methyldopa (Aldomet), and tricyclic antidepressants, such as amitriptyline (Elavil).

Enhanced central nervous system depression follows the use of certain drugs in combination. Alcohol potentiates the depressant effects of barbiturates. Phenothiazines, when combined with rauwolfia alkaloids, barbiturates, bromides, narcotic analgesics, or alcohol, result in increased central depression. The hypnotic effects of barbiturates and chloral hydrate are enhanced by monamine oxidase inhibitors. Patients being given monamine oxidase inhibitors will experience a prolonged and deep anesthetic effect from general anesthesia.[86]

Mepivacaine (Carbocaine), a local anesthetic used for paracervical block, and caudal and lumbar epidural obstetrical anesthesia, can lead to fetal intoxication with resultant bradycardia, cyanosis, apnea, limpness, unresponsiveness, coma, seizures, and death. Intoxication occurs either from maternal absorption of the anesthetic which then passes across the placenta into the fetal circulation and is poorly detoxified in the newborn, or from accidental direct injection into the fetus. The latter route of administration has been corroborated by observation of puncture marks in the scalp of the newborn. Treatment consists of general supportive measures and exchange transfusions.[121,296,330]

Coma, unaccompanied by localizing neurological signs, should always be considered as possibly drug-induced. Large doses of various drugs that can cause coma often are ingested in suicide attempts. Hypnotics, sedatives, and psychoactive drugs are often implicated. Salicylate poisoning can lead to coma, especially in children, usually with Kussmaul's respiration. Overdoses of morphine, heroin, and other narcotics cause coma accompanied by pinpoint pupils and depressed respiration. Narcotic antagonists such as nalorphine (Nalline) or naloxone (Narcan) produce prompt reversal of these narcotic depressant effects. Narcotic analgesics used in patients who are receiving monamine oxidase inhibitors can lead to potentiation of narcotic central depression. Narcotic effects are also enhanced in patients with hypothyroidism, severe liver disease, and adrenocortical insufficiency.

Hypoglycemic coma can result from excess doses of insulin or of oral hypoglycemic drugs. Coma may be accompanied by seizures. Rare instances of hypothermic myxedema coma in hypothyroid patients have been precipitated by chlorpromazine (Thorazine) and imipramine (Tofranil).[238] Acute alcohol intoxication probably remains the most common cause of hospital admission for coma.

Stroke and Intracerebral Bleeding

Women taking oral contraceptives have a risk of cerebral ischemia or thrombosis that is nine times greater than those not using oral contraceptives.[69] Carotid artery thrombosis, middle cerebral artery occlusion, thalamic infarction, and superior sagittal sinus thrombosis have been attributed to the use of oral contraceptives.[322]

Fatal intracerebral hemorrhage has resulted from the hypertensive crisis that occurs when patients receiving monamine oxidase inhibitors are treated at the same time with other monamine oxidase inhibitors, tricyclic antidepressants, sympathomimetic amines, or foods rich in tyramine[86] (see the section on cardiovascular manifestations).

Anticoagulant therapy can lead to intracerebral and subarachnoid hemorrhage, notably in hypertensive patients.[305] Moreover, in patients receiving anticoagulants, trivial head trauma has resulted in subdural hematomas.

Increased Intracranial Pressure

Benign increased intracranial pressure (pseudotumor cerebri) is occasionally drug-induced (see Table 4–59). Most affected persons are children or young women who appear well but complain of headache and are found to have papilledema. The cerebrospinal fluid pressure is elevated without increased numbers of cells or elevated protein

TABLE 4-59. *Drugs Known to Cause Benign Increased Intracranial Pressure (Pseudotumor Cerebri).*

Hypervitaminosis A
Corticosteroids
Oral contraceptives
Tetracyclines
Nalidixic acid
Lead or arsenic poisoning

---

levels. Ventriculograms show normal sized or small ventricles. The mechanism by which this syndrome is produced is unknown.

Hypervitaminosis A, although an uncommon condition, often causes increased intracranial pressure. Large doses (41,000 to 100,000 IU daily) taken for two months to nine years for treatment of acne or in vitamin preparations have caused this syndrome. Symptoms clear when vitamin A ingestion is stopped.[259]

On rare occasions prolonged corticosteroid treatment,[65] corticosteroid withdrawal,[90] and oral contraceptives[358] have been associated with the production of pseudotumor cerebri. The syndrome has been caused by therapy with tetracyclines (usually in infants but occasionally in adults,[205] by nalidixic acid (NegGram),[36] and by lead and arsenic poisoning.

Spinal Cord Lesions

Drugs rarely injure the spinal cord. The previous use of thorium dioxide (Thorotrast) as a contrast medium in myelography caused progressive cauda equina lesions.[86] Intraspinal injection of amphotericin B has led to arachnoiditis with resultant flaccid paraplegia, which usually is reversible.[229] On occasion, anticoagulant therapy causes intraspinal and spinal epidural hemorrhage.[6] Hypercalcemia, including that induced by the milk-alkali syndrome and vitamin D intoxication, can cause increased cerebrospinal fluid (CSF) protein without pleocytosis or elevated CSF pressure. The increased CSF protein level does not correlate with the serum calcium level, but returns to normal after correction of the hypercalcemia.[208]

Other Neurological Disorders

ATAXIA. Ataxia with nystagmus is a frequent toxic effect of diphenylhydantoin therapy. The antituberculous drugs isoniazid, para-aminosalicylic acid, and cycloserine interfere with the metabolism of diphenylhydantoin, leading to a greater incidence of diphenylhydantoin toxicity.[211] Ataxia also often follows the use of high doses of chlordiazepoxide (Librium), especially when the drug is used parenterally and in elderly patients.[84] Colistin (Coly-Mycin) can cause ataxia in patients with renal insufficiency, or if given in excessive doses.[374] Piperazine (Antepar), used in the treatment of pinworms and ascaris, has caused vertigo, tremor, incoordination, poor balance, muscle weakness, visual disturbances, and memory deficit associated with electroencephalographic abnormalities. These effects are enhanced by decreased renal function.[21,255]

MIGRAINE HEADACHES. Oral contraceptives can exacerbate or result in the *de novo* appearance of migraine headaches. Standard therapy for migraine is relatively ineffective while oral contraceptives are continued, but relief occurs when they are discontinued.[322,323]

WITHDRAWAL SYNDROMES. Withdrawal syndromes occur when addicting drugs are suddenly discontinued. Withdrawal from opiates, such as morphine and heroin, is characterized by initial anorexia, lacrimation, rhinorrhea, sweating, irritability, and restlessness followed by tremor, nausea, vomiting, diarrhea, and abdominal cramps. A similar syndrome occurs if prolonged administration of pentazocine (Talwin) is abruptly stopped. Addiction to propoxyphene (Darvon), a nonnarcotic analgesic structurally similar to methadone, occurs but is rare. Withdrawal symptoms have followed the discontinuance of propoxyphene in patients taking up to 2,300 mg daily.[372] Withdrawal of barbiturates, ethychlorvynol (Placidyl), and glutethimide (Doriden) leads to anorexia, insomnia, tremor, and irritability which can progress to delirium and seizures.[130] Lesser withdrawal symptoms can occur with abrupt cessation of long-term use of chloral hydrate, meprobamate, and paraldehyde. Termination of the nontherapeutic use of alcohol can precipitate delirium tremens.

Kernicterus is discussed in the section on liver manifestations.

Antituberculous therapy with isoniazid during pregnancy has resulted in the birth of infants with myoclonia, convulsions, and mental retardation. These abnormalities were felt to be caused by the interference of isoniazid with the metabolism of pyridoxine in the nervous system.[363]

14. BEHAVIORAL MANIFESTATIONS

Drug therapy can induce emotional changes as a desired therapeutic effect or as an untoward reaction. Undesired effects range from symptoms of anxiety and depression to psychosis that can culminate in suicide. Delirium and withdrawal reactions are considered in the section on neurologic manifestations.

Drug-Induced Anxiety

A sense of anxiety accompanied by apprehension, nervousness, tremor, tachycardia, palpitations, and sweating can result from the use of sympathomimetic amines, with strong beta-adrenergic stimulatory effects. Parenterally administered epinephrine and inhalers containing isoproterenol (Isuprel) used to treat asthma are common examples of drugs which produce these effects. Weight-reducing preparations containing amphetamines often have a similar effect. Rapidly developing hypoglycemia produced by insulin or sulfonylurea compounds causes the release of endogenous epinephrine as a means of reestablishing glucose homeostasis. Thus, anxiety, weakness, and hunger occur as typical concomitants of hypoglycemia.

Nervousness, tremor, and sweating accompany hyperthyroidism which can be induced by excessive amounts of exogenous thyroid hormone, by discontinuing iodide treatment of hyperthyroidism, and by release of stored thyroid hormone by radio-iodine treatment.[47,62] Tricyclic antidepressants such as amitriptyline (Elavil) may cause anxiety, restlessness, and insomnia.

Paradoxical anxiety can result from the use of barbiturates in young children and the elderly. Previous use of rauwolfia alkaloids in the treatment of psychiatric disorders occasionally produces a similar effect. Other drugs and drug combinations capable of producing central excitation, with anxiety as a component, are discussed in the section on neurologic disorders.

Drug-Induced Euphoria

Although the desired therapeutic effect of psychoactive drugs is to improve the patient's mood, this does not include a reaction of euphoria. Elevation of mood, elation, an exaggerated sense of well-being, increased initiative and confidence, and greater motor and speech activity can occur with the use of amphetamines and corticosteroids. Amphetamines are habituating, and although euphoria is initially a pleasant sensation, long-term intoxication can lead to psychosis, and withdrawal can lead to depression. Corticosteroid therapy is often associated with a heightened sense of well-being which can progress to euphoria ("steroid jag") that is not correlated with the improvement of the underlying disease process. Instances have been recorded in which patients used subterfuge to obtain corticosteroids for their euphoric effects and developed depression when these drugs were discontinued.[236]

Drug-Induced Depression

Oral contraceptives, because of their wide use, are the most common cause of drug-induced depression. A history of previous depression is an important predisposing factor. Between 5 and 30 per cent of all women taking the birth control pill experience irritability, tension, and depression, while 10 to 20 per cent have an improved mental state because of relief from premenstrual tension. Depression is correlated with the progestin content of combined preparations and occurs more often with combination preparations than with sequential drugs.[86] Some depressed women who take oral contraceptives develop biochemical evidence of pyridoxine deficiency. Depression in these women responds to pyridoxine therapy, but no such response occurs in women without evidence of pyridoxine deficiency.[2] The best treatment is discontinuing the oral contraceptives.

Although euphoria is the usual mood change produced by corticosteroids, depression also occurs, especially with a previous history of such illness.[86] Depression has followed withdrawal of corticosteroids taken for their euphoric effects.[236] Immunosuppressive therapy with corticosteroids and azathioprine (Imuran) has led to severe depression.[253]

Amphetamine withdrawal after large doses or prolonged use can often precipitate depression. The use of minor tranquilizers, for example chlordiazepoxide (Librium) and diazepam (Valium), in patients who are depressed can worsen depression. Rauwolfia alkaloids, when used in high doses to treat psychoses, have led to depression. This is less likely with smaller doses used to treat hypertension, but depression does occur and may be severe enough to lead to suicide.

Drug-Induced Psychoses

Corticosteroids can induce manic-depressive psychoses with suicidal tendencies and schizophrenic-type reactions. These psychoses are not dose-related but correlate with the patient's previous mental state. However, apparently emotionally stable individuals can be affected. Psychotic reactions may not occur with the first course of corticosteroid therapy but with subsequent treatment periods.[355]

Depressive and schizoaffective psychoses with mania occasionally have occurred in women starting oral contraceptives, usually the sequential variety, in the postpartum period. Psychosis has also followed withdrawal of large-dose oral contraceptives. The premorbid personality of the patient is an important contributing factor.[85]

Psychoses induced by toxicity occur from overdoses of anticholinergic drugs. Preparations of scopolamine in sleeping pills have caused hallucinations, both auditory and visual, delusions, confusion, and disorientation.[27]

On rare occasion, akinetic mutism has been caused by prochlorperazine (Compazine): patients become mute and unable to move their extremities, a state resembling catalepsy.[151] Carbamazepine (Tegretol) has been reported to activate psychoses in the elderly.[80] Infrequent instances of psychosis have resulted from disulfram (Antabuse) alone or in combination with metronidazole (Flagyl), which is characterized by confusion, paranoid delusions, and auditory and visual hallucinations.[303]

Isoniazid can affect the nervous system by producing peripheral neuritis and seizures; psychosis occurs rarely.[355] Toxicity-induced psychosis has been attributed to ampicillin.[355]

Digitalis intoxication, especially in elderly arteriosclerotic patients and in those with aortic valve lesions, infrequently produces an acute confusional psychosis and delirium.[174] Propranolol (Inderal) has caused confusion and hallucinations.[258a]

Prolonged amphetamine intoxication can lead to a psychosis similar to schizophrenia, with paranoia, confused ideas of reference, delusions, and hallucinations.

Withdrawal syndromes associated with abrupt cessation of barbiturates, diazepam (Valium), and other sedatives may comprise elements of psychotic behavior.[355]

The drugs mescaline and lysergide (LSD), often abused for their intoxicating and hallucinogenic effects, have induced psychotic behavior.[355]

15. MULTISYSTEM MANIFESTATIONS

The clinical effects of some drug reactions cannot be localized to one organ or organ system, but produce manifestations that are constitutional or involve many organ systems. Drug fever, vasculitis, systemic lupus erythematosus, serum sickness, and anaphylaxis, all drug-induced reactions that have no single target organ or organ system, will be discussed in this section.

Drug Fever

The term "drug fever" is generally used to signify fever as the only or the most prominent clinical feature of a drug reaction. Fever, however, can also be a secondary result of drug therapy. In past years, intravenous fluids produced fever because of contamination with bacterial pyrogens. A sterile abscess formed at the site of intramuscular injection can result in fever until it is drained. Drugs have been contaminated with microorganisms that produced infection. The Herxheimer reaction, which occurs following antibiotic treatment of secondary syphilis, is accompanied by fever. Any drug reaction that causes acute tissue injury, for example hemolysis in G-6-PD deficiency, is often accompanied by fever. Uncoupling of oxidative phosphorylation by dinitrophenol and general anesthetics leads to an increased rate of tissue metabolism and fever. Increases in body temperature occasionally occur from decreased heat loss as a result of peripheral vasoconstriction induced by epinephrine and norepinephrine. Lysergide, amphetamines, atropine, caffeine, cocaine, picrotoxin, and strychnine, usually in toxic doses, may produce fever by a central effect. Etiocholanolone, pollen extracts, vaccines, kaolin, and dextran also can produce fever.[63]

Fever accompanies other drug-induced states as a secondary phenomenon. This is noted in serum sickness, systemic lupus erythematosus, hepatitis, agranulocytosis, vasculitis, and other drug reactions.

Fever as the major manifestation of drug allergy can be produced by almost any drug, although certain drugs tend to do so more often than others (see Table 4-60).[63,138,194,245,356]

Some drugs, such as digitalis, chloramphenicol, tetracyclines, and insulin rarely if ever produce fever.

Fever may be the only sign of drug allergy, but often other signs of allergy, such as urticaria, rash, or eosinophilia, are present. Fever tends to appear progressively seven to ten days after a drug has been started. There may be accompanying chill, headache, and arthralgias. The fever may be sustained or remittent, but persists as long as the drug is taken. Once the drug is discontinued, fever abates in one or two days, except in instances in which there is slow drug excretion. In a sensitized person, there is an accelerated reaction if the drug is given again, and fever appears within one to two hours after readministration.[63]

Drug fever should be suspected clinically: if the patient is receiving almost any drug, but especially those listed in Table 4-60; if the patient appears less ill than the fever would indicate; if other manifestations of drug allergy are present; and if fever is unexpected, especially if the patient's clinical state is improving. One of the more frequently encountered examples of drug fever occurs in patients being treated with penicillin for pneumonia. After a few days the patient defervesces, but on about the seventh day of illness, when he is clinically improved, fever recurs. Instead of having the typical toxic appearance of a patient with a suppurative complication, such as empyema, he appears relatively well. If penicillin is discontinued, defervescence occurs promptly.

If drug fever is suspected in a patient receiving many drugs, all drugs should be discontinued to determine whether the fever is drug-induced. In order to determine which was the offending drug, each drug may be reintroduced separately to see which one will produce a fever. If it is not possible to discontinue all drugs simultaneously, each drug should be discontinued for a two- or three-day period to see if the patient's temperature falls. In the rare instances in which the patient must continue to take the drug that is causing fever, concomitant use of corticosteroids will suppress the fever, while antihistamines will not.[63]

Fever also may occur from an overdose of amphetamines or monamine oxidase inhibitors. The combination of monamine oxidase inhibitors with dextroamphetamine and imipramine (Tofranil) in normal doses has resulted in hyperpyrexia.[209]

TABLE 4-60. *Drugs Known to Cause Fever Alone without Other Manifestations**

Penicillin	Barbiturates
Cephalothin (Keflin)	Cocaine derivatives
Cephaloridine (Loridine)	Coumarin
Streptomycin	Diphenylhydantoin (Dilantin)
Novobiocin	Dextran iron complex (Imferon)
Isoniazid	Iodides
Para-aminosalicylic acid	Mercurials
Amphotericin B	Methyldopa (Aldomet)
Mithramycin	Diazoxide
Sulfonamides	Procainamide
Allopurinol (Zyloprim)	Quinidine
Antihistamines	Salicylates
Atropine	Propylthiouracil

* Underlined drugs are a relatively frequent cause of drug fever.

Drugs rarely produce hypothermia. Febrile patients treated with salicylates may become mildly hypothermic and hypotensive during defervescence. Phenothiazines may also depress body temperature. Instances of hypothermia (93.4° F and 94.6° F) have been attributed to tetracyclines. Normal body temperature was restored by discontinuing the drug and administering corticosteroids.[72]

Drug-Induced Systemic Lupus Erythematosus

A syndrome clinically indistinguishable from systemic lupus erythematosus (SLE) has been induced by many structurally unrelated drugs. Severity may range from only a positive lupus erythematosus cell preparation to serious illness. It has been estimated that 3 to 12 per cent of cases of SLE are drug-induced.[219] The most frequent clinical findings are arthralgias and arthritis, pleuritic chest pain, fever, pericarditis, myalgias, lymph node enlargement, hepatomegaly, splenomegaly, and rash. Renal involvement, however, is notably absent in most cases. Blood studies show findings that are similar to those occurring in spontaneous SLE (elevated erythrocyte sedimentation rate, positive lupus erythematosus cell preparation, and positive antinuclear antibody), except that serum complement levels are not depressed.

The syndrome usually appears with conventional drug doses and is usually related to prolonged drug exposure. Hydralazine (Apresoline) therapy is an exception to this rule in that large doses (more than 500 mg per day) are an important factor in eliciting the SLE reaction.[219] In most instances, symptoms abate after the offending drug is discontinued, but lingering symptoms can be managed with salicylates or corticosteroids. However, symptoms may persist for

TABLE 4–61. *Drugs Known to Cause SLE**

Hydralazine (Apresoline)	Streptomycin
Procainamide	Tetracyclines
Isoniazid	Quinidine
Anticonvulsants:	Para-aminosalicylic acid
Diphenylhydantoin (Dilantin)	Phenylbutazone (Butazolidin)
Mephenytoin (Mesantoin)	Propylthiouracil
Primidone (Mysoline)	Methylthiouracil
Trimethadione (Tridione)	Phenothiazines:
Ethosuximide (Zarontin)	Chlorpromazine (Thorazine)
Methsuximide (Celontin)	Methotrimeprazine (Levoprome)
Barbiturates	Perphenazine (Trilafon)
Griseofulvin	Promazine (Sparine)
Sulfonamides	Methyldopa (Aldomet)
Penicillin	Reserpine

* Underlined drugs indicate frequent cause of reaction.

prolonged periods of time. Studies have shown that family members of patients with drug-induced SLE have a high incidence of drug sensitivity and other allergic manifestations. On this basis, it has been postulated that there is a lupus diathesis that is uncovered by certain drugs.

Some drugs cause SLE (Table 4-61) with regularity (hydralazine, procainamide, isoniazid, and diphenylhydantoin), while the rest do so sporadically.[4,5,32,70,77,215,219,277]

A syndrome misinterpreted as SLE may result from the complications of prolonged corticosteroid therapy. Patients develop arthralgias, myalgias, proteinuria, edema, and hypertension. These symptoms are exacerbated by increasing drug doses and ameliorated by reducing or discontinuing corticosteroids.[160]

Drug-Induced Vasculitis

Drugs can produce reactions that primarily affect small blood vessels resulting in vasculitis or angiitis (Table 4-62). Clinically, these reactions may resemble periarteritis nodosa, nonspecific vasculitis, or allergic (Henoch-Schönlein) purpura. Many instances have been associated with serum sickness.

A syndrome resembling periarteritis nodosa, in which small vessels show inflammation but usually without the formation of aneurysms, has been caused most often by penicillin, sulfonamides, and propylthiouracil, and less often by iodides, phenylbutazone (Butazolidin), quinidine, chlorpromazine (Thorazine), diphenylhydantoin (Dilantin), serum, organic arsenicals, mercurials, gold salts, and the insecticide DDT.[346]

Other clinical forms of vasculitis, with associated arthralgias, dependent purpura, low-grade fever, dermatitis, and subcutaneous nodules, have resulted from therapy with penicillin, phenylbutazone, sulfonamides, barbiturates, and anticonvulsants.[198,237] Vasculitis with cool cyanotic fingers, splinter hemorrhages, and positive lupus

TABLE 4-62. *Drugs Known to Cause Vasculitis**

Penicillin	Organic arsenicals
Sulfonamides	Mercurials
Propylthiouracil	Gold salts
Iodides	DDT
Phenylbutazone (Butazolidin)	Barbiturates
Quinidine	Procainamide
Quinine	Chlorothiazide (Diuril)
Chlorpromazine (Thorazine)	Tetracyclines
Diphenylhydantoin (Dilantin)	Salicylates
Serum	

* Underlined drugs indicate frequent cause of reaction.

erythematosus cell preparation without other systemic signs has been caused by procainamide.[301]

A syndrome resembling allergic (Henoch-Schönlein) purpura has been attributed to penicillin, ampicillin, barbiturates, chlorothiazide (Diuril), tetracyclines, salicylates, quinine, quinidine, and gold salts.[86,346]

It has been reported that thrombotic thrombocytopenic purpura has been caused by sulfonamides, penicillin, arsenicals, iodides, and chlorpropamide (Diabinese).[346]

Drug-Induced Serum Sickness

Serum sickness results from an allergic reaction to a foreign protein, most often horse serum, or to a drug. Symptoms usually appear seven to ten days after exposure, but may take up to three weeks to appear. With previous sensitization, reactions appear in a shorter time and an immediate reaction may occur with anaphylaxis. Concomitant with the appearance of symptoms, there is a rise in complement-fixing serum antibody levels. Illness begins with pruritus, followed by skin eruptions, usually urticaria, fever, and arthralgias or arthritis. Other common findings include lymphadenopathy, angioneurotic edema, myalgias, and renal involvement with proteinuria, casts, and microscopic hematuria. Less frequently, peripheral neuropathy and cardiac involvement may occur. There may be an elevated white blood cell count and mild eosinophilia.

Symptoms usually last from one to three weeks. Urticaria responds to treatment with epinephrine or antihistamines. Most other

TABLE 4-63. *Drugs Known to Cause Serum Sickness**

Serums (esp. horse serum)	Insulin
Penicillins	Iodides
Streptomycin	Iodinated contrast media
Sulfonamides	Isoniazid
Propylthiouracil	Mercurials
ACTH	Oxytetracycline
Arsenicals	Phenolphthalein
Barbiturates	Phenylbutazone (Butazolidin)
Bismuth	Probenecid (Benemid)
Cinchophen	Procainamide
Digitalis	Quinidine
Diphenylhydantoin (Dilantin)	Quinine
Erythromycin	Salicylates
Griseofulvin	Streptomycin
Heparin	Tripelennamine (Pyribenzamine)
Hydralazine (Apresoline)	Vaccines
Dextran iron complex (Imferon)	Viomycin (Viocin)

* Underlined drugs indicate frequent cause of reactions.

symptoms are relieved by aspirin. In severe cases, a brief course of corticosteroid therapy may be required.

Penicillin and its congeners, i.e., methicillin (Staphcillin) and ampicillin, are the most frequent causative drugs. A list of many of the drugs that have caused serum sickness is given in Table 4–63.[17,122,245]

Drug-Induced Anaphylaxis

Anaphylaxis consists of an acute, potentially fatal, drug reaction. It is more likely to occur if a drug is given parenterally, but it may also follow oral administration. Within 1 to 30 minutes after a drug is received, the patient rapidly develops a wide variety of symptoms:

TABLE 4–64. *Drugs Known to Produce Anaphylaxis**

Antisera (nonhuman)
Allergens used in desensitization
Enzymes:
Chymotrypsin
Penicillinase (Neutrapen)
Antimicrobials:
Penicillin
Cephalothin (Keflin)
Cephaloridine (Loridine)
Tetracyclines
Chlortetracycline (Aureomycin)
Demethylchlortetracycline (Declomycin)
Nitrofurantoin (Furadantin)
Streptomycin
Sulfonamides
Other drugs:
Procaine (Novocain)
Bromsulfalein (BSP)
Sodium dehydrocholate (Decholin)
Dextrans
Dextran iron complex (Imferon)
ACTH
Insulin
Relaxin (Releasin)
Thiamine
Folic acid
Salicylates
Aminopyrine
Probenecid (Benemid)
Heparin
Iodinated contrast media
Meprobamate
Tripelennamine (Pyribenzamine)
Triphenylmethane (dye to determine burn depth)

* Underlined drugs indicate frequent cause of reactions.

CLINICAL MANIFESTATIONS 203

weakness, dyspnea (due to either bronchospasm with wheezing or angioedema of the larynx), cough, tightness in the chest, sweating, tachycardia, pallor, cyanosis, pruritus (usually of the face, palms, and soles), and urticaria. Hypotension may lead to vascular collapse and death.

Penicillin is probably the drug that most frequently produces anaphylaxis. Penicillin anaphylaxis is more common in individuals with a history of atopy,[335] and in those who have had previous minor allergic reactions, such as a rash, to this drug. In addition to parenteral administration, penicillin anaphylaxis has occurred with oral, topical, and conjunctival therapy. Anaphylaxis has also followed oral therapy with demethylchlortetracycline (Declomycin), chlortetracycline (Aureomycin), nitrofurantoin (Furadantin), folic acid, salicylates, aminopyrine, iodinated contrast media, meprobamate, and tripelennamine (Pyribenzamine).[122,126]

Dextrans used as plasma expanders cause a higher number of cases of anaphylaxis than has been generally realized. About 10 per cent of patients receiving dextrans have other symptoms suggestive of allergic reactions, such as pruritus, urticaria, and joint pains.[254]

Therapy consists of epinephrine and support of respiration and circulation, if necessary. If the injection site permits (e.g., upper arm), a tourniquet may be used to retard drug absorption. Corticosteroids are of little value, since they do not take effect for up to six hours, and will not prevent anaphylaxis even if given before the drug.

A list of drugs that have produced anaphylaxis is given in Table 4–64.[122,126,168,245]

16. INFECTIONS

Certain drugs can alter the normal microbial flora or host defense mechanisms so that infections may supervene or be disseminated as a result of their use. Antimicrobial agents suppress the normal bacterial flora and allow overgrowth of resistant, potentially pathogenic organisms. Corticosteroids, immunosuppressive agents, and antineoplastic drugs impair normal host defenses against microbial invasion. Resultant infections can be due to bacteria, mycobacteria, fungi, viruses, protozoa, or worms.

Bacterial Infections

The use of antimicrobial agents for the treatment of bacterial infections has led to the emergence of organisms that are resistant to drugs to which they were previously sensitive. Staphylococci can develop rapid resistance to erythromycin. Penicillin-sensitive staphylococci do not become resistant to penicillin, but the use of penicillin allows initially penicillin-resistant organisms to flourish. Group A beta-hemolytic streptococci are now found to be resistant to tetracycline, making this drug no longer acceptable for treatment of infection caused by this organism. Tetracycline-resistant pneumococci have developed in patients given prolonged treatment with this antibiotic. Subsequently, tetracycline-resistant pneumococcal pneumonia has appeared. Penicillin-resistant staphylococci have proliferated, and staphylococci that are resistant to vancomycin and methicillin have appeared. Gonococci have become decreasingly sensitive to penicillin. Consequently, the effective dose of penicillin in gonococcal infections has had to be increased. Sulfonamide-resistant strains of meningococci, mostly group B but some group C, are found in almost one-third of infected patients. Penicillin has now supplanted the sulfonamides as the preferred drug in treating these infections.[136,220]

The use of antibiotics, especially large doses of penicillin and broad-spectrum antibiotics such as tetracycline, chloramphenicol, cephalothin (Keflin), and others, may lead to superinfection with resistant organisms, such as resistant staphylococci and gram-negative bacteria. The normal bacterial flora is suppressed by antibiotic treatment, and the host's own resistant organisms, or those introduced from the environment, often the hospital, take hold and constitute a new microbial flora. Furthermore, during antibiotic therapy naturally resistant strains of bacteria increase in number as sensitive strains are suppressed, and resistant mutants may appear.[136] Children treated with penicillin may have penicillin-resistant *Streptococcus viridans* in their throats. This finding may influence the use of penicillin alone as chemoprophylaxis for endocarditis during dental procedures in children with valvular heart lesions.[343] The use of nafcillin (Unipen) in the treatment of penicillin-resistant staphylococcal infections has led to superinfection with enterococci and gram-negative organisms (klebsiella, *Escherichia coli,* proteus, pseudomonas, and herellea).[108]

Pseudomembranous and staphylococcal colitis became more prevalent during the antibiotic era. They can be precipitated by treatment with tetracycline, oral neomycin, lincomycin, or other broad-spectrum antibiotics.[314]

Oral contraceptives produce relaxation of smooth muscle in the urinary tract that may predispose the patient to cystitis or pyelonephritis.[86]

The use of corticosteroids and immunosuppressive drugs, usually prednisone and azathioprine (Imuran), in patients with renal transplants, and the use of antineoplastic drugs in other patients, have led to infections with bacteria, viruses, fungi, and protozoa. At autopsy, almost one-half of renal transplant patients have an infection.[169] Bacteria that often produce infection in patients treated with corticosteroids, immunosuppressive drugs, and antineoplastic agents include pseudomonas, paracolon, klebsiella, *E. coli,* staphylococcus, herellea, serratia, and listeria.[44,169]

An unusual instance of pneumococcal sepsis and disseminated intravascular coagulation has been reported in a patient who had previously received thorium dioxide (Thorotrast). Overwhelming sepsis was felt to be due to reticuloendothelial blockade.[23]

Mycobacterial Infections

Corticosteroids may lead to the reactivation of tuberculosis, which may then become disseminated. At the same time, the clinical signs of infection can be masked by these drugs.[232] Azathioprine (Imuran) has also exacerbated tuberculous infection.[74]

Fungal Infections

Candidiasis is the most frequently drug-induced fungal infection. Candida is a normal saprophyte that can produce infections of the skin, mouth, intestines, peritoneum, gall bladder, lungs, pleura, and vagina. Instances of invasive infection and sepsis occur infrequently. Treatment with antibiotics, corticosteroids, immunosuppressive agents, and antineoplastic drugs predispose to fungal infection.[318] Patients with renal transplants often have local or disseminated fungal infection.[169,306] The use of oral contraceptives is often associated with the appearance of candida vaginitis, which may not respond to treatment until these drugs are discontinued.[86]

Opportunistic fungal infections often result from corticosteroid and immunosuppressive therapy in patients with renal transplants. Infections with aspergillus, nocardia, and candida occur most frequently. The lungs, gastrointestinal tract, central nervous system, and kidneys are involved in decreasing order of frequency. Aspergillus has a predilection for the lungs and central nervous system. Concomitant bacterial, viral, and parasitic infections usually occur.[169,293] Cryptococcus infections have been associated with the use of corticosteroids.[86]

Viral Infections

Corticosteroids increase susceptibility to certain viral infections and can lead to a protracted, severe course and disseminated infection. Ocular herpes simplex infections may be aggravated by the use of local corticosteroids. Chickenpox may develop in children during corticosteroid therapy, and may be fatal. In adults receiving corticosteroids, chickenpox may lead to hemorrhagic varicella pneumonia.[232] Herpes zoster also may become disseminated in patients receiving corticosteroids. Reportedly, increased susceptibility to poliomyelitis occurs during treatment with corticosteroids.[86]

Patients receiving immunosuppressive therapy and corticosteroids have developed infections with cytomegalovirus,[166,185] herpes zoster, and herpes simplex.[306] Prolonged and disseminated herpes zoster infection has resulted from treatment with cytosine arabinoside in patients with advanced lymphomas.[341]

Protozoal Infections

Pneumocystis carinii pneumonia is associated with corticosteroid, immunosuppressive, and antineoplastic therapy in patients with renal transplants and in those with leukemia and lymphomas.[169,334] Infections with *Toxoplasma gondii,* often involving the central nervous system or heart, tend to occur in patients with hematologic malignancies treated with corticosteroids and antineoplastic drugs.[58,365] Amebic dysentery has appeared during corticosteroid therapy.[110] Adrenocorticotropic hormone therapy has produced increased parasitemia in induced malaria.

Instances of fatal strongyloidiasis have occurred in patients receiving corticosteroids for a variety of illnesses.[82]

17. OCULAR MANIFESTATIONS

Systemically administered and topically applied drugs can produce adverse effects on the eye. In addition, topical ophthalmic preparations occasionally lead to systemic effects due to excessive absorption. Of the many known drug-induced eye disorders, those which are particularly important will be discussed.

External Disorders

Long-term, high dose corticosteroid therapy can lead to *exophthalmos,* which is also found in six to eight per cent of patients with Cushing's disease. Discontinuing treatment reverses the condition.[86] Hyperthyroidism produced by excessive amounts of exogenous thyroid hormone can produce exophthalmos and conjunctival congestion. Unilateral and bilateral exophthalmos have occurred with pharmacologic doses of lithium carbonate used in the therapy of manic-depressive psychosis. In a few of these patients with exophthalmos, hypothyroidism developed. Eye changes regressed when the drug was discontinued.[319]

Conjunctivitis is a part of the syndrome of drug-induced erythema multiforme (see section on dermatologic manifestations for causative drugs). Subconjunctival hemorrhage may occur as a result of anticoagulant therapy.[291]

Extraocular Muscle Disorders

Diplopia is the cardinal symptom of *extraocular muscle paresis.* Intoxication from many drugs, principally barbiturates, diphenylhydantoin (Dilantin), meprobamate, and bromides, can result in diplopia. Furaltadone (Altafur) neuropathy has been associated with bilateral paresis of the lateral rectus eye muscles.[249] Drugs that cause neuromuscular blockade, for example, polymyxin B and colistin (Coly-Mycin), can lead to external ophthalmoplegia.[228]

The *oculogyric crisis* caused by phenothiazines, most often prochlorperazine (Compazine), is characterized by a brief fixed stare followed by upward or lateral deviation of the eyes requiring tilting of the head in order to see. Dramatic relief is produced by treatment with parenteral antihistamines, barbiturates, and antiparkinsonian drugs.[100]

Disorders of the Cornea

The use of topical corneal anesthetic agents, such as tetracaine, proparacaine, and butacaine, at frequent intervals for days or weeks to relieve the discomfort of minor eye injuries, can lead to severe *keratitis* and even permanently decreased visual acuity. Excessive use of these anesthetics causes loss of the corneal epithelium with resultant greater discomfort; this leads to even more frequent use of these agents, ending in a cyclical problem of corneal damage. Edema of the cornea, opacification, and inflammatory changes in the anterior segment of the eye soon follow. Treatment consists of discontinuing the use of these agents.[114]

Acute keratitis has occurred when triacetoxyanthracene, used in the topical treatment of psoriasis, has gotten into the eyes. Prednisolone and atropine eye drops produced relief.[250] Topical corticosteroids may exacerbate herpetic keratitis and are therefore contraindicated in this disorder. In addition, topical application of excessive amounts of idoxuridine (Stoxil) in the treatment of herpetic keratitis has resulted in ulceration and perforation of the cornea.[226] Long-term chlorpromazine (Thorazine) therapy can lead to the deposition of a granular, brown pigment in the cornea.[93]

Disorders of the Lens of Anterior Chamber and Vitreum

CATARACTS. Lenticular deposits can occur from systemic phenothiazine and corticosteroid therapy, and from topical treatment of glaucoma with anticholinesterase eye drops. Prolonged phenothiazine therapy, usually with chlorpromazine (Thorazine), can cause cutaneous pigmentation and lenticular and corneal opacities. A yellow or light brown granular material that is probably a drug metabolite is deposited on the posterior surface of the cornea and on the anterior capsular and subcapsular portion of the lens. Stellate anterior lenticular opacities composed of the same material occur less often. These changes are thought to be caused by accumulation of the drug or one of its metabolites in the anterior chamber of the eye. Light exposure probably plays a role in producing granular deposition.[86,93]

Posterior subcapsular cataracts that usually do not impair vision can result from systemic corticosteroid therapy, most often in patients with rheumatoid arthritis. The formation of cataracts is related both to the dose and the duration of treatment: the greater the total amount of corticosteroids received, the greater the incidence of cataracts. The pathogenesis of corticosteroid-induced cataracts is not understood.[344] The appearance of similar cataracts has followed the use of oral contraceptives.[86]

Anticholinesterase (e.g., phospholine iodide) eye drops used in the treatment of glaucoma have caused anterior subcapsular lenticular opacities without visual impairment that tend to disappear with cessation of therapy.[10]

Drugs known to cause cataracts can be found in Table 4–65.

*TABLE 4-65. Drugs
Known to Cause
Cataracts*

Phenothiazines
Corticosteroids
Oral contraceptives
Anticholinesterase eye drops

GLAUCOMA. Both topical and systemic drug therapy can lead to glaucoma by increasing intraocular pressure (Table 4-66). Local mydriatics can precipitate attacks of narrow-angle glaucoma in susceptible individuals by dilating the pupil and impeding the egress of aqueous humor. The most commonly used mydriatics are anticholinergics (atropine and homatropine) or sympathomimetic amines (phenylephrine [Neo-Synephrine]). Systemic use of anticholinergics, and less often of sympathomimetic amines (ephedrine, epinephrine, and amphetamines), can produce similar but less marked effects on the pupil and induce glaucoma attacks.

Corticosteroid therapy can raise intraocular pressure by blocking the outflow of aqueous humor. This effect may occur weeks after topical therapy and months after systemic therapy. Glaucoma is reversible if the drug is discontinued.[86] Phenothiazines may also increase intraocular pressure.[86]

RETROLENTAL FIBROPLASIA. Excessive administration of oxygen to newborns, especially premature infants, leads to the development of retrolental fibroplasia. Ophthalmic lesions vary in severity. Ophthalmologic examination may show retinal pallor, growth of new capillaries, peripheral retinal separation, vitreous hemorrhages, neovascularization, vitreous strands, and partial or complete retrolental membranes. Visual impairment correlates with the degree of pathologic ocular changes. Myopia in proportion to the extent of disease also occurs, but is correctable with glasses.[379]

*TABLE 4-66. Drugs
That Can Precipitate
Glaucoma*

Topical:
  Mydriatics
  Corticosteroids
Systemic:
  Anticholinergics
  Sympathomimetic amines
  Corticosteroids
  Phenothiazines

Disorders of the Retina

The anti-inflammatory properties of certain antimalarial drugs, principally chloroquine (Aralen) and hydroxychloroquine (Plaquenil), have led to their use in the treatment of discoid and systemic lupus erythematosus, scleroderma, rheumatoid arthritis, and petit mal epilepsy. Prolonged, high-dose therapy with these drugs can lead to severe, usually irreversible retinal damage with marked visual impairment. Retinopathy may progress after these drugs have been discontinued, or may appear as late as three to five years after cessation of therapy.

Ocular findings consist of granular or stippled hyperpigmentation of the macula, surrounded by a clear zone of depigmentation which is encircled by another ring of hyperpigmentation. This is the so-called doughnut or bull's-eye lesion. There may be no symptoms or severe visual loss. An early sign is paracentral scotoma, followed by a pericentral ring scotoma which interferes with reading. Poor color vision and night blindness may occur. Other visual symptoms may occur which are independent of the retinopathy. Blurred vision and glare halos follow the deposition of chloroquine in the cornea, which in itself is harmless. A myopathy of the accommodative and extraocular muscles may lead to blurred vision and diplopia.

Chloroquine and hydroxychloroquine are bound to melanin, which is found in large quantity in the uveal tract and retinal pigment epithelium. Attached to melanin, these drugs may be retained in the body for many years. The mechanism by which retinal damage is produced is unknown. Periodic eye examinations for patients receiving long-term chloroquine and hydroxychloroquine therapy are mandatory. These drugs should be discontinued at the earliest sign of retinal damage, although, as mentioned, lesions may progress or appear after treatment is terminated. Corneal deposits clear after cessation of the drugs.[46]

Phenothiazines in large doses, especially thioridazine (Mellaril), but also prochlorperazine (Compazine) and chlorpromazine (Thorazine), accumulate in the pigment cells of the retina and can cause an illness resembling retinitis pigmentosa with defective central vision, night blindness, and narrowed retinal arterioles. Pigment aggregates, however, occur in large clumps rather than as the bone-corpuscle configuration type seen in retinitis pigmentosa.[222]

Disorders of the Optic Nerve

The major symptom of *optic neuritis* is loss of vision. Also, there is usually some discomfort, especially with movement of the eyes, and scotomas or constricted visual fields. Examination may reveal papillitis with edema of the optic disc, dilated vessels, and if severe,

TABLE 4-67. *Drugs Known to Cause Optic Neuritis*

Chloramphenicol
Streptomycin
Isoniazid
Ethambutol (Myambutol)
Pheniprazine (Catron)
Penicillamine
Quinine
Digitalis
Oral contraceptives
Arsenic compounds

retinal edema with a macular star, hemorrhages, and exudates. If inflammation affects the retrobulbar portion of the optic nerve, no visible changes are noted in examining the eye but symptoms are the same. Varying degrees of optic atrophy follow resolution of optic neuritis. There are changes in visual fields and decreased vision, with pallor of the optic disc.

Most drugs that have induced optic neuritis have done so after long-term or high-dose therapy (Table 4-67). Chloramphenicol-induced optic neuritis is not always reversible. Streptomycin has been reported to cause optic neuritis, especially when used intrathecally to treat tuberculous meningitis.[357] Isoniazid, which can cause peripheral neuritis and convulsions, also produces optic neuritis that may be the result of pyridoxine deficiency.[226] The antituberculous drug ethambutol (Myambutol) has also led to optic neuritis.[53]

Pheniprazine (Catron), a monamine oxidase inhibitor that has been withdrawn from the market, caused optic neuritis after several weeks of therapy.[226] Prolonged penicillamine therapy used in the treatment of Wilson's disease has led to optic neuritis that can be prevented and treated with pyridoxine.[226]

Quinine toxicity has frequently led to optic atrophy (quinine amblyopia).[150] Digitalis is a rare cause of transient or permanent visual loss and retrobulbar neuritis.[222] Oral contraceptives have caused bilateral optic neuritis, including retrobulbar neuritis, which has cleared after the drug was discontinued and returned when oral contraceptives were reinstituted.[358] Arsenic compounds may cause optic nerve damage and blindness. Sodium arsanilate (Axotyl), a drug previously used to treat trypanosomiasis, has been withdrawn from use because it often caused optic neuritis.[150]

Papilledema is one of the manifestations of benign increased intracranial pressure (pseudotumor cerebri). This disorder has been caused by hypervitaminosis A, prolonged corticosteroid therapy, corticosteroid withdrawal, oral contraceptives, tetracycline, and nalidixic acid (NegGram). (See section on neurologic manifestations.)

Other Ocular Disorders

VASCULAR LESIONS. Oral contraceptives have been associated with the occurrence of thrombosis of the retinal artery or one of its branches, and less often with central retinal vein thrombosis. Sudden loss of vision, which is permanent, is the cardinal symptom.

SYMPTOMS INDUCED BY DIGITALIS INTOXICATION. Visual symptoms from digitalis intoxication are more frequent and more varied than is generally recognized. Ocular symptoms occur in about 25 per cent of patients with digitalis toxicity; in 10 per cent of cases they precede other symptoms. These symptoms are often overlooked because patients neglect to mention them, physicians forget to ask about them, and because concern generally is focused on the more dramatic cardiovascular effects. Photophobia, flashes, sparks, silvery streaks, flickering, and blurred vision may be noted by the patient. Chromatopsia is usually manifested by yellow or green vision and less often by red, brown, blue, or white vision. White halos may surround dark objects and objects may appear to be covered with snow or frost. Transient scotomata, loss of vision, retrobulbar neuritis, and diplopia produced by oculomotor palsies may also occur.[143,222]

CONGENITAL OCULAR MALFORMATIONS. Thalidomide-induced congenital lesions of the limbs have received great publicity and resulted in the withdrawal of the drug from the market. This drug also has produced ocular malformations. Thalidomide has caused congenital oculomotor paralyses, bilateral aplasia of the macula, coloboma of the choroid, microphthalmos, anophthalmos, and epiphora (excessive tearing).[380]

18. EAR MANIFESTATIONS

Drugs that affect the ear can produce vertigo or tinnitus and deafness, depending on whether the vestibular or the auditory portion of the eighth cranial nerve is affected predominantly. There are only a few other drug-induced ear problems: bleeding from the ear has been caused by anticoagulant therapy,[195] and otitis externa has been produced by either pseudomonas or proteus following the use of broad-spectrum antibiotics.[122]

Vestibular Damage

Streptomycin affects the eighth nerve primarily by producing vestibular damage. The patient experiences giddiness, and sudden movement produces vertigo. The danger of nerve damage is heightened by large drug doses, decreased renal function, and increasing age. Deafness is rarely caused by streptomycin, except in cases of tuberculous meningitis in which cerebrospinal fluid concentrations of streptomycin are increased.[86]

Auditory Damage

TINNITUS AND DEAFNESS. The aminoglycoside antibiotics, with the exception of streptomycin and gentamicin, primarily cause tinnitus and deafness (Table 4-68). Streptomycin, however, can cross the placental barrier and lead to deafness without vestibular damage in the fetus.[363] Gentamicin has rarely produced deafness.

Dihydrostreptomycin was withdrawn from use because it led to a high incidence of deafness, even after therapy had been discontinued.[86]

Neomycin, kanamycin (Kantrex), and viomycin (Viocin) can all lead to deafness. Neomycin is not used parenterally because of its ototoxic and nephrotoxic effects. Insignificant amounts are absorbed from the intestine when the drug is used as a bowel disinfectant.

TABLE 4-68. Drugs Known to Cause Deafness

Dihydrostreptomycin
Neomycin
Kanamycin (Kantrex)
Viomycin (Viocin)
Furazolidone (Furoxone)
Ethacrynic acid (Edecrin)
Furosemide (Lasix)
Quinine
Salicylates

Ulcerative lesions of the bowel, however, can lead to greater drug absorption and in the presence of decreased renal function can produce high blood concentrations of the drug and result in deafness.[86] The use of neomycin in combination with polymyxin B via a plastic catheter to irrigate an osteomyelitic lesion has caused deafness.[193]

Deafness caused by kanamycin is particularly likely to occur with high dose or prolonged therapy, or in the presence of decreased renal function. Deafness may appear or progress but persists after the drug has been discontinued.[86] Viomycin, an antituberculous drug, mainly produces deafness but can also affect vestibular function. Furazolidone (Furoxone) is a considerably less frequent cause of tinnitus and deafness.[86]

Ethacrynic acid (Edecrin), usually when given intravenously but also after oral therapy in uremic patients, has caused transient vertigo, a sensation of fullness in the ears, tinnitus, and deafness. Permanent deafness has followed both oral and intravenous therapy.[283] Moderate to severe permanent hearing loss has occurred in uremic patients treated with ethacrynic acid and small doses of streptomycin. The synergistic effect of these two drugs may have been the cause of the permanent deafness.[251]

Transient vertigo, tinnitus, and hearing loss have also occurred with high-dose, intravenously administered furosemide (Lasix) therapy in patients with impaired renal function.[313]

High blood levels of quinine and salicylates can lead to cinchonism, which is characterized by headache, vertigo, tinnitus, hearing loss, blurred vision, and nausea and vomiting. These symptoms abate with cessation of the use of these drugs.[264] Some degree of tinnitus and hearing loss occurs frequently with high-dose aspirin treatment for rheumatoid arthritis or acute rheumatic fever. When salicylic acid is used in the treatment of psoriasis, enough salicylate may be absorbed through the skin to lead to transient hearing loss. Salicylate absorption is dependent on the pathological state of the skin and the type of base in which salicylic acid is dissolved.[276]

REFERENCES

1. Abbruzzese, A., and Swanson, J.: Jaundice after therapy with chlordiazepoxide hydrochloride. New Eng. J. Med., 273:321, 1965.
2. Adams, P. W., Wynn, V., Rose, D. P., et al.: Effect of pyridoxine hydrochloride (vitamin B_6) upon depression associated with oral contraceptives. Lancet, 1:897, 1973.
3. Aggeler, P. M., O'Reilly, R. A., Leong, L., and Kowitz, P. E.: Potentiation of anticoagulant effect of warfarin by phenylbutazone. New Eng. J. Med., 276:496, 1967.
4. Alarcón-Segovia, D.: Drug-induced lupus syndromes. Mayo Clin. Proc., 44:664, 1969.
5. Alarcón-Segovia, D., Worthington, J. W., Ward, L. E., and Wakim, K. G.: Lupus diathesis and the hydralazine syndrome. New Eng. J. Med., 272:462, 1965.

6. Alderman, D. B.: Extradural spinal-cord hematoma: Report of a case due to dicumarol and review of the literature. New Eng. J. Med., 255:839, 1956.
7. Ambani, L. M., and Van Woert, M. H.: Start hesitation—a side effect of long-term levodopa therapy. New Eng. J. Med., 288:1113, 1973.
8. Arseneau, J. C., Bagley, C. M., Anderson, T., and Canellos, S. P.: Hyperkalemia, a sequel to chemotherapy of Burkitt's lymphoma. Lancet, 1:10, 1973.
9. Aviram, A., Pfau, A., Czaczkes, J. W., and Ullmann, T. D.: Hyperosmolality with hyponatremia, caused by inappropriate administration of mannitol. Am. J. Med., 42:648, 1967.
10. Axelsson, U., and Hoemberg, A.: The frequency of cataract after miotic therapy. Acta Ophthalmol., 44:421, 1966.
11. Azen, E. A., Bryan, G. T., Shahidi, N. T., Rossi, E. C., and Clatanoff, D. V.: Obscure hemolytic anemia due to analgesic abuse: Does enterogenous cyanosis exist? Am. J. Med., 48:724, 1970.
12. Babior, B. M., and Davidson, C. S.: Hepatitis: Drug or viral? Am. J. Med., 41:491, 1966.
13. Baer, R. L., and Schwarzchild, L.: Selected allergic skin diseases in older persons. Geriatrics, 10:265, 1955.
14. Baldwin, D. S., Levine, B. B., McCluskey, R. T., and Gallo, G. R.: Renal failure and interstitial nephritis due to penicillin and methicillin. New Eng. J. Med., 279:1245, 1968.
15. Bartter, F. C.: The syndrome of inappropriate secretion of antidiuretic hormone (SIADH). DM, November, 1973.
16. Baum, J. K., Holtz, F., Brookstein, J. J., and Klein, E. W.: Possible association between benign hepatomas and oral contraceptives. Lancet, 2:926, 1973.
17. Becker, C. E., MacGregor, R. R., Walker, K. S., and Jandl, J. H.: Fatal anaphylaxis after intramuscular iron-dextran. Ann. Intern. Med., 65:745, 1966.
18. Beeson, P. B., and McDermott, W., eds.: Textbook of Medicine, 13th ed., Philadelphia, W. B. Saunders Co., 1971.
19. Belkin, G.: Cocktail purpura: An unusual case of quinine sensitivity. Ann. Intern. Med., 66:583, 1967.
20. Beller, B. M., Trevino, A., and Urban, E.: Pitressin-induced myocardial injury and depression in a young woman. Am. J. Med., 51:675, 1971.
21. Belloni, C., and Rizzoni, G.: Neurotoxic side-effects of piperazine. Lancet, 2:369, 1967.
22. Benedek, T. G.: Goiter formation as a result of therapy with phenylbutazone and vitamin A. J. Clin. Endocrinol. Metab., 22:959, 1962.
23. Bensinger, T. A., Keller, A. R., Merrell, L. F., and O'Leary, D. S.: Thorotrast-induced reticuloendothelial blockade in man: Clinical equivalent of the experimental model associated with patent pneumococcal septicemia. Am. J. Med., 51:663, 1971.
24. Berger, S., Downey, J. L., Traisman, H. S., and Metz, R.: Mechanism of the cortisone-modified glucose tolerance test. New Eng. J. Med., 274:1460, 1966.
25. Bergman, L. A., Ellison, M. R., and Dunea, G.: Acute renal failure after drip-infusion pyelography. New Eng. J. Med., 279:1277, 1968.
26. Berkowitz, S., Parrish, J. E., and Field, J. B.: Factitious hypoglycemia: Why not diagnose before laparotomy? Am. J. Med., 51:669, 1971.
27. Bernstein, S., and Leff, R.: Toxic psychosis from sleeping medicines containing scopolamine. New Eng. Med. J., 277:638, 1967.
28. Beutler, E.: Drug-induced hemolytic anemia. Pharmacol. Rev., 21:73, 1969.
29. Bialostozky, D., Contreras, R., Tinajeros, C. A., et al.: Gastrointestinal hemorrhagic necrosis: Report of ten cases. Am. J. Med., 46:90, 1969.
30. Bianchine, J. R., Macaraeg, P. V. J., Lasagna, L., et al.: Drugs as etiologic factors in the Stevens-Johnson syndrome. Am. J. Med., 44:390, 1968.
31. Blereau, R. P., and Weingarten, C. M.: Diabetic acidosis secondary to steroid therapy. New Eng. J. Med., 271:836, 1964.
32. Blomgren, S. E., Condemi, J. J., and Vaughan, J. H.: Procainamide-induced lupus erythematosus: Clinical and laboratory observations. Am. J. Med., 52:338, 1972.
33. Bloom, M. E., Mintz, D. H., and Field, J. B.: Insulin-induced posthypoglycemic hyperglycemia as a cause of "brittle" diabetes: Clinical clues and therapeutic implications. Am. J. Med., 47:891, 1969.

34. Bodman, S. F., and Condemi, J. J.: Mediastinal widening in iatrogenic Cushing's syndrome. Ann. Intern. Med., 67:399, 1967.
35. Bohnen, R. F., Ultmann, J. E., Gorman, J. G., et al.: The direct Coomb's test: Its clinical significance: Study in a large university hospital. Ann. Intern. Med., 68:19, 1968.
36. Boréus, L. O., and Sundström, B.: Intracranial hypertension in a child during treatment with nalidixic acid. Br. Med. J., 2:744, 1967.
37. Boulos, B. M., and Davis, L. E.: Hazard of simultaneous administration of phenothiazine and piperazine. New Eng. J. Med., 280:1245, 1969.
38. Bowie, E. J. W., Todd, M., Thompson, J. H., et al.: Anticoagulant malingerers (the "Dicumarol-Eaters"). Am. J. Med., 39:855, 1965.
39. Brauer, M. J., and Dameshek, W.: Hypoplastic anemia and myeloblastic leukemia following chloramphenicol therapy: Report of three cases. New Eng. J. Med., 277:1003, 1967.
40. Breckenridge, A., Dollery, C. T., Worlledge, S. M., et al.: Positive direct Coombs' tests and antinuclear factor in patients treated with methyldopa. Lancet, 2:1365, 1967.
41. Breckenridge, A., Welborn, T. A., Dollery, C. T., et al.: Glucose tolerance in hypertensive patients on long term diuretic therapy. Lancet, 1:61, 1967.
42. Brennan, M. F., Clarke, A. M., and Macbeth, W. A. A. G.: Infarction of the midgut associated with oral contraceptives. New Eng. J. Med., 279:1213, 1968.
43. Brookler, M. I.: Vascular bruits and oral contraceptives. New Eng. J. Med., 276:1386, 1967.
44. Buchner, L. H., and Schneierson, S. S.: Clinical and laboratory aspects of Listeria monocytogenes infections. Am. J. Med., 45:904, 1968.
45. Burgess, J. L., and Birchall, R.: Nephrotoxicity of amphotericin B, with emphasis on changes in tubular function. Am. J. Med., 53:77, 1972.
46. Burns, R. P.: Delayed onset of chloroquine retinopathy. New Eng. J. Med., 275:693, 1966.
47. Burrows, B., Niden, A. H., and Barclay, W. R.: Goiter and myxedema due to iodide administration. Ann. Intern. Med., 52:858, 1960.
48. Burton, J. R., Lichtenstein, N. S., Colvin, R. B., et al.: Acute interstitial nephritis from oxacillin. Johns Hopkins Med. J., 134:58, 1974.
49. Buskop, J. J., Price, M., and Molnar, I.: Untoward effects of diazepam. New Eng. J. Med., 277:316, 1967.
50. Canada, A. T., and Burka, E. R.: Aplastic anemia after indomethacin. New Eng. J. Med., 278:743, 1968.
51. Canfield, C. J., and Bates, R. W.: Nonpuerperal galactorrhea. New Eng. J. Med., 273:897, 1965.
52. Carey, R. M., Coleman, M., and Feder, A.: Pericardial tamponade: A major manifestation of hydralazine-induced lupus syndrome. Am. J. Med., 54:84, 1973.
53. Carr, R. E., and Henkind, P.: Ocular manifestations of ethambutol. Arch. Ophthalmol., 67:566, 1962.
54. Carson, P. E., and Frischer, H.: Glucose-6-phosphate dehydrogenase deficiency and related disorders of the pentose phosphate pathway. Am. J. Med., 41:744, 1966.
55. Carter, S. A.: Potentiation of the effect of orally administered anticoagulants by phenyramidol hydrochloride. New Eng. J. Med., 273:423, 1965.
56. Cassileth, P. A.: Monocytosis in chlorpromazine-associated agranulocytosis. Am. J. Med., 43:471, 1967.
56a. Catz, C. S., and Abuelo, D.: Drugs and pregnancy. Drug Ther., April:79, 1974.
57. Charytan, C., and Purtilo, D.: Glomerular capillary thrombosis and acute renal failure after epsilon-amino caproic acid therapy. New Eng. J. Med., 280:1102, 1969.
58. Cheever, A. W., Valsamis, M. D., and Rabson, A. S.: Necrotizing toxoplasmic encephalitis and herpetic pneumonia complicating treated Hodgkin's disease. New Eng. J. Med., 272:26, 1965.
59. Chernoff, R. W., Wallen, M. H., and Müller, O. F.: Cardiac toxicity of methylphenidate: Report of two cases. New Eng. J. Med., 266:400, 1962.
60. Chokas, W. V.: Bilateral adrenal hemorrhage complicating dicoumarol therapy for myocardial infarction. Am. J. Med., 24:454, 1958.

61. Clinicopathological Conference: Generalized seizures following isoniazid therapy for tuberculosis in a patient with uremia. Am. J. Med., 53:765, 1972.
62. Clinicopathological Conference: Thyroid storm shortly after ^{131}I therapy of a toxic multinodular goiter. Am. J. Med., 52:786, 1972.
63. Cluff, L. E., and Johnson, J. E.: Drug fever. Progr. Allergy, 8:149, 1964.
64. Cohen, A. B.: Hyperkalemic effect of triamterene. Ann. Intern. Med., 65:521, 1966.
65. Cohn, G. A.: Pseudotumor cerebri in children secondary to administration of adrenal steroids. J. Neurosurg., 20:784, 1963.
66. Cohen, M. I., Winslow, P. R., and Boley, S. J.: Intestinal obstruction associated with cholestyramine therapy. New Eng. J. Med., 280:1285, 1969.
67. Cohen, R. J., Sachs, J. R., Wicker, D., et al.: Methemoglobinemia provoked by malerial chemoprophylaxis in Vietnam. New Eng. J. Med., 279:1127, 1968.
68. Cohen, T., and Creger, W. P.: Acute myeloid leukemia following seven years of aplastic anemia induced by chloramphenicol. Am. J. Med., 43:762, 1967.
68a. Cohlan, S. Q., Bevelander, G., and Tiamsic, T.: Growth inhibition of prematures receiving tetracycline. Am. J. Dis. Child., 105:453, 1963.
69. Collaborative Group for the Study of Stroke in Young Women: Oral contraception and increased risk of cerebral ischemia or thrombosis. New Eng. J. Med., 288:871, 1973.
70. Condemi, J. J., Moore-Jones, D., Vaughan, J. H., et al.: Antinuclear antibodies following hydralazine toxicity. New Eng. J. Med., 276:486, 1967.
71. Conn, R. D.: Diphenylhydantoin sodium in cardiac arrhythmias. New Eng. J. Med., 272:277, 1965.
72. Copperman, I. J.: Hypersensitivity to tetracycline. Lancet, 2:610, 1967.
73. Corcino, J. J., Waxman, S., and Herbert, V.: Absorption and malabsorption of vitamin B_{12}. Am. J. Med., 48:562, 1970.
74. Corley, C. C., Lessner, H. E., and Larsen, W. E.: Azathioprine therapy of "autoimmune diseases." Am. J. Med., 41:404, 1966.
75. Cotzias, G. C., Papavasiliou, P. S., and Gellene, R.: Modification of parkinsonism – chronic treatment with L-dopa. New Eng. J. Med., 280:337, 1969.
76. Covey, G. W., and Whitlock, H. H.: Intoxication resulting from the administration of massive doses of vitamin D. Ann. Intern. Med., 25:508, 1946.
77. Cram, D. L.: Life-threatening drug eruptions. Drug Ther., December:31–39, 1973.
78. Crammer, J. L., and Elkes, A.: Agranulocytosis after desipramine. Lancet, 1:105, 1967.
79. Cranswick, E. H., Simpson, G. M., and Nies, A.: An abnormal thyroid finding produced by a phenothiazine. J.A.M.A., 181:554, 1962.
80. Crill, W. E.: Carbamazepine. Ann. Intern. Med., 79:844, 1973.
81. Croft, J. D., Swisher, S. N., Gilliland, B. C., et al.: Coombs'-test positivity induced by drugs: Mechanisms of immunologic reactions and red cell destruction. Ann. Intern. Med., 68:176, 1968.
82. Cruz, T., Reboucas, G., and Rocha, H.: Fatal strongyloidiasis in patients receiving corticosteroids. New Eng. J. Med., 275:1093, 1966.
83. Cunliffe, W. J., and Shuster, S.: Effect of thiabendazole on muscle. Lancet, 1:579, 1967.
84. Current Concepts in Therapy: Tranquilizers, III: Meprobamate, phenaglycodol and chlordiazepoxide. New Eng. J. Med., 264:870, 1961.
85. Daly, R. J., Kane, F. J., and Ewing, J. A.: Psychosis associated with the use of a sequential contraceptive. Lancet, 2:444, 1967.
86. D'Arcy, P. F., and Griffin, J. P.: Iatrogenic Diseases. London, Oxford University Press, 1972.
87. Da Silva, Horta J., Abbott, J. D., Cayolla da Motta, L., et al.: Malignancy and other late effects following administration of thorotrast. Lancet, 2:201, 1965.
88. Davidoff, F., Tishler, S., and Rosoff, C.: Marked hyperlipidemia and pancreatitis associated with oral contraceptive therapy. New Eng. J. Med., 289:552, 1973.
88a. Davidson, M. B., Bozarth, W. R., Challoner, D. R., et al.: Phenformin, hypoglycemia and lactic acidosis. New Eng. J. Med., 275:886, 1966.
89. Davies, D. M., and Cavanagh, J.: Jaundice from potassium p-aminobenzoate. Lancet, 1:896, 1967.

90. Dees, S. C., and McKay, H. W.: Occurrence of pseudotumor cerebri (benign intracranial hypertension) during treatment of children with asthma by adrenal steroids. Pediatrics, 23:1143, 1959.
91. De Fronzo, R. A., Braine, H., Colvin, O. M., et al.: Water intoxication in man after cyclophosphamide therapy. Ann. Intern. Med., 78:861, 1973.
92. De Moura, M. C., Correia, J. P., and Madeira, F.: Clinical alcohol hypoglycemia. Ann. Intern. Med., 66:893, 1967.
93. Dencker, S. J., and Enoksson, P.: Ocular changes produced by chlorpromazine. Acta Ophthalmol., 44:397, 1966.
94. Doak, P. B., Montgomerie, J. Z., North, J. D. K., et al.: Reticulum cell sarcoma after renal transplantation and azathioprine and prednisone therapy. Br. Med. J., 4:746, 1968.
95. Dobkin, A. B., Israel, J. S., and Pieloch, P. A.: The metabolic response to pentazocine as a supplement to balanced anesthesia for major abdominal surgery. Canad. Anaesth. Soc. J., 17:485, 1970.
96. Doherty, J. E.: Digitalis glycocides. Pharmacokinetics and their clinical implications. Ann. Intern. Med., 79:229, 1973.
97. Domar, M., and Juhlin, L.: Allergic dermatitis produced by oral clioquinol. Lancet, 1:1165, 1967.
98. Dougan, L., and Woodliff, H. J.: Acute leukemia associated with phenylbutazone treatment: A review of the literature and report of a further case. Med. J. Aust., 1:217, 1965.
99. Douglas, J. B., and Healy, J. K.: Nephrotoxic effects of amphotericin B, including renal tubular acidosis. Am. J. Med., 46:154, 1969.
100. Drug Therapy: Neurologic syndromes associated with antipsychotic drug use. New Eng. J. Med., 289:20, 1973.
101. Dujovne, C. A., Chan, C. H., and Zimmerman, H. J.: Sulfonamide hepatic injury: Review of the literature and report of a case due to sulfamethoxazole. New Eng. J. Med., 277:785, 1967.
102. Duvernoy, W. F. C.: Positive phentolamine test in hypertension induced by a nasal decongestant. New Eng. J. Med., 280:877, 1969.
103. Earley, L. E.: Diuretics. New Eng. J. Med., 276:1023, 1967.
104. Ebert, R. V.: Oral anticoagulants and drug interactions. Arch. Intern. Med., 121:373, 1968.
104a. Editorial: Neonatal thrombocytopenia and thiazide drugs. Br. Med., J., 1:1395, 1964.
105. Editorial: Aspirin and gastrointestinal bleeding. Lancet, 2:460, 1967.
106. Editorial: Lithium-induced diabetes insipidus. Br. Med. J., 1:726, 1972.
107. Editorial: Liver tumors and steroid hormones. Lancet, 2:1481, 1973.
108. Eickhoff, T. C., Kislak, J. W., and Finland, M.: Clinical evaluation of nafcillin in patients with severe staphylococcal disease. New Eng. J. Med., 272:699, 1965.
109. Eipe, J., Johnson, S. A., Kiamko, R. T., et al.: Hypoparathyroidism following ^{131}I therapy for hyperthyroidism. Arch. Intern. Med., 121:270, 1968.
110. Eisert, J., Hannibal, J. E., and Sanders, S. L.: Fatal amebiasis complicating corticosteroid management of pemphigus vulgaris. New Eng. J. Med., 261:843, 1959.
111. Eisner, E. V., and Kasper, K.: Immune thrombocytopenia due to a metabolite of para-aminosalicylic acid. Am. J. Med., 53:790, 1972.
112. Elkington, S. G., Goffinet, J. A., and Conn, H. O.: Renal and hepatic injury associated with methoxyflurane anesthesia. Ann. Intern. Med., 69:1229, 1968.
113. Emmer, M., and DeVita, V. T.: Pneumocystis carinii pneumonia and pentamidine isethionate toxicity. Ann. Intern. Med., 69:637, 1968.
114. Epstein, D. L., and Paton, D.: Keratitis from misuse of corneal anesthetics. New Eng. J. Med., 279:396, 1968.
115. Epstein, E. L., and Braunwald, W.: Beta-adrenergic receptor blockade: Propranolol and related drugs. Ann. Intern. Med., 67:1333, 1967.
116. Erlanger, H.: Cardiac arrhythmias in relationship to anesthesia: Past and present concepts. Am. J. Med. Sci., 243:651, 1962.
117. Erslev, A. J.: Drug-induced blood dyscrasias: I. Aplastic anemia. J.A.M.A., 188:531, 1964.
118. Eyster, M. E.: Melphalan (Alkeran) erythrocyte agglutinin and hemolytic anemia. Ann. Intern. Med., 66:573, 1967.

119. Fell, S. C., Rubin, I. L., Enselberg, C. D., et al.: Anticoagulant-induced hemopericardium with tamponade: Its occurrence in the absence of myocardial infarction or pericarditis. New Eng. J. Med., 272:670, 1965.
120. Field, J. B., Ohta, M., Boyle, C., et al.: Potentiation of acetohexamide hypoglycemia by phenylbutazone. New Eng. J. Med., 277:889, 1967.
121. Finster, M., and Poppers, P. J.: Fetal intoxication after local anesthesia during delivery. New Eng. J. Med., 272:696, 1965.
122. Fitzpatrick, T. B., Arndt, K. A., Clark, W. H., et al.: Dermatology in General Medicine. New York, McGraw-Hill Book Co., 1971.
123. Fleischer, N., Brown, H., Graham, D. Y., et al.: Chronic laxative-induced hyperaldosteronism and hypokalemia simulating Bartter's syndrome. Ann. Intern. Med., 70:791, 1969.
124. Fries, J., and Siraganian, R.: Sulfonamide hepatitis: Report of a case due to sulfamethoxazole and sulfisoxazole. New Eng. J. Med., 274:95, 1966.
125. Fulop, M., and Drapkin, A.: Potassium-depletion syndrome secondary to nephropathy apparently caused by "outdated tetracycline." New Eng. J. Med., 272:986, 1965.
126. Furey, W. W., and Tan, C.: Anaphylactic shock due to oral demethylchlortetracycline. Ann. Intern. Med., 70:357, 1969.
127. Furuyama, M. and Matsuda, I.: Chloramphenicol and jaundice in a baby. Lancet, 2:366, 1967.
128. Gams, R. A., Neal, J. A., and Conrad, F. G.: Hydantoin-induced pseudopseudolymphoma. Ann. Intern. Med., 69:557, 1968.
129. Gangarosa, E. J., Johnson, T. R., and Ramos, H. S.: Ristocetin-induced thrombocytopenia: Site and mechanism of action. Arch. Intern. Med., 105:83, 1960.
130. Gardner, A. J.: Withdrawal fits in barbiturate addicts. Lancet, 2:337, 1967.
131. Gault, M. H., Blennerhassett, J., and Muehrcke, R. C.: Analgesic nephropathy: A clinicopathologic study using electron microscopy. Am. J. Med., 51:740, 1971.
132. Gazes, P. C., Holmes, C. R., Moseley, V., et al.: Acute hemorrhage and necrosis of the intestines associated with digitalization. Circulation, 23:358, 1961.
133. Gazzaniga, A. B., and Stewart, D. R.: Possible quinidine-induced hemorrhage in a patient on warfarin sodium. New Eng. J. Med., 280:711, 1969.
134. Gesztes, T.: Prolonged apnoea after suxamethonium injection associated with eye drops containing an anticholinesterase agent. Br. J. Anaesth., 38:408, 1966.
135. Gianelly, R., vonder Groeben, J. O., Spivack, A. P., et al.: Effect of lidocaine on ventricular arrhythmias in patients with coronary heart disease. New Eng. J. Med., 277:1215, 1967.
136. Gill, F. A., and Hook, E. W.: Changing patterns of bacterial resistance to antimicrobial drugs. Am. J. Med., 39:780, 1965.
137. Gipstein, R. M., and Boyle, J. D.: Hypernatremia complicating prolonged mannitol diuresis. New Eng. J. Med., 272:1116, 1965.
138. Glontz, G. E., and Saslaw, S.: Methyldopa fever. Arch. Intern. Med., 122:445, 1968.
139. Gold, G. N., and Richardson, A. P.: An unusual case of neuromuscular blockade seen with therapeutic blood levels of colistin methanesulfonate (Coly-Mycin). Am. J. Med., 41:316, 1966.
140. Goldfischer, J. D.: Acute myocardial infarction secondary to ergot therapy. New Eng. J. Med., 262:860, 1960.
141. Goldstein, M. J., and Rothenberg, A. J.: Jaundice in a patient receiving acetohexamide. New Eng. J. Med., 275:97, 1966.
142. Gollub, M. J.: Myocardial infarction after the phentolamine test. New Eng. J. Med., 273:37, 1965.
143. Gomes de Carvalho, A.: Where the vision fails. New Eng. J. Med., 273:168, 1965.
144. Good, A. E., Green, R. A., and Zarofonetis, C. J. D.: Rheumatic symptoms during tuberculosis therapy: A manifestation of isoniazid toxicity? Ann. Intern. Med., 63:800, 1965.
145. Goss, J. E., and Dickhaus, D. W.: Increased bishydroxycoumarin requirements in patients receiving phenobarbital. New Eng. J. Med., 273:1094, 1965.
146. Gott, P. H.: Drug reactions simulating tetanus. New Eng. J. Med., 274:167, 1966.
147. Gowans, J. D. C., and Granieri, P. A.: Septic arthritis: Its relation to intra-articular injections of hydrocortisone acetate. New Eng. J. Med., 261:502, 1959.

148. Graf, M., and Tarlov, A.: Agranulocytosis with monohistiocytosis associated with ampicillin therapy. Ann. Intern. Med., 69:91, 1968.
149. Graham, J. R., Suby, H. I., Le Compte, P. R., et al.: Fibrotic disorders associated with methysergide therapy for headache. New Eng. J. Med., 274:359, 1966.
150. Granström, K. O.: Ocular complications of some older drugs: A historical glimpse. Acta Ophthalmol., 44:279, 1966.
151. Greaves, A. A., Larmon, W. A., and Mier, M.: Akinetic mutism after prochlorperazine. New Eng. J. Med., 272:1297, 1965.
152. Greene, M. L., Fujimoto, W. Y., and Seegmiller, J. E.: Urinary xanthine stones — a rare complication of allopurinol therapy. New Eng. J. Med., 280:426, 1969.
153. Gregg, W. I.: Galactorrhea after contraceptive hormones. New Eng. J. Med., 274:1432, 1966.
154. Griffith, G. C., Nichols, G., Asher, J. D., et al.: Heparin osteoporosis. J.A.M.A., 193:91, 1965.
155. Gross, L.: Oxyphenbutazone-induced parotitis. Ann. Intern. Med., 70:1229, 1969.
156. Gutman, R. A., Brunell, J. M., and Solak, F.: Paraldehyde acidosis. Am. J. Med., 42:435, 1967.
157. Gynn, T. N., Messmore, H. L., and Friedman, I. A.: Drug-induced thrombocytopenia. Med. Clin. North Am., 56:65, 1972.
158. Hadden, J. W., and Metzner, R. J.: Pseudoketosis and hyperacetaldehydemia in paraldehyde acidosis. Am. J. Med., 47:642, 1969.
159. Halsted, C. H., and McIntyre, P. A.: Intestinal malabsorption caused by aminosalicylic acid therapy. Arch. Intern. Med., 130:935, 1972.
160. Hardin, J. G.: Steroid-induced morbidity mimicking active systemic lupus erythematosus. Ann. Intern. Med., 78:558, 1973.
161. Harris, P. W. R.: Malignant hypertension associated with oral contraceptives. Lancet, 2:466, 1969.
162. Harris, W. S.: Toxic effects of aerosol propellants on the heart. Arch. Intern. Med., 131:162, 1973.
163. Harris, W. S., and Goodman, R. M.: Hyper-reactivity to atropine in Down's syndrome. New Eng. J. Med., 279:407, 1968.
164. Hazzard, W. R., Spiger, M. J., Bagdade, J. D., et al.: Studies on the mechanism of increased plasma triglyceride levels induced by oral contraceptives. New Eng. J. Med., 280:471, 1969.
165. Heckman, B. A., and Walsh, J. H.: Hypernatremia complicating sodium sulfate therapy for hypercalcemia crisis. New Eng. J. Med., 276:1082, 1967.
166. Hedley-Whyte, E. T., and Craighead, J. E.: Generalized cytomegalic inclusion disease after renal homotransplantation. New Eng. J. Med., 272:473, 1965.
167. Henderson, B. E., Benton, B. D. A., Weaver, P. T., et al.: Stilbestrol and urogenital-tract cancer in adolescents and young adults. New Eng. J. Med., 288:354, 1973.
168. Hepps, S., and Dollinger, M.: Anaphylactic death after administration of a triphenylmethane dye to determine burn depth. New Eng. J. Med., 272:1281, 1965.
169. Hill, R. B., Dahrling, B. E., Starzl, T. E., et. al.: Death after transplantation: An analysis of sixty cases. Am. J. Med., 42:327, 1967.
170. Hilton, J. G., and Kessler, E.: Toxic reactions to ethacrynic acid, a new oral diuretic. J. New Drugs, 4:93–97, 1964.
171. Hoefnagel, E.: Toxic effects of atropine and homatropine eyedrops in children. New Eng. J. Med., 264:168, 1961.
172. Hudgson, P., Foster, J. B., and Walton, J. N.: Methysergide and coronary artery disease. Lancet, 1:444, 1967.
173. Hunton, R. B., Wells, M. V., and Skipper, E. W.: Hypothyroidism in diabetics treated with sulphonylurea. Lancet, 2:449, 1965.
174. Hurst, J. W., and Logue, R. B.: The Heart, 2nd ed., New York, McGraw-Hill Book Co., 1970, pp. 463–466.
175. Ingall, D., Sherman, J. D., Cockburn, F., et al.: Amelioration by ingestion of phenylalanine of toxic effects of chloramphenicol on bone marrow. New Eng. J. Med., 272:180, 1965.
176. Irons, G. V., Ginn, W. N., and Orgain, E. S.: Use of a beta adrenergic receptor blocking agent (propranolol) in the treatment of cardiac arrhythmias. Am. J. Med., 43:161, 1967.
177. Ison, A. E., and Tucker, J. B.: Photosensitivity from soaps. New Eng. J. Med., 278:81, 1968.

178. Jaffe, I. A., Treser, G., Suzuki, Y., et al.: Nephropathy induced by D-penicillamine. Ann. Intern. Med., 69:549, 1968.
179. Janower, M. L., Sidel, V. W., Baker, W. H., et al.: Late clinical and laboratory manifestations of thorotrast administration in cerebral arteriography: A follow-up study of thirty patients. New Eng. J. Med., 279:186, 1968.
180. Johnson, B. F.: Hemochromatosis resulting from prolonged oral iron therapy. New Eng. J. Med., 278:1100, 1968.
181. Johnson, F. L., Feagler, J. R., Lerner, K. G., et al.: Association of androgenic-anabolic steroid therapy with development of hepatocellular carcinoma. Lancet, 2:1273, 1972.
182. Johnson, H. K., and Waterhouse, C.: Lactic acidosis and phenformin: Report of two successfully treated patients. Arch. Intern. Med., 122:367, 1968.
183. Jones, C. C.: Megaloblastic anemia associated with long-term tetracycline therapy. Ann. Intern. Med., 78:910, 1973.
184. Kalowski, S., Nanra, R. S., Mathew, T. H., et al.: Deterioration in renal function in association with co-trimoxazole therapy. Lancet, 1:394, 1973.
185. Kanich, R. E., and Craighead, J. E.: Cytomegalovirus infection and cytomegalic inclusion disease in renal homotransplant recipients. Am. J. Med., 40:874, 1966.
186. Kaplan, J. M., and Barrett, O.: Reversible pseudo-Pelger anomaly related to sulfisoxazole therapy. New Eng. J. Med., 277:421, 1967.
187. Kaplan, K., Reisberg, B., and Weinstein, L.: Cephaloridine: Studies of therapeutic activity and untoward effects. Arch. Intern. Med., 121:17, 1968.
188. Kass, E. H., Geiman, Q. M., and Finland, M.: Effects of ACTH on induced malaria in man. New Eng. J. Med., 245:1000, 1951.
189. Kastor, J. A., and Yurchak, P. M.: Recognition of digitalis intoxication in the presence of atrial fibrillation. Ann. Intern. Med., 67:1045, 1967.
190. Kattus, A. A., Bicoe, B. W., Dashe, A. M., et al.: Spurious heart disease induced by digitalis-containing reducing pills. Arch. Intern. Med., 122:298, 1968.
191. Kawanishi, H., Rudolph, E., and Bull, F. E.: Azathioprine-induced acute pancreatitis. New Eng. J. Med., 289:357, 1973.
192. Keighley, J. F.: Iatrogenic asthma associated with adrenergic aerosols. Ann. Intern. Med., 65:985, 1966.
193. Kelly, D. R., Nilo, E. R., and Berggren, R. B.: Deafness after topical neomycin wound irrigation. New Eng. J. Med., 280:1338, 1969.
194. Kennedy, B. J.: Metabolic and toxic effects of mithramycin during tumor therapy. Am. J. Med., 49:494, 1970.
195. Keyes, J. W., Drake, E. H., and Smith, F. J.: Survival rates after acute myocardial infarction and long-term anticoagulant therapy. Circulation, 14:254, 1956.
196. Kilpatrick, Z. M., Silverman, J. F., Betancourt, E., et al.: Vascular occlusion of the colon and oral contraceptives: Possible relation. New Eng. J. Med., 278:438, 1968.
197. Kincaid-Smith, P.: Pathogenesis of the renal lesion associated with the abuse of analgesics. Lancet, 1:859, 1967.
198. Kirshbaum, B. A., Beerman, H., and Stahl, E. B.: Drug eruptions: A review of some of the recent literature. Am. J. Med. Sci., 240:512, 1960.
199. Klatskin, G.: Toxic and drug-induced hepatitis. In Schiff, L., ed., Diseases of the Liver, 3rd ed., Philadelphia, J. B. Lippincott Co., 1969.
200. Klatskin, G., and Kimberg, D. V.: Recurrent hepatitis attributable to halothane sensitization in an anesthetist. New Eng. J. Med., 280:515, 1969.
201. Knight, A. H., and Parkinson, T.: Diuretic induced hyperkalemia. Lancet, 1:446, 1967.
202. Kochar, M. S., and Wang, R. I. H.: Considerations in the prevention and care of drug-induced liver damage. Drug Ther., 3:90, 1973.
203. Koch-Weser, J.: Coumarin necrosis. Ann. Intern. Med., 68:1365, 1968.
204. Koch-Weser, J.: Quinidine-induced hypoprothrombinemic hemorrhage in patients on chronic warfarin therapy. Ann. Intern. Med., 68:511, 1968.
205. Koch-Weser, J., and Gilmore, E. B.: Benign intracranial hypertension in an adult after tetracycline therapy. J.A.M.A., 200:345, 1967.
206. Kontos, H. A.: Myopathy associated with chronic colchicine toxicity. New Eng. J. Med., 266:38, 1962.
207. Koutsoulieris, E.: Granulopenia and thrombocytopenia after ethosuximide. Lancet, 2:310, 1967.

208. Krawitt, E. L., and Bloomer, A. A.: Increased cerebrospinal-fluid protein secondary to hypercalcemia of the milk-alkali syndrome. New Eng. J. Med., 273:154, 1965.
209. Krisko, I., Lewis, E., and Johnson, J. E.: Severe hyperthermia due to tranylcypromine-amphetamine toxicity. Ann. Intern. Med., 70:559, 1969.
210. Kunelis, C. T., Peters, J. L., and Edmondson, H. A.: Fatty liver of pregnancy and its relationship to tetracycline therapy. Am. J. Med., 38:359, 1965.
211. Kutt, H., Winter, W., and McDowell, F. H.: Depression of parahydroxylation of diphenylhydantoin by antituberculosis chemotherapy. Neurology, 16:594, 1966.
212. Kyle, R. A., Schwartz, R. S., Oliner, H. L., et al.: A syndrome resembling adrenal cortical insufficiency associated with long term busulfan (Myleran) therapy. Blood, 18:497, 1961.
213. Lampe, W. T.: Hypoglycemia due to acetohexamide. Arch. Intern. Med., 120:239, 1967.
214. Langer, T., and Levy, R. I.: Acute muscular syndrome associated with administration of clofibrate. New Eng. J. Med., 279:856, 1968.
215. Lappat, E. J., and Cawein, M. J.: A familial study of procainamide-induced systemic lupus erythematosus. Am. J. Med., 45:846, 1968.
216. Laragh, J. H.: The proper use of newer diuretics. Ann. Intern. Med., 67:606, 1967.
217. Laszlo, M. H.: Constrictive pericarditis as a sequel to hemopericardium: Report of a case following anticoagulant therapy. Ann. Intern. Med., 46:403, 1957.
218. Lederman, R. J., Davis, F. B., and Davis, P. J.: Exchange transfusion as treatment of acute hepatic failure to antituberculosis drugs. Ann. Intern. Med., 68:830, 1968.
219. Lee, S. L., Rivero, I., and Siegel, M.: Activation of systemic lupus erythematosus by drugs. Arch. Intern. Med., 117:620, 1966.
220. Leedom, J. M., Ivler, D., Mathies, A. W., et al.: Importance of sulfadiazine resistance in meningococcal disease in civilians. New Eng. J. Med., 273:1395, 1965.
221. Leonards, J. R., Levy, G., and Niemczura, R.: Gastrointestinal blood loss during prolonged aspirin administration. New Eng. J. Med., 289:1020, 1973.
222. Leopold, I. H.: Ocular complications of drugs: Visual changes. J.A.M.A., 205:631, 1968.
223. Levine, P. H., and Weintraub, L. R.: Pseudoleukemia during recovery from dapsone-induced agranulocytosis. Ann. Intern. Med., 68:1060, 1968.
224. Levine, R. J., and Strauch, B. S.: Hypertensive responses to methyldopa. New Eng. J. Med., 275:946, 1966.
225. Lieberman, F. L., and Bateman, J. R.: Megaloblastic anemia possibly induced by triamterene in patients with alcoholic cirrhosis: Two case reports. Ann. Intern. Med., 68:168, 1968.
226. Liljestrand, A.: Ocular side effects of new drugs: Some viewpoints. Acta Ophthalmol., 44:283, 1966.
227. Lindenbaum, J., and Hargrove, R. L.: Thrombocytopenia in alcoholics. Ann. Intern. Med., 68:526, 1968.
228. Lindesmith, L. A., Baines, R. D., Bigelow, D. B., et al.: Reversible respiratory paralysis associated with polymyxin therapy. Ann. Intern. Med., 68:318, 1968.
229. Littman, M. L.: Cryptococcosis (Torulosis): Current concepts and therapy. Am. J. Med., 27:976, 1959.
230. Lo Buglio, A. F., and Jandl, J. H.: The nature of the alpha-methyldopa red-cell antibody. New Eng. J. Med., 276:658, 1967.
231. Lockey, R. F., Rucknagel, D. L., and Vanselow, N. A.: Familial occurrence of asthma, nasal polyps, and aspirin intolerance. Ann. Intern. Med., 78:57, 1973.
232. Logan, G. B.: Use of steroids in allergic respiratory diseases in children. Pediatr. Clin. North Am., 6:745, 1959.
233. Lopes, V. M.: Cyclophosphamide nephrotoxicity in man. Lancet, 1:1060, 1967.
234. Loughnan, P. M., Gold, H., and Vance, J. C.: Phenytoin teratogenicity in man. Lancet, 1:70, 1973.
235. Lucena, G. E., Bennett, W. M., and Pierre, R. V.: "Dewlap," a corticosteroid induced episternal fatty tumor. New Eng. J. Med., 275:834, 1966.
236. McCawley, A.: Cortisone habituation—a clinic note. New Eng. J. Med., 273:976, 1965.
237. McCombs, R. P., Patterson, J. F., and MacMahon, H. E.: Syndromes associated with "allergic" vasculitis. New Eng. J. Med., 255:251, 1956.

238. McGrath, M. D., and Paley, R. G.: Hypothermia induced in a myxoedematous patient by imipramine hydrochloride. Br. Med. J., 2:1364, 1960.
239. McMillan, D. E., and Freeman, R. B.: The milk alkali syndrome: A study of the acute disorder with comments on the development of the chronic condition. Medicine, 44:485, 1965.
240. McQueen, A.: Skin diseases. In D'Arcy, P. F., and Griffin, J. P., Iatrogenic Diseases, London, Oxford University Press, 1972.
241. Macoul, K. L.: Hepatitis due to sulfamethoxazole. New Eng. J. Med., 275:39, 1966.
242. Maddrey, W. C., and Boitnott, J. K.: Isoniazid hepatitis. Ann. Intern. Med., 79:1, 1973.
243. Mailloux, L., Schwartz, C. D., Capizzi, R., et. al.: Acute renal failure after administration of low-molecular weight dextran. New Eng. J. Med., 277:1113, 1967.
244. Main, R. A.: Polymorphic light eruptions. Practitioner, 196:654, 1966.
245. Mandell, G. L.: Cephaloridine. Ann. Intern. Med., 79:561, 1973.
246. Manninen, V., Apajalahti, A., Melin, J., et al.: Altered absorption of digoxin in patients given propantheline and metoclopramide. Lancet, 1:398, 1973.
247. Marco, J., Calle, C., Roman, D., et al.: Hyperglucaganism induced by glucocorticoid treatment in man. New Eng. J. Med., 288:128, 1973.
248. Martinez-Maldonado, M., and Torrell, J.: Lithium carbonate-induced nephrogenic diabetes insipidus and glucose intolerance. Arch. Intern. Med., 132:881, 1973.
249. Mast, W. H.: Neuropathy due to furaltadone. New Eng. J. Med., 263:963, 1960.
250. Mathalone, M. B. R., and Easty, D. L.: Acute keratitis in psoriatic patients using triacetoxyanthracene. Lancet, 2:195, 1967.
251. Mathog, R. H., and Klein, W. J.: Ototoxicity of ethacrynic acid and aminoglycoside antibiotics in uremia. New Eng. J. Med., 280:1223, 1969.
252. Mengel, C. E., Frei, E., and Nachman, R., eds.,: Hemotology: Principles and Practice. Chicago, Year Book Medical Publishers, Inc., 1972.
253. Michael, A. F., Vernier, R. L., Drummond, K. N., et al.: Immunosuppressive therapy of chronic renal disease. New Eng. J. Med., 276:817, 1967.
254. Michelson, E.: Anaphylactic reaction to dextrans. New Eng. J. Med., 278:552, 1968.
255. Miller, C. G., and Carpenter, R.: Neurotoxic side-effects of piperazine. Lancet, 1:895, 1967.
256. Miller, J. J., Williams, G. F., and Leissring, J. C.: Multiple late complications of therapy with cyclophosphamide, including ovarian destruction. Am. J. Med., 50:530, 1971.
257. Molthan, L., Reidenberg, M. M., and Eichman, M. F.: Positive direct Coombs' test due to cephalothin. New Eng. J. Med., 277:123, 1967.
258. Monson, R. R., Rosenberg, L., Hartz, S. C., et al.: Diphenylhydantoin and selected congenital malformations. New Eng. J. Med., 289:1049, 1973.
258a. Morrelli, H. F.: Propranolol. Ann. Intern. Med., 78:913, 1973.
259. Muenter, M. D., Perry, H. D., and Ludwig, J.: Chronic vitamin A intoxication in adults. Am. J. Med., 50:129, 1971.
260. Muller, S. A.: Hirsutism. Am. J. Med., 46:803, 1969.
261. Murray, I. P. C., and Stewart, R. D. H.: Iodine goiter. Lancet, 1:922, 1967.
262. Murray, M. J., and Kronenberg, R.: Pulmonary reactions simulating pulmonary edema caused by nitrofurantoin. New Eng. J. Med., 273:1185, 1965.
263. Mustala, O. and Toivonen, S.: Glucose tolerance and diuretics. Lancet, 1:901, 1967.
264. Myers, E. N., Berstein, J. M., and Fostiropolous, G.: Salicylate ototoxicity: A clinical study. New Eng. J. Med., 273:587, 1965.
265. Nagle, R. E., and Pilcher, J.: Respiratory and circulatory effects of pentazocine. Br. Heart J., 34:244, 1972.
266. Nash, G., Blennerhasset, J. B., and Pontoppidan, H.: Pulmonary lesions associated with oxygen therapy and artificial ventilation. New Eng. J. Med., 276:368, 1967.
267. Nicklaus, T. M., and Snyder, A. B.: Nitrofurantoin pulmonary reaction: A unique syndrome. Arch. Intern. Med., 121:151, 1968.
268. Ockner, R. K., and Davidson, C. S.: Hepatic effects of oral contraceptives. New Eng. J. Med., 276:331, 1967.
269. Oravetz, J., and Slodki, S. J.: Recurrent ventricular fibrillation precipitated by quinidine. Arch. Intern. Med., 122:63, 1968.

270. O'Reilly, R. A.: Interaction of sodium warfarin and disulfiram (Antabuse) in man. Ann. Intern. Med., 78:73, 1973.
271. Ortuño, J., and Botella, J.: Recurrent acute renal failure induced by phenazone hypersensitivity. Lancet, 2:1473, 1973.
272. Parfitt, A. M.: Acetazolamide and sodium bicarbonate induced nephrocalcinosis and nephrolithiasis. Arch. Intern. Med., 124:736, 1969.
273. Parfitt, A. M.: Chlorothiazide-induced hypercalcemia in juvenile osteoporosis and hyperparathyroidism. New Eng. J. Med., 281:55, 1969.
274. Parry, E. H. O., Bryceson, A. D. M., and Leithead, C. S.: Acute hemodynamic changes during treatment of louse-borne relapsing fever. Lancet, 1:81, 1967.
275. Penman, H. G.: Lymphadenopathy after phenylbutazone. Lancet, 1:513, 1967.
276. Perlman, L. V.: Salicylate intoxication from skin application. New Eng. J. Med., 274:164, 1966.
277. Perry, H. M.: Late toxicity to hydralazine resembling systemic lupus erythematosus or rheumatoid arthritis. Am. J. Med., 54:58, 1973.
278. Peters, R. L., Edmondson, H. A., Reynolds, T. B., et al.: Hepatic necrosis associated with halothane anesthesia. Am. J. Med., 47:748, 1969.
279. Peterson, H. D.: Association of trimethadione therapy and myasthenia gravis. New Eng. J. Med., 274:506, 1966.
280. Petz, L. D., and Fudenberg, H. H.: Coombs'-positive hemolytic anemia caused by penicillin administration. New Eng. J. Med., 274:171, 1966.
281. Pickering, D.: Hepatic necrosis after chlordiazepoxide therapy. New Eng. J. Med., 274:1449, 1966.
282. Pilewski, R. M., Ellis, L. D., Sapira, J. D., et al.: Oxyphenbutazone and aplastic anemia. Am. J. Med., 53:693, 1972.
283. Pillay, V. K. G., Schwartz, F. D., Aimi, K., et al.: Transient and permanent deafness following treatment with ethacrynic acid in renal failure. Lancet, 1:77, 1969.
284. Plunkett, T. G., Haslock, D. I., and Golding, J. R.: Lymphadenopathy after phenylbutazone. Lancet, 1:448, 1967.
285. Pollack, H.: Nicotinic acid and diabetes. Diabetes, 11:144, 1962.
286. Poole, G. W., and Schneeweiss, J.: Peripheral neuropathy due to ethionamide. Am. Rev. Resp. Dis., 84:890, 1961.
287. Propp, R. P., and Stillman, J. S.: Agranulocytosis and hydroxychloroquine. New Eng. J. Med., 277:492, 1967.
288. Rabinowitz, H., and Halpern, S. R.: Drug allergy in pediatric practice. J. Pediatr., 56:75, 1960.
289. Raskin, N. H., and Fishman, R. A.: Pyridoxine-deficiency neuropathy due to hydralazine. New Eng. J. Med., 273:1182, 1965.
290. Ricker, R. B., and Hynes, H. E.: Pure red blood cell aplasia associated with chlorpropamide therapy. Arch. Intern. Med., 123:445, 1969.
291. Reussi, C., Schiavi, J. E., Altman, R., et al.: Unusual complications in the course of anticoagulant therapy. Am. J. Med., 46:460, 1969.
292. Reyes, M. P., Palutke, M., and Lerner, A. M.: Granulocytopenia associated with carbenicillin: Five episodes in two patients. Am. J. Med., 54:413, 1973.
293. Rifkind, D., Marchioro, T. L., Schneck, S. A., and Hill, R. B.: Systemic fungal infections complicating renal transplantation and immunosuppressive therapy. Am. J. Med., 43:28, 1967.
294. Rizzuto, V. J., Inglesby, T. V., and Grace, W. J.: Probenecid (Benemid) intoxication with status epilepticus. Am. J. Med., 38:646, 1965.
295. Rose, M. S.: Vinca alkaloids and salivary gland pain. Lancet, 1:213, 1967.
296. Rosefsky, J. B., and Petersiel, M. E.: Perinatal deaths associated with mepivacaine paracervical-block anesthesia in labor. New Eng. J. Med., 278:530, 1968.
297. Rosenberg, M. S., and Graettinger, J. S.: Digitalis intoxication—management and prevention. DM, 1:61, 1962.
298. Rosenblum, D., Wessler, S., and Avioli, L. A.: Drug-induced blood dyscrasias. Arch. Intern. Med., 131:750, 1973.
299. Rosenow, E. C.: The spectrum of drug-induced pulmonary disease. Ann. Intern. Med., 77:977, 1972.
300. Rosenow, E. C., DeRemee, R. A., and Dines, D. E.: Chronic nitrofurantoin pulmonary reaction: Report of five cases. New Eng. J. Med., 279:1258, 1968.
301. Rosin, J. M.: Vasculitis following procainamide therapy. Am. J. Med., 42:625, 1967.

302. Rosman, M., and Bertino, J. R.: Azathioprine. Ann. Intern. Med., 79:694, 1973.
303. Rothstein, E., and Clancy, D. D.: Toxicity of disulfiram with metronidazole. New Eng. J. Med., 280:1006, 1969.
304. Rubenstein, C. J.: Peripheral polyneuropathy caused by nitrofurantoin. J.A.M.A., 187:647, 1964.
305. Russek, H. I., and Zohman, B. L.: Anticoagulant therapy in acute myocardial infarction. Am. J. Med. Sci., 225:8, 1953.
306. Russell, P. S.: Kidney transplantation. Am. J. Med., 44:776, 1968.
307. Russell, R. P., and Sullivan, M. A.: The pill and hypertension. Johns Hopkins Med. J., 127:287, 1970.
308. Sabath, L. D., Gerstein, D. A., and Finland, M.: Serum glutamic oxalacetic transaminase: False elevations during administration of erythromycin. New Eng. J. Med., 279:1137, 1968.
309. Schaff, M., and Payne, C. A.: Dystonic reactions to prochlorperazine in hypoparathyroidism. New Eng. J. Med., 275:991, 1966.
310. Schneeweiss, J., and Poole, G. W.: Hyperuricemia due to pyrazinamide. Br. Med. J., 2:830, 1960.
311. Schoonmaker, F. W., Osteen, R. T., and Greenfield, J. C.: Thioridazine (Mellaril)-induced ventricular tachycardia controlled with an artificial pacemaker. Ann. Intern. Med., 65:1076, 1966.
312. Schreiner, G. E., and Maher, J. F.: Toxic nephropathy. Am. J. Med., 38:409, 1965.
313. Schwartz, G. H., David, D. S., Riggio, R. R., et al.: Ototoxicity induced by furosemide. New Eng. J. Med., 282:1413, 1970.
314. Scott, A. J., Nicholson, G. I., and Kerr, A. R.: Lincomycin as a cause of pseudomembranous colitis. Lancet, 2:1232, 1973.
315. Scott, J. L., Cartwright, G. E., and Wintrobe, M. M.: Acquired aplastic anemia: An analysis of thirty-nine cases and review of the pertinent literature. Medicine, 38:119, 1959.
316. Scott, J. L., Finegold, S. M., Belkin, G. A., et al.: A controlled doubleblind study of the hematologic toxicity of chloramphenicol. New Eng. J. Med., 272:1137, 1965.
317. Seamans, K. B., Gloor, P., Dobell, A. R. C., et al.: Penicillin-induced seizures during cardiopulmonary bypass: A clinical and electroencephalographic study. New Eng. J. Med., 278:861, 1968.
318. Seelig, M. S.: The role of antibiotics in the pathogenesis of Candida infections. Am. J. Med., 40:887, 1966.
319. Segal, R. L., Rosenblatt, S., and Eliasoph, I.: Endocrine exophthalmos during lithium therapy of manic-depressive psychosis. New Eng. J. Med., 289:136, 1973.
320. Shackney, S., and Hasson, J.: Precipitous fall in serum calcium, hypotension, and acute renal failure after intravenous phosphate therapy for hypocalcemia: Report of two cases. Ann. Intern. Med., 66:906, 1967.
321. Shafer, N.: Hypotension due to nitroglycerin combined with alcohol. New Eng. J. Med., 273:1169, 1965.
322. Shafey, S., and Scheinberg, P.: Neurological syndromes occurring in patients receiving synthetic steroids (oral contraceptives). Neurology, 16:205, 1966.
323. Shafey, S., and Scheinberg, P.: Vascular headaches and oral contraceptives. Ann. Intern. Med., 65:863, 1966.
324. Shanklin, D. R., and Wolfson, S. L.: Therapeutic oxygen as a possible cause of pulmonary hemorrhage in premature infants. New Eng. J. Med., 277:833, 1967.
325. Sharpe, A. R.: Inhibition of thyroidal I^{131} uptake by parabromdylamine maleate. J. Clin. Endocrinol. Metab., 21:739, 1961.
325a. Shepard, T. H.: Teratogenicity from drugs; An increasing problem. DM, June, 1974.
326. Sherins, R. J., and DeVita, V. T.: Effect of drug treatment for lymphoma on male reproductive capacity: Studies of men in remission after therapy. Ann. Intern. Med., 79:216, 1973.
327. Sherlock, S., Senewiratne, B., Scott, A., et al.: Complications of diuretic therapy in hepatic cirrhosis. Lancet, 1:1049, 1966.
328. Sherwood, L. M.: Hypernatremia during sodium sulfate therapy. New Eng. J. Med., 277:314, 1967.

329. Shorey, J., Schenker, S., Suki, W. N., et al.: Hepatotoxicity of mercaptopurine. Arch. Intern. Med., *122*:54, 1968.
330. Sinclair, J. C., Fox, H. A., Lentz, J. F., et al.: Intoxication of the fetus by a local anesthetic: A newly recognized complication of maternal caudal anesthesia. New Eng. J. Med., *273*:1173, 1965.
331. Singer, I., and Rotenberg, D.: Demeclocycline-induced nephrogenic diabetes insipidus. Ann. Intern. Med., *79*:679, 1973.
332. Sise, H. S.: Potentiation of tolbutamide by dicumarol. Ann. Intern. Med., *67*:460, 1967.
333. Sjöberg, S., and Perers, D.: Leukemia after oxyphenylbutazone. Lancet, *2*:441, 1965.
334. Smith, E., and Gáspár, I. A.: Pentamidine treatment of Pneumocystis carinii pneumonitis in an adult with lymphatic leukemia. Am. J. Med., *44*:626, 1968.
335. Smith, J. W., Johnson, J. E., and Cluff, L. E.: Studies on the epidemiology of adverse drug reactions. II. An evaluation of penicillin allergy. New Eng. J. Med., *274*:998, 1966.
336. Snijder, J. A. M., and Nieweg, H. O.: Acetylsalicylic acid as a cause of pancytopenia from bone marrow damage. Lancet, *2*:768, 1966.
337. Sollaccio, P. A., Ribaudo, C. A., and Grace, W. J.: Subacute pulmonary infiltration due to nitrofurantoin. Ann. Intern. Med., *65*:1284, 1966.
338. Steinberg, A. D.: Pulmonary edema following ingestion of hydrochlorothiazide. J.A.M.A., *204*:825, 1968.
339. Steinberg, M., Brauer, M. J., and Necheles, T. F.: Acute hemolytic anemia associated with erythrocyte glutathione-peroxidase deficiency. Arch. Intern. Med., *125*:302, 1970.
340. Stevens, A. R.: Agranulocytosis induced by sulfaguanidine. Arch. Intern. Med., *123*:428, 1969.
341. Stevens, D. A., Jordan, G. W., Waddell, T. F., et al.: Adverse effect of cytosine arabinoside on disseminated zoster in a controlled trial. New Eng. J. Med., *289*:873, 1973.
342. Stewart, R. B., and Cluff, L. E.: Gastrointestinal manifestations of adverse drug reactions. Am. J. Dig. Dis., *19*:1, 1974.
343. Stirland, R. M., and Shotts, N.: Antibiotic resistant streptococci in the mouths of children treated with penicillin. Lancet, *1*:405, 1967.
344. Sundmark, E.: The cataract-inducing effect of systemic corticosteroid therapy. Acta Ophthalmol., *44*:291, 1966.
344a. Sutherland, J. M., and Light, I. J.: The effect of drugs upon the developing fetus. Ped. Clin. North Am., *12*:781, 1965.
345. Swanson, M. A., Channougan, D., and Schwartz, R. S.: Immunohemolytic anemia due to antipenicillin antibodies. New Eng. J. Med., *274*:178, 1966.
346. Symmers, W. S.: The occurrence of angiitis and of other generalized diseases of connective tissues as a consequence of the administration of drugs. Proc. R. Soc. Med., *55*: 20, 1962.
347. Tobias, H., and Auerbach, R.: Hepatotoxicity of long-term methotrexate therapy for psoriasis. Arch. Intern. Med., *132*:391, 1973.
348. Turkington, R. W.: Prolactin secretion in patients treated with various drugs. Arch. Intern. Med., *130*:349, 1972.
348a. Underwood, P., Hester, L. L., Laffitte, T., and Gregg, K. V.: The relationship of smoking to the outcome of pregnancy. Am. J. Obstet. Gynecol., *91*:270, 1965.
349. Updike, S. J., and Harrington, A. R.: Acute diabetic ketoacidosis—a complication of intravenous diazoxide treatment for refractory hypertension. New Eng. J. Med., *280*:768, 1969.
350. Utz, J. P.: Antimicrobial therapy in systemic fungal infections. Am. J. Med., *39*:826, 1965.
351. Vagenakis, A. G., Cote, R., Miller, M. E., et al.: Enhancement of warfarin-induced hypoprothrombinemia by thyrotoxicosis. Johns Hopkins Med. J., *131*:69, 1972.
352. Vanselow, N. A., and Smith, J. R.: Bronchial asthma induced by indomethacin. Ann. Intern. Med., *66*:568, 1967.
352a. Villasanta, V.: Thromboembolic disease in pregnancy. Am. J. Obstet. Gynecol., *93*:142, 1965.

353. Vivacqua, R. J., Haurani, F. I., and Erslev, A. J.: "Selective" pituitary insufficiency secondary to busulfan. Ann. Intern. Med., 67:380, 1967.
354. Vogler, W. R., Bain, J. A., Huguley, C. M., et al.: Metabolic and therapeutic effects of allopurinol in patients with leukemia and gout. Am. J. Med., 40:548, 1966.
355. Wahl, C. W., Golden, J. S., Liston, E. H., et al.: Toxic and functional psychoses: Diagnosis and treatment in medical setting. Ann. Intern. Med., 66:989, 1967.
356. Wales, J. K., and Wolff, F.: Hematological side effects of diazoxide. Lancet, 1:53, 1967.
357. Walker, G. F.: Blindness during streptomycin and chloramphenicol therapy. Br. J. Ophthalmol., 45:555, 1961.
358. Walsh, F. B., Clark, D. B., Thompson, R. S., et al.: Oral contraceptives and neuro-ophthalmologic interest. Arch. Ophthalmol., 74:628, 1965.
359. Warne, G. L., Fairley, K. F., Hobbs, J. B., et al.: Cyclophosphamide-induced ovarian failure. New Eng. J. Med., 289:1159, 1973.
360. Waxman, S., Corcino, J. J., and Herbert, V.: Drugs, toxins and dietary amino acids affecting vitamin B_{12} or folic acid absorption or utilization. Am. J. Med., 48:599, 1970.
361. Waxman, S., and Herbert V.: Mechanism of pyrimethamine-induced megaloblastosis in human bone marrow. New Eng. J. Med., 280:1316, 1969.
362. Webb, D. I., Chodos, R. B., Mahar, C. Q., et al.: Mechanism of vitamin B_{12} malabsorption in patients receiving colchicine. New Eng. J. Med., 279:845, 1968.
363. Weinstein, L., and Dalton, A. C.: Host determinants of response to antimicrobial agents. New Eng. J. Med., 279:467, 524, 580, 1968.
364. Wintrobe, M. M.: Clinical Hematology. 6th ed., Philadelphia, Lea Febiger, 1967.
365. Wertlake, P. T., and Winter, T. S.: Fatal toxoplasma myocarditis in an adult patient with acute lymphocytic leukemia. New Eng. J. Med., 273:438, 1965.
366. Whelton, M. J., and Pope, F. M.: Azure lunules in argyria: Corneal changes resembling Kayser-Fleischer rings. Arch. Intern. Med., 121:267, 1968.
367. Williams, C. L., Beckwith, J. R., and Wood, J. E.: Hemorrhagic pericardial fluid in acute benign nonspecific pericarditis: Report of a case and review of the literature. Ann. Intern. Med., 52:914, 1960.
368. Williams, E. D., and Doniach, I.: The antithyroid activity of the anticoagulant phenyldanedione. J. Endocrinol., 21:421, 1961.
369. Williams, J. O., Mengel, C. E., Sullivan, L. W., et al.: Megaloblastic anemia associated with chronic ingestion of an analgesic. New Eng. Med. J., 280:312, 1969.
370. Winter, S. L., and Boyer, J. L.: Hepatic toxicity from large doses of vitamin B_3 (nicotinamide). New Eng. J. Med., 289:1180, 1973.
371. Wolfe, J. D., Metzger, A. L., and Goldstein, R. C.: Aspirin hepatitis. Ann. Intern. Med., 80:74, 1974.
372. Wolfe, R. C., Reidenberg, M., and Vispo, R. H.: Propoxyphene (Darvon) addiction and withdrawal syndrome. Ann. Intern. Med., 70:773, 1969.
373. Wolff, J.: Iodide goiter and the pharmacologic effects of excess iodide. Am. J. Med., 47:101, 1969.
374. Wolinsky, E., and Hines, J. D.: Neurotoxic and nephrotoxic effects of colistin in patients with renal failure. New Eng. J. Med., 266:759, 1962.
375. Woods, J. W.: Oral contraceptives and hypertension. Lancet, 2:653, 1967.
376. Yaffee, H. S., and Grots, I.: Moniliasis due to norethynodrel with mestranol. New Eng. J. Med., 272:647, 1965.
376a. Yerushalmy, J., and Milkovich, L.: Evaluation of the teratogenic effect of meclizine in man. Am. J. Obstet. Gynecol., 93:553, 1965.
377. Young, R. C., Nachman, R. L., and Horowitz, H. I.: Thrombocytopenia due to digitoxin demonstration of antibody and mechanisms of action. Am. J. Med., 41:605, 1966.
378. Yunis, A. A., Arimura, G. K., Lutcher, C. L., et al.: Biochemical lesion in Dilantin-induced erythroid aplasia. Blood, 30:587, 1967.
379. Zacharias, L., Chisholm, J. F., and Chapman, R. B.: Visual and ocular damage in retrolental fibroplasia. Am. J. Ophthalmol., 53:337, 1962.
380. Zetterström, B.: Ocular malformations caused by thalidomide. Acta Ophthalmol., 44:391, 1966.

CHAPTER 5

INDIVIDUAL DRUGS AND THEIR ADVERSE EFFECTS

This list of known adverse reactions to drugs is intended to serve as a quick guide to common drug reactions. It is not a comprehensive listing of either drugs or drug reactions. The reactions of nausea and vomiting have not been included unless they occur very commonly or are severe, since these effects can follow the use of nearly every drug. In order to provide a more general reference, at times the reader is referred from a specific drug listed in the table to a general or prototypical drug in that class for information on adverse effects. It should be understood that the adverse effects of the specific and the prototype may not be identical, and that the reference should serve only as a guide. Appropriate examples of common trade names have also been included. The classification of drugs is similar to that used by the American Hospital Formulary Service.

TABLE 5-1. *Individual Drugs and Their Adverse Effects*

DRUG	REACTIONS	REFERENCES
Antihistamines		
Brompheniramine maleate (Dimetane) Chlorpheniramine maleate (Chlor-Trimeton, Teldrin) Diphenhydramine hydrochloride (Benadryl) Tripelennamine citrate (Pyribenzamine) Triprolidine hydrochloride (Actidil)	Central nervous system actions include sedation, dizziness, tinnitus, fatigue, blurred vision, nervousness, insomnia, and tremors. Anticholinergic actions may cause dryness of the mouth, constipation, or dysuria. Hypersensitivity after topical administration may occur.	4, 50, 130, 133
PHENOTHIAZINE ANTIHISTIMINES:		
Promethazine hydrochloride (Phenergan)	See under Central Nervous System Drugs – Phenothiazines.	
Trimeprazine tartrate (Temaril)	See under Central Nervous System Drugs – Phenothiazines.	
Anti-Infective Agents		
ANTHELMINTICS:		
Piperazine citrate (Antepar)	Gastrointestinal side effects include nausea, vomiting, and diarrhea. Neurological disturbances include blurred vision, vertigo, and muscle weakness. Cataracts have been reported.	4, 159
Pyrvinium pamoate (Povan)	Nausea, vomiting, and gastrointestinal cramping after large doses. Drug colors the stool and vomitus red.	4, 28, 57
Quinacrine hydrochloride (Atabrine)	Gastrointestinal symptoms and temporary yellow discoloration of the skin.	4
Thiabendazole (Mintezol)	Frequent anorexia, nausea, and vomiting. Central effects include dizziness and insomnia.	89, 170

TABLE 5-1 *continued on following page.*

TABLE 5-1. (Continued)

DRUG	REACTIONS	REFERENCES
ANTIFUNGAL ANTIBIOTICS:		
Amphotericin B (Fungizone)	Frequent side effects include fever, tremor, anorexia, and generalized pain. This drug is nephrotoxic in nearly all patients. Normochromic anemia and hypokalemia are commonly observed.	4, 27, 54, 188, 206
Flucytosine (Ancobon)	Toxic effects occur in rapidly dividing tissues, resulting in bone marrow depression. Toxicity to the gastrointestinal lining also has been reported. Hepatic dysfunction and euphoria also may occur.	4, 202
Griseofulvin (Fulvicin)	Side effects of angioneurotic edema, urticaria, and leukopenia. Interferes with porphyrin metabolism. Central effects include drowsiness, fatigue, depression, insomnia, and frequent headaches.	4, 155, 137
Nystatin (Mycostatin)	Few side effects occur with this drug since it is not absorbed from the gastrointestinal tract. Gastrointestinal side effects occur rarely.	4
ANTIBIOTICS:		
Ampicillin	The incidence of allergic reactions (approx. 10%) to this drug is higher than observed with other antibiotics, and usually present as a maculopapular rash or urticaria. Serum sickness, fever, and anaphylactoid reactions have been reported. Bone marrow depression has occurred, but it is rare. Ampicillin may promote the occurrence of superinfections by bacteria, yeast, and mycotic organisms. Gastrointestinal side effects are frequent, including nausea, vomiting, diarrhea, and glossitis.	113, 180

Drug	Adverse Effects	References
Carbenicillin (Geopen)	Severe nausea and vomiting have been reported as effects of the oral form of the drug. The allergic reactions that occur are common to other penicillins. Severe hypokalemia and disturbances of platelet function have been reported, as well as elevated serum glutamic oxaloacetic transaminase (SGOT) levels, elevated serum glutamic pyruvic transaminase (SGPT) levels, and azotemia.	4, 21, 94, 129, 134
Cephalexin monohydrate (Keflex)	Allergic reactions in the form of urticaria and rash have been observed. Diarrhea is a common side effect.	4, 76
Chloramphenicol	Bone marrow depression is the most severe effect of this drug. Mortality from aplastic anemia has been estimated at 80%. Allergic reactions, including Stevens-Johnson syndrome and toxic epidermal necrolysis, have been reported.	4, 142
Clindamycin (Cleocin)	Anorexia and diarrhea commonly occur. Rash and urticaria are common hypersensitivity reactions. Transient leukopenia and elevations of serum alkaline phosphatase and serum transaminase levels also have been observed. *Colitis*.	4, 67, 190
Cloxacillin sodium (Tegopen)	Allergic symptoms are similar to those produced by penicillin, and include skin rash, urticaria, and drug fever.	4
Colistimethate sodium (Coly-Mycin)	Like other polymyxins, this drug causes nephrotoxicity. Circumoral and peripheral paresthesias and other neurotoxic effects are common. Febrile reactions and gastrointestinal effects also occur.	4, 25
Demeclocycline (Declomycin)	See under Tetracycline. Photosensitivity reactions are much more common with this tetracycline.	18
Doxycycline (Vibramycin)	See under Tetracycline.	
Erythromycin	Nausea, vomiting, dyspepsia, and diarrhea are common. Allergic reactions such as rash are uncommon but have occurred. Hepatic dysfunction is common (2–4%), especially with the estolate salt, and is most often cholestatic.	4, 34, 214

TABLE 5–1 continued on following page.

TABLE 5-1. (Continued)

DRUG	REACTIONS	REFERENCES
Gentamicin (Garamycin)	The most important toxic effect of this drug occurs in the eighth cranial nerve, which causes dizziness, tinnitus, and hearing loss. Nephrotoxicity manifested by oliguria, granular casts in the urine, or increased blood urea nitrogen (BUN) may occur in approximately 2% of the patients. Allergic reactions are uncommon; however, cross-allergy with other aminoglycoside antibiotics appears with high frequency.	4, 7, 20, 59, 156
Kanamycin (Kantrex)	Ototoxicity to the auditory and vestibular function of the eighth cranial nerve is the most important effect. Allergic reactions are rare, but cross-sensitization with other aminoglycosides is common. Nephrotoxicity is a common complication but is usually reversible. Neuromuscular paralysis has been reported. Elevated SGOT or SGPT levels occur.	4, 134, 156
Lincomycin (Lincocin)	Allergic reactions are rare. Diarrhea may occur in a high percentage (10%) of patients receiving the drug orally. Cardiac arrest has been reported in patients receiving rapid intravenous administration in large doses.	4, 126, 144
Methicillin sodium (Staphcillin)	See under Penicillin G.	
Minocycline (Minocin)	See under Tetracycline. Headache and dizziness occur frequently.	84
Penicillin G	Allergic reactions include anaphylaxis, edema, urticaria, serum sickness, hemolytic anemia, fever, and exfoliative dermatitis. Cholestatic hepatitis may occur. Hematologic reactions may include eosinophilia and hemolytic anemia. Anemia results only after large intravenous doses. Central nervous system toxicity results in encephalopathy and convulsive seizures.	4, 119, 213

INDIVIDUAL DRUGS AND THEIR ADVERSE EFFECTS 233

Penicillin G procaine	See under Penicillin G. Accidental intravascular injection may produce a pseudo-anaphylactic reaction exhibited by tachycardia, hypertension, and acute psychotic reactions.	199
Spectinomycin (Trobicin)	Urticaria, fever, chills, and insomnia have been observed.	4
Streptomycin sulfate	The most serious toxic effect of streptomycin occurs in the auditory and vestibular branches of the eighth cranial nerve. Allergic reactions, including rash and edema, are common; however, anaphylactic reactions are rare. Like other aminoglycosides, the drug has neuromuscular blocking properties.	4, 19, 152
Tetracycline hydrochloride	Hypersensitivity reactions may include morbilliform rashes, urticaria, and exfoliation. Intestinal symptoms of anorexia, dyspepsia, nausea, vomiting, and diarrhea are common. Phototoxicity will appear with this drug, but is less frequent than with demethylchlortetracycline. Hepatic and nephrotoxic effects have been documented. This drug may cause discoloration and damage of the teeth of the fetus or child when given at any time from the fourth month of gestation to the eighth year of life. Superinfections by tetracycline-resistant organisms are common.	4, 126
ANTITUBERCULOUS DRUGS:		
Aminosalicylic acid (P.A.S.)	Nausea, vomiting, and diarrhea are common. Liver damage and jaundice occasionally occur.	4, 68
Ethambutol hydrochloride (Myambutol)	Retrobulbar neuritis is the most common side effect and is dose-related.	48, 118
Isoniazid (INH)	Toxic reactions in the nervous system include peripheral neuritis, hyperreflexia, convulsions, and psychosis. These symptoms can usually be prevented by the administration of pyridoxine. Hepatic reactions include elevated SGOT and SGPT levels, and hepatitis. Hypersensitivity reactions, while rare, have included fever, chills, rashes, and lymphadenopathy, as well as a lupus erythematosus-like syndrome.	4, 97, 181

TABLE 5–1 continued on following page.

TABLE 5-1. (Continued)

DRUG	REACTIONS	REFERENCES
Rifampin	Reactions are few and usually minor, but may include gastrointestinal symptoms, headache, and hepatic reactions.	4, 43
ANTIMALARIALS:		
Chloroquine phosphate (Aralen)	Blood dyscrasias appear, including agranulocytosis and neutropenia. Retinopathy is a common complication, especially after high doses over a prolonged period of time. Toxicity to the auditory nerve has been observed.	4, 29, 197, 201
Primaquine phosphate	Hemolytic anemia in patients with G-6-PD deficiency.	4
Quinine sulfate	Toxic hematologic effects include hemolytic anemia and thrombocytopenia. Cinchonism effects of diarrhea, vomiting, nausea, tinnitus, vertigo, and visual disturbances may occur.	4, 15, 86
SULFONAMIDES: Side effects of sulfonamides are shared by all the individual agents in this category and differ primarily in degree and frequency. Therefore, individual sulfonamides will not be listed separately.	Allergic reactions include rashes, fever, periarteritis nodosa, erythema nodosum, and photosensitivity. Suppression of bone marrow may result in pancytopenia, leukopenia, agranulocytosis, or thrombocytopenia. Renal toxicity occurs more frequently from less soluble sulfonamides as a result of crystalluria. Gastrointestinal symptoms of nausea and vomiting appear frequently. Hemolytic anemia may occur in patients with G-6-PD deficiency.	4
TRICHOMONACIDES:		
Metronidazole (Flagyl)	Gastrointestinal symptoms of anorexia, nausea, vomiting, and diarrhea are common. Central nervous system side effects include blurred vision, headache, confusion, and depression. Leukopenia has been observed in some patients.	4, 201

INDIVIDUAL DRUGS AND THEIR ADVERSE EFFECTS 235

URINARY GERMICIDES:		
Methenamine mandelate	Side effects are rare but may be evidenced by gastrointestinal distress, dysuria, or rashes.	4
Nalidixic acid (NegGram)	Most common side effects are gastrointestinal. Rashes and photosensitivity may occur.	4, 16, 26
Nitrofurantoin (Furadantin)	Allergic rashes and fever may occur. Acute allergic reactions of sudden severe dyspnea with pulmonary infiltration and effusion are common. Gastrointestinal side effects of dyspepsia and anorexia occur in a high percentage of patients. Severe cases of neuropathy characterized by demyelination of peripheral nerve fibers and spinal cord have been reported.	4, 153, 169
Phenazopyridine hydrochloride (Pyridium)	Methemoglobinemia and hemolytic anemia have been reported.	4
ANTINEOPLASTICS:		
Azathioprine (Imuran)	Bone marrow suppression with leukopenia, anemia, and thrombocytopenia. Gastrointestinal side effects are common. Infection is a common hazard.	2, 4, 45
Chlorambucil (Leukeran)	Gastrointestinal side effects occur in nearly one-half of the patients and include nausea, vomiting, diarrhea, oral ulcerations, and intractable emesis. Leukopenia and thrombocytopenia are common.	4, 74, 141
Cyclophosphamide (Cytoxan)	Alopecia occurs in a high percentage of patients. Bone marrow suppression results in leukopenia and thrombocytopenia. Hemorrhagic cystitis is a common side effect. Nausea and vomiting are commonly observed.	4
Cytarabine hydrochloride (Cytosar)	Bone marrow suppression with leukopenia, thrombocytopenia, and anemia are common. Nausea, vomiting, and diarrhea also present frequently. Vascular spasm at the site of injection may occur.	151, 203

TABLE 5–1 continued on following page.

TABLE 5-1. (*Continued*)

Drug	Reactions	References
Fluorouracil (5-FU)	Nausea, vomiting, stomatitis, diarrhea, and gastrointestinal hemorrhage are common reactions. Bone marrow suppression with leukopenia, thrombocytopenia, and anemia. Alopecia also has been reported.	4, 6, 140
Mechlorethamine hydrochloride (Nitrogen mustard)	Thrombophlebitis may occur at the injection site. Severe nausea and vomiting are common. Bone marrow suppression with granulocytopenia, thrombocytopenia, and lymphocytopenia. Amenorrhea, weakness, and headache also result.	4, 64
Mercaptopurine (6-MP)	The major side effects are found in the GI tract and hematopoietic system. Leukopenia and thrombocytopenia are reported side effects.	56, 139
Methotrexate	The main side effects are bone marrow suppression with leukopenia, thrombocytopenia, and anemia. Gastrointestinal side effects are common and include stomatitis. Hepatic dysfunction is common with chronic therapy, and may be irreversible. Pneumonitis and renal tubular toxicity have been reported.	4, 65
Procarbazine hydrochloride (Matulane)	Frequent nausea and vomiting have been observed. Bone marrow suppression with anemia, leukopenia, and thrombocytopenia. Central nervous system side effects are frequent, including paresthesias, neuropathies, mental depression, psychosis, and euphoria.	4, 178, 183
Thioguanine	Reactions are similar to other antimetabolites, including bone marrow suppression with pancytopenia and oral lesions.	4, 157

Vinblastine sulfate (Velban)	Observed effects are leukopenia, thrombocytopenia, nausea, vomiting, diarrhea, alopecia, and stomatitis. Neurological toxic effects include mental depression, psychosis, and paresthesias.	4, 66
Vincristine sulfate (Oncovin)	A wide variety of neurological and neuromuscular side effects are common with this drug, including paresthesias, loss of deep-tendon reflex, muscle weakness, ataxia, and ptosis. Gastrointestinal side effects are common, with constipation being a common complaint. Alopecia and leukopenia also have been reported.	4, 35, 98

Autonomic Nervous System Drugs

PARASYMPATHOMIMETICS (CHOLINERGICS):

Bethanechol chloride (Urecholine)	Cholinergic response may include gastrointestinal cramping, flushing of the skin or sweating, salivation, diarrhea, asthmatic attacks, and hypotension.	4
Neostigmine bromide (Prostigmin)	See under Bethanechol.	

PARASYMPATHOLYTICS:

Atropine sulfate	Side effects are a result of the drug's antimuscarinic action and include dryness of the mouth, blurred vision, mydriasis, photophobia, tachycardia, and decreased sweating. It may reduce the tone of the gastrointestinal tract and urinary bladder, resulting in constipation and urinary retention, respectively. Central nervous system effects include disorientation, irritability, restlessness, and hallucinations. Hypersensitivity reactions affect the skin, and in rare instances exfoliation may occur.	4, 92, 171

TABLE 5-1 continued on following page.

TABLE 5-1. (Continued)

DRUG	REACTIONS	REFERENCES
The following parasympatholytic drugs have actions and side effects similar to those of atropine, which vary only in degree. Additional side effects are reported next to the specific drug.		
Benztropine methanesulfonate (Cogentin)		4, 148
Glycopyrrolate (Robinul)		
Isopropamide iodide (Darbid)	Sedation	
Propantheline bromide (Pro-Banthine)		
Trihexyphenidyl hydrochloride (Artane)		168
SYMPATHOMIMETICS:		
Ephedrine sulfate	Effects may include nervousness, insomnia, tremors, psychotic reactions, arrhythmias, and sweating.	4
Isoproterenol hydrochloride (Isuprel)	Activity of the drug on beta receptors results in tachycardia, palpitation, arrhythmias, headache, and flushing of the skin. Death may occur after excessive use of inhalers.	4, 46, 204
Levarterenol bitartrate (Levophed)	Headache, hypersensitivity, and bradycardia.	4
Phenylpropanolamine (Propadrine)	Insomnia, restlessness, tachycardia, and headache.	4
SYMPATHOLYTICS:		
Azapetine phosphate (Ilidar)	Postural hypotension, malaise, nasal congestion, and drug fever.	4
Ergotamine tartrate	Nausea and vomiting frequently occur, and vasoconstriction of the extremities resulting in gangrene. May precipitate angina pectoris.	4, 100, 106
Methysergide maleate (Sansert)	Tachycardia, postural hypotension, coronary insufficiency, claudication, leg cramps, and edema of the extremities are reported effects. Prolonged therapy may result in retroperitoneal fibrosis or fibrotic lesions elsewhere. Dizziness, drowsiness, vertigo, confusion, headache, and nightmares also occur.	4, 77, 114

INDIVIDUAL DRUGS AND THEIR ADVERSE EFFECTS 239

Phenoxybenzamine hydrochloride (Dibenzyline)	Nasal congestion, postural hypotension, miosis, reflex tachycardia, dryness of the mouth, and interference with ejaculation have been observed. Respiratory effects may include wheezing, rales, and rhonchi.	4, 14, 165
SKELETAL MUSCLE RELAXANTS:		
Carisoprodol (Soma)	Sedation, weakness, vertigo, and rashes.	4
Chlorzoxazone (Paraflex)	Dizziness, paresthesias, and lethargy have been reported.	4, 182
Methocarbamol (Robaxin)	Headache, anorexia, vertigo, fever, and skin eruptions.	4
Iron Preparations		
Dextran iron complex (Imferon)	Headache, fever, nausea, vomiting, arthralgia, and regional lymphadenopathy. Staining of the skin at the site of injection. Anaphylactic reactions.	4, 13
Ferrous sulfate	Gastrointestinal side effects occur in 15–20% of patients.	4, 125
Anticoagulants		
Bishydroxycoumarin (Dicumarol)	The most frequent adverse effect of anticoagulants is hemorrhage. Hemorrhage has been reported from nearly every site.	4, 120
Heparin sodium	The major side effect is bleeding. Hypersensitivity reactions may occur, with chills, fever, urticaria, arthralgia, and anaphylaxis. Alopecia and osteoporosis also have been known to occur.	4, 222
Warfarin sodium (Coumadin)	See under Bishydroxycoumarin.	

TABLE 5–1 continued on following page.

TABLE 5-1. (Continued)

DRUG	REACTIONS	REFERENCES
Cardiovascular Drugs		
DIGITALIS GLYCOSIDES:	Gastrointestinal effects include nausea, vomiting, and diarrhea. Digitalis may produce nearly all types of cardiac arrhythmias, including premature ventricular contractions, interference dissociation, atrial tachycardia, nodal tachycardia, atrioventricular blocks, atrial fibrillation, atrial flutter, ventricular tachycardia, and ventricular fibrillation. Central nervous system effects include drowsiness, weakness, irritability, hallucinations, and visual disorders. Gynecomastia has been reported.	4, 222
Digitoxin	See under Digitalis Glycosides.	
Digoxin	See under Digitalis Glycosides.	
Lidocaine hydrochloride (Xylocaine)	Central nervous system effects include drowsiness, disorientation, euphoria, visual disturbances, and paresthesias. Muscle twitching, convulsions, and respiratory distress and arrest may also occur. With high doses, cardiac effects of hypotension, conduction defects, heart block, and bradycardia have been reported.	4, 197
Procainamide hydrochloride (Pronestyl)	Toxic effects on the heart include depression of atrioventricular and intraventricular conduction, bradycardia, complete heart block, and ventricular tachycardia or fibrillation. Drug-induced lupus erythematosus with fever, rash, arthralgia pleuritis, and splenomegaly. Allergic reactions with fever and rash. Agranulocytosis has been reported.	4, 58, 209

TABLE 5-1. (Continued)

DRUG	REACTIONS	REFERENCES
Propranolol hydrochloride (Inderal)	The effects of this drug may precipitate congestive heart failure. Hypotension, circulatory collapse, asystole, and bradycardia are reported reactions. Bronchospasm, dyspnea, and wheezing are respiratory effects. Hypoglycemia. Rashes. Central nervous system effects include confusion or giddiness. Other effects include nausea, vomiting, and diarrhea	4, 179
Quinidine	A high percentage (20–40%) of patients experience gastrointestinal effects, including anorexia, nausea, vomiting, and diarrhea. Allergic reactions may include drug fever, rash, thrombocytopenia, hemolytic anemia, and anaphylactic shock. Prolongation of ventricular action potential and decreased intraventricular conduction. Bradycardia, heart block, asystole, atrial flutter, ventricular flutter, and fibrillation. Cinchonism effects include tinnitus, visual disturbances, vertigo, and convulsions.	4, 179
ANTILIPEMICS:		
Clofibrate (Atromid-S)	Muscle aches, cramps and elevated levels of creatine phosphokinase.	4, 100, 115
HYPOTENSIVES:		
Diazoxide	Hypotension, hyperglycemia, and hyperuricemia.	135
Guanethidine sulfate (Ismelin)	Orthostatic hypotension, dizziness, syncope, impotence, failure of ejaculation, and ptosis. Blurring of vision, bradycardia, depression, and severe diarrhea. Edema and sodium retention.	4, 184
Hydralazine hydrochloride (Apresoline)	Postural hypotension, tachycardia, severe headache, dizziness and nausea. Peripheral neuropathies and paresthesias. Rheumatic and febrile reactions, including arthritis or arthralgia, lupus erythematosus factor, and fever.	

TABLE 5-1 continued on following page.

TABLE 5-1. (Continued)

DRUG	REACTIONS	REFERENCES
Methyldopa (Aldomet)	Sedation is the most frequent side effect. Orthostatic hypotension, bradycardia, nasal stuffiness and failure of ejaculation have also been reported. Drug fever and hemolytic anemia may occur. Positive reactions to Coombs' test occur in 10-20% of patients receiving the drug.	4, 47, 39
Pargyline (Eutonyl)	This is a monamine oxidase inhibitor and as such produces side effects common to this group, including insomnia, nightmares, and interaction with catecholamines and tyramine. Postural hypotension, dry mouth, and impotence.	4
Phentolamine hydrochloride (Regitine)	Tachycardia, orthostatic hypotension, nasal stuffiness, and gastrointestinal symptoms.	4, 37
Reserpine (Sandril, Serpasil)	Reactivation of peptic ulcerations. Hypotension and bradycardia. Depression also may occur, with suicidal tendencies. Nightmares, blurred vision, and ptosis.	4, 122
Rescinnamine (Moderil)	See under Reserpine.	
VASODILATORS:		
Cyclandelate (Cyclospasmol)	Flushing and tingling of the extremities, and headache.	17
Dipyridamole (Persantin)	Nausea, vomiting, and headache.	24
Glyceryl trinitrate (Nitroglycerin)	Headache and flushing.	4, 96
Isosorbide dinitrate (Isordil)	Headache, and increased intraocular pressure.	4
Isoxuprine hydrochloride (Vasodilan)	Nausea, vomiting, and palpitations.	4
Nicotinyl alcohol (Roniacol)	Flushing of face or neck, paresthesias, and gastrointestinal disorders.	4, 147

Central Nervous System Drugs

ANALGESICS AND ANTIPYRETICS:

Drug	Effects	Ref
Acetaminophen (Tylenol)	Few side effects, but these may include nausea or urticaria.	182
Acetophenetidin (Phenacetin)	Methemoglobinemia and hemolytic reactions occur in susceptible patients. Renal papillary necrosis occurs in abusers of the drug. Gastrointestinal disturbances have been noted.	4
Aspirin	The most important effects occur in the gastrointestinal tract, causing dyspepsia, gastric erosion, and massive hemorrhage. Effects of salicylism include ringing in the ears, mental confusion, and sweating. Hypersensitivity reactions include urticaria, asthma, and angioedema.	4, 71, 128, 196
Codeine	The major unwanted effect is dependence. Respiratory depression, and a high incidence of nausea, vomiting, and constipation.	4
Colchicine	Dyspepsia, nausea, vomiting, and diarrhea. Hematuria and oliguria.	4
Dipyrone (Pyralgin)	Blood dyscrasias, including leukopenia and agranulocytosis.	4
Hydromorphone hydrochloride (Dilaudid)	See under Codeine.	
Indomethacin (Indocin)	Central nervous system effects include headache, disturbances in equilibrium, depersonalization, and mental confusion. Gastrointestinal effects may be severe, with dyspepsia, nausea, vomiting, and diarrhea. Gastrointestinal ulcerations may occur. Pruritus, skin rash, and erythema nodosum. Bone marrow depression. Respiratory distress and asthma may present in hypertensive patients.	4, 85
Meperidine hydrochloride (Demerol)	Respiratory depression, sedation, euphoria, and dependence. Nausea and vomiting.	4, 177
Methadone hydrochloride (Dolophine)	Nausea, vomiting, lightheadedness, drowsiness, and dependence.	4

TABLE 5-1 continued on following page.

TABLE 5-1. (Continued)

DRUG	REACTIONS	REFERENCES
Morphine sulfate	Dependence. Hypotension may be caused by decreased systemic arterial pressure. Respiratory depression. Mental clouding, euphoria, and sedation are central nervous system effects. Nausea, vomiting, and constipation.	4, 62, 132
Pentazocine hydrochloride (Talwin)	Dependence. Nausea, vertigo, fatigue, sedation, and constipation. Allergic reactions. Hypotension or hypertension. Dizziness and lightheadedness.	4, 108, 215
Phenylbutazone (Butazolidin)	Hypersensitivity reactions of rashes, fever, lymphadenopathy, hepatic damage and Stevens-Johnson syndrome. Anemia, pancytopenia, and agranulocytosis. Leukemoid reactions. Nausea, dyspepsia, and vomiting, as well as gastrointestinal bleeding. Headache, psychosis, depression, and vertigo.	4, 109, 186, 191
Propoxyphene hydrochloride (Darvon)	Nausea, vomiting, and constipation. Central nervous system effects include headache and sedation.	33
Nalorphine hydrochloride (Nalline)	Lethargy, nausea, respiratory depression, euphoria, hallucinations, and disorientation.	4
Naloxone hydrochloride (Narcan)	Depression and irritability.	4
ANTICONVULSANTS:		
Diphenylhydantoin (Dilantin)	Gingival hyperplasia, lymphadenopathy, and systemic lupus erythematosus. Hypersensitivity reactions include rashes and exfoliative dermatitis. Gastrointestinal effects are dyspepsia, nausea, and vomiting. Ataxia, extrapyramidal reactions, psychosis, and confusion may occur. Numerous blood dyscrasias may appear, including aplastic and megaloblastic anemia, leukopenia, eosinophilia, and thrombocytopenia. Hepatic damage. Electrocardiographic changes.	4, 88

INDIVIDUAL DRUGS AND THEIR ADVERSE EFFECTS 245

Drug	Adverse Effects	References
Ethosuximide (Zarontin)	Gastrointestinal effects, headache, and sedation. Leukopenia.	26, 82, 210
Methsuximide (Celontin)	Anorexia, vomiting, and diarrhea. Drowsiness, ataxia, and rash.	4
Primidone (Mysoline)	Drowsiness and ataxia.	4
Trimethadione (Tridione)	Gastric irritation, nausea, rashes, and photosensitivity. Aplastic anemia, nephrotic syndrome, and teratogenic effects.	4, 69, 93
ANTIDEPRESSANTS:		
Amitriptyline (Elavil)	Anticholinergic effects of constipation, dysuria, dryness of the mouth, blurred vision, and tachycardia. Paralytic ileus has been reported. Drowsiness and ataxia. Palpitations, orthostatic hypotension.	9, 123, 207
Doxepin (Sinequan)	Anticholinergic effects of dryness of the mouth, dysuria, and constipation. Drowsiness and orthostatic hypotension.	4
Imipramine hydrochloride (Tofranil)	Anticholinergic effects of dryness of the mouth, blurred vision, constipation, urinary retention, and tachycardia. Parkinson's syndrome. Hypotension. Seizures in epileptic patients. Arrhythmias have occurred. Central nervous system effects of drowsiness and weakness and headache.	4, 9, 73, 95, 207
Nortriptyline hydrochloride (Aventyl)	See under Amitriptyline.	
Tranylcypromine sulfate (Parnate)	Hypertensive crisis, occipital headache, palpitations. Intracranial bleeding.	38, 207
TRANQUILIZERS:		
Chlordiazepoxide (Librium)	Somnolence, ataxia, dry mouth.	12, 111, 164
Chlorpromazine (Thorazine)	Dryness of the mouth, blurred vision, constipation, nasal stuffiness. Hypersensitivity reactions of cholestatic jaundice, rashes, photosensitivity, eosinophilia, and contact dermatitis. Blood disorders of agranulocytosis, leukopenia, endocrine disorders, and ocular changes including deposition of particulate matter in the lens and the cornea. Extrapyramidal syndromes of parkinsonian dystonia, dyskinesia, and akathisia symptoms. Hypotension, tachycardia, and syncope.	4, 44, 103, 160

TABLE 5–1 continued on following page.

TABLE 5-1. (Continued)

Drug	Reactions	References
Diazepam (Valium)	See under Chlordiazepoxide.	
Fluphenazine (Prolixin)	Extrapyramidal effects of akinesia, dyskinesia, akathisia, and parkinsonism. Drowsiness, fatigue, and depression.	
Haloperidol (Haldol)	Extrapyramidal effects. Depression, apprehension, anxiety, and euphoria. Anticholinergic effects of dryness of the mouth, constipation, urinary retention, and blurred vision.	4, 121, 172, 200
Hydroxyzine (Atarax, Vistaril)	Drowsiness and dryness of the mouth.	4, 193
Perphenazine (Trilafon)	See under Chlorpromazine.	
Prochlorperazine (Compazine)	See under Chlorpromazine.	
Thioridazine (Mellaril)	See under Chlorpromazine.	
Thiothixene (Navane)	Extrapyramidal effects. Drowsiness and insomnia. Seizures, orthostatic hypotension, dryness of the mouth, constipation, tachycardia, and dermatitis. Electrocardiographic changes.	4, 189, 218
Trifluoperazine (Stelazine)	See under Chlorpromazine.	
CEREBRAL STIMULANTS:		
Dextroamphetamine sulfate (Dexedrine)	Dependency, psychosis, or neurosis. Tachycardia, arrhythmias, and hypertension. Anorexia and dryness of the mouth. Nervousness, headache.	4, 36, 150
Methamphetamine hydrochloride (Desoxyn)	See under Dextroamphetamine.	
Methylphenidate hydrochloride (Ritalin)	Nervousness, insomnia, headache, and palpitations. Seizures. Hypertension.	4, 163, 216

SEDATIVES AND HYPNOTICS:

Drug	Adverse Effects	Refs
Amobarbital (Amytal)	See under Phenobarbital.	
Butabarbital sodium (Butisol)	See under Phenobarbital.	
Chloral hydrate (Noctec)	Nausea, vomiting, and gastrointestinal irritation. Ataxia and confusion.	4, 136
Ethchlorvynol (Placidyl)	Excitement, confusion, vertigo, and headache.	4
Flurazepam hydrochloride (Dalmane)	See under Diazepam.	
Methaqualone (Quaalude)	Drowsiness and headache.	49
Methyprylon (Noludar)	Nausea, vomiting, constipation, headache, and rashes.	4
Pentobarbital sodium (Nembutal)	See under Phenobarbital.	
Phenobarbital (Luminal)	Depression, confusion, and delirium. Skin rashes are the most frequent side effect. Respiratory depression.	4, 70
Secobarbital (Seconal)	See under Phenobarbital.	
Sodium bromide	Confusion, disorientation, acneiform rash.	194

Diuretics

Drug	Adverse Effects	Refs
Acetazolamide (Diamox)	Allergic reactions of skin rash. Hyperuricemia, drowsiness, and acidosis.	
Chlorothiazide (Diuril)	Skin rashes including photosensitivity. Hemorrhagic pancreatitis. Orthostatic hypotension. Hyperglycemia, hypokalemia, hyperuricemia, and gout.	4, 75, 162, 212
Chlorthalidone (Hygroton)	Hypokalemia, hyponatremia, hyperglycemia, and hyperuricemia. Skin rashes. Orthostatic hypotension.	4
Ethacrynic acid (Edecrin)	Nausea, dyspepsia, and diarrhea. Parenteral administration may induce gastrointestinal hemorrhage. Ototoxicity. Hyperglycemia and hyperuricemia. Agranulocytosis. Orthostatic hypotension.	4, 116, 208, 219

TABLE 5-1 continued on following page.

TABLE 5-1. (Continued)

DRUG	REACTIONS	REFERENCES
Furosemide (Lasix)	Nausea. Hypokalemia and hyperuricemia. Orthostatic hypotension. Dermatitis.	131, 211
Hydrochlorothiazide (Hydrodiuril, Esidrix)	See under Chlorothiazide.	
Spironolactone (Aldactone)	Hyperkalemia, gynecomastia, generalized weakness, and rash.	32, 40, 91
Triamterene (Dyrenium)	Nausea, vomiting, and diarrhea. Hyperkalemia.	4
Drugs in Gout		
Allopurinol (Zyloprim)	Hypersensitivity reactions of fever, leukopenia, and rashes.	101, 187
Probenecid (Benemid)	Rashes, hypersensitivity reactions, and gastrointestinal distress.	4, 167
Gastrointestinal Drugs		
Diphenoxylate	Nausea, vomiting, and abdominal cramps. Headache, tachycardia, and paresthesias.	4, 174
Bisacodyl (Dulcolax)	Abdominal cramps and diarrhea.	166
Dioctyl sodium sulfosuccinate (Colace)	Diarrhea.	195
Trimethobenzamide hydrochloride (Tigan)	Hypotension after parenteral administration. Symptoms resemble those of Parkinson's disease.	4
Gold		
Gold sodium thiomalate (Myochrysine)	Pruritis, rashes, urticaria, and exfoliative dermatitis. Leukopenia, agranulocytosis, thrombocytopenia, eosinophilia. Proteinuria and hematuria. Stomatitis.	4, 22, 117

Hormones and Synthetic Substitutes

ADRENALS:

Betamethasone (Celestone)	See under Prednisone.	
Dexamethasone (Decadron)	See under Prednisone.	87
Methylprednisolone (Medrol)	See under Prednisone.	224
Prednisone	Cushing's syndrome of moon faces, acne, muscular weakness, cervicothoracic hump, hypertension, osteoporosis, edema, and leukocytosis. Viral, fungal, and bacterial infections of the skin may result. Peptic ulceration. Central nervous effects include euphoria and psychosis. Increased ocular pressure. Hyperglycemia.	4, 52, 127
Triamcinolone (Aristocort, Kenalog)	See under Prednisone.	

ANDROGENS:

Fluoxymesterone (Halotestin)	See under Methyltestosterone.	
Methandrostenolone (Dianabol)	See under Methyltestosterone.	
Methyltestosterone (Metandren)	Acne and hirsutism, and priapism. Cholestatic jaundice, hypercalcemia, and edema.	4, 63, 138

ESTROGENS:

Diethylstilbestrol (Stilbestrol)	Nausea, gynecomastia, and edema. Adenocarcinoma of vagina in offspring of mothers treated with this drug in pregnancy.	4, 112

ORAL CONTRACEPTIVES:

Progestogen-estrogen combinations	Gastrointestinal symptoms primarily of nausea. Acne, alopecia, and increased pigmentation. Hepatic dysfunction and jaundice. Thromboembolism. Hypertension. Nervousness, irritability, and depression. Edema and breast changes. Increased incidence of candidiasis. Megaloblastic anemia.	4, 81, 102, 145, 158, 185

INSULINS AND ANTIDIABETICS:

Chlorpropamide (Diabinese)	Hypoglycemia, jaundice, and cutaneous reactions. Agranulocytosis.	4, 30

TABLE 5-1 continued on following page.

TABLE 5-1. (Continued)

Drug	Reactions	References
Phenformin hydrochloride (D.B.I.)	A high incidence of nausea, vomiting, and diarrhea. Hypoglycemia. Lactic acidosis.	53, 104
Tolbutamide (Orinase)	Hypoglycemia. Hypersensitivity reactions including erythema, urticaria, and photosensitization. Cholestatic jaundice.	4, 11, 80
Insulin injection (regular insulin)	Hyperinsulinism resulting in hypoglycemia. Reactions of itching, redness, and swelling at the injection site occur in approximately one-fourth of patients. Atrophy or hypertrophy at the site of injection. Allergic and anaphylactic reactions.	4, 154
PITUTARY:		
Corticotropin (ACTH)	Allergic reactions to preparations of animal origin. See also Prednisone.	198, 217
THYROID AND ANTITHYROID:		
Levothyroxine sodium (Synthroid)	See under Thyroid.	
Liothyronine sodium (Cytomel)	See under Thyroid.	
Methimazole (Tapazole)	Agranulocytosis, leukopenia, and thrombocytopenia. Rashes. Arthritis.	4, 55, 60
Propylthiouracil	Agranulocytosis, thrombocytopenia, and leukopenia. Hypersensitivity reactions of rashes and fever.	4, 79
Thyroid	Palpitations, angina, headache, diarrhea, and restlessness. Allergic cutaneous reactions.	4, 171
Local Anesthetics		
Dibucaine hydrochloride (Nupercaine)	Central nervous system stimulation. Hypersensitivity reactions.	4

Mepivacaine hydrochloride (Carbocaine)	Nausea, vomiting, drowsiness, headache, apnea, arrhythmias, and hypotension. Hypersensitivity reactions.	4, 83
Procaine hydrochloride (Novocain)	Central nervous system stimulation. Hypersensitivity reactions.	4, 72
Tetracaine hydrochloride (Pontocaine)	Central nervous system stimulation. Hypersensitivity reactions.	4, 107

Oxytocics

Oxytocin (Pitocin)	Water intoxication if administered intravenously. Uterine rupture. Hypotension, hypertension, and electrocardiographic changes.	8, 90

Vitamins

Vitamin A	Chronic ingestion of high doses may produce dry skin, rash, pruritis, hair loss, weakness, bone and joint pain, anorexia, headache, and weight loss. Papilledema and diplopia.	146
Vitamin D	Hypercalcemia. Anorexia, diarrhea, polydipsia, and polyuria. Tiredness, hallucinations, ataxia, and headache.	4

Unclassified Agents

Disulfiram (Antabuse)	Shock and myocardial infarction. Confusion, disorientation, and psychosis. Peripheral neuropathy, agranulocytosis, and thrombocytopenia.	3, 41, 173
Levodopa (Larodopa)	Nausea, diarrhea, cardiac changes, orthostatic hypotension, ataxia, and dyskinesias. Psychic changes include euphoria, dementia, depression, and hallucinations. Urinary retention	51, 78, 176

REFERENCES

1. Alarcon-Segovia, D., Wakim, K. G., Worthington, J. W., and Ward, L. E.: Clinical and experimental studies in the hydralazine syndrome and its relationship to systemic lupus erythematosus. Medicine (Baltimore), 46:1–33, 1967.
2. Alwall, N., Halldorson, T., Kjellstrand, C. M., Lindholm, T., and Ahlstrom, C. G.: On corticosteroid and azathioprine treatment of glomerular renal diseases: A study of 90 cases, treated 1964–1969. Acta Med. Scand., 192:455–463, 1972.
3. Amador, E., and Gazdar, A.: Sudden death during disulfiram-alcohol reaction. Q. J. Stud. Alcohol, 28:649–654, 1967.
4. American Hospital Formulary Service. Washington, D.C., American Society of Hospital Pharmacists, 1972.
5. Angus, J. W. S., and Simpson, G. M.: Fluphenazine enanthate in the treatment of chronic schizophrenia. Pharmakopsychiat. Neuropsychopharm., 2:60, 1969.
6. Ansfield, F. J., Ramirez, G., Skibba, J. L., Bryan, G. T., Davis, H. L., Jr., and Wirtanen, G. W.: Intrahepatic arterial infusion with 5-fluorouracil. Cancer, 28:1147–1151, 1971.
7. Arcieri, G. M., Falco, F. G., Smith, H. M., and Hobson, L. B.: Clinical research experience with gentamicin. Med. J. Aust., 1:30–34, 1970.
8. Awais, G. M., and Lebherz, T.: Ruptured uterus, a complication of oxytocin induction and high parity. Obstet. Gynecol., 34:465–472, 1970.
9. Ayd, F. J.: Amitriptyline: Reappraisal after six years experience. Dis. Nerv. Syst., 26:719–727, 1965.
10. Ayd, F. J.: Fluphenazine: Twelve years experience. Dis. Nerv. Syst., 29:744–747, 1968.
11. Balodimos, M. C., Camerini-Davalos, R. A., and Marble, A.: Nine years experience with tolbutamide in the treatment of diabetes. Metabolism, 15:957–970, 1966.
12. Ban, T. A.: The benzodiazepines—Part II. Appl. Ther., 9:677–680, 1967.
13. Becker, C. E., MacGregor, R. R., Walker, K., and Jandi, J. H.: Fatal anaphylaxia after intramuscular iron dextran. Ann. Intern. Med., 65:745–748, 1966.
14. Beilin, L. J., and Juel-Jenson, B. E.: Alpha- and beta-adrenergic blockade in hypertension. Lancet, 1:979–982, 1972.
15. Bennett, J. M., and Desforges, J. F.: Quinine-induced haemolysis: Mechanism of action. Br. J. Haematol., 13:706–712, 1967.
16. Birkett, D. A., Garrett, S. M., and Stevenson, C. J.: Phototoxic bullous eruptions due to nalidixic acid. Br. J. Dermatol., 81:342–344, 1969.
17. Birkett, D. P.: Vasodilators in geriatric psychiatry. J. Med. Soc. N.J., 68:619–623, 1971.
18. Blank, H., Cullen, S. I., and Catalano, P. M.: Photosensitivity studies with demethylchlortetracycline and doxycycline. Arch. Dermatol., 97:1–2, 1968.
19. Boman, G.: Rifampin-isoniazid compared with PAS-isoniazid—streptomycin in initial treatment of pulmonary tuberculosis. A controlled cooperative trial. Chest, 61:533–538, 1972.
20. Boxerbaum, B., Pittman, S., Doershuk, C. F., Stern, R. C., and Matthews, L. W.: Use of gentamicin in children with cystic fibrosis. J. Infect. Dis., 124, Suppl.:293–295, 1971.
21. Bran, J. L., Karl, D. M., and Kaye, D.: Human pharmacology and clinical evaluation of an oral carbenicillin preparation. Clin. Pharmacol. Ther., 12:525–530, 1971.
22. Today's Drugs: Drugs for rheumatoid disorders. Br. Med. J., 1:545–546, 1964.
23. Brown, P. C. C., Donaghy, M. C., Dootson, P. H., Titcombe, D. H. M., and Maclaren, D. M.: Sulphadimidine and nalidixic acid therapy in urinary tract infections in general practice. Practitioner, 207:819–826, 1971.
24. Browse, N. L., and Hall, J. H.: Effects of dipyridamole on the incidence of clinically detectable deep vein thrombosis. Lancet, 2:718–720, 1969.
25. Brumfitt, W., Black, M., and Williams, J. D.: Colestin in Pseudomonas pyocyanea infections and its effects on renal function. Br. J. Urol., 38:495–500, 1966.
26. Buchanan, R., Kinkel, A., and Smith, T.: The absorption of ethosuximide. Int. J. Clin. Pharmacol., 7:213–218, 1973.
27. Busey, J. F.: Blastomycosis III: A comparative study of 2-hydroxystilbamidine and amphotericin B therapy. Am. Rev. Resp. Dis., 105:812–818, 1972.

28. Carney, D. F., O'Reilly, B. J., and Tweddell, E. D.: Pyrantel embonate in the treatment of enterobiasis. Med. J. Aust., 2:254–256, 1971.
29. Carr, R. E., Paul, H., Rothfield, N., and Siegel, I. M.: Ocular toxicity of antimalarial drugs: Long-term follow-up. Amer. J. Opthalmol., 66:738–744, 1968.
30. Cervantes-Amezena, A., Naldjian, S., Camerini-Davalos, R., and Marble, A.: Long-term use of chlorpropamide in diabetes. J.A.M.A., 193:759–762, 1965.
31. Church, G., Schamroth, L., Schwartz, N. L., and Marriott, H. J. L.: Deliberate digitalis intoxication. Ann. Intern. Med., 57:946–956, 1962.
32. Clark, E.: Spironolactone therapy and gynecomastia. J.A.M.A., 193:163–164, 1965.
33. Cohen, A., Corgill, D. A., Abruzzi, W., Ligon, C. W., and De Felice, E. A.: Double blind comparison of namoxyrate and d-propoxyphene; A co-operative clinical trial. J. New Drugs, 6:38–44, 1966.
34. Cohen, P. G., and Romansky, M. J.: Factors influencing the trend in antimicrobial therapy. Med. Ann. D.C., 37:575–587, 1968.
35. Colarizi, A., Stegagno, G., and Multari, G.: Therapy with vincristine. Minerva Med., 63:1423–1429, 1972.
36. Connell, P. H.: Amphetamine psychosis. In Maudsley Monograph Series, no. 5, Oxford, Oxford University Press, 1958.
37. Coodley, E. L.: Newer istropic agents in the management of arrhythmias associated with cardiac failure. Angiology, 23:260–266, 1972.
38. Cooper, A. J., Magnus, R. V., and Rose, M. J.: A hypertensive syndrome with tranylcypromine medication. Lancet, 1:527–529, 1964.
39. Coull, D. C., Crooks, J., Davidson, J. F., Gallon, S. C., and Weir, R. D.: A method of monitoring drugs for adverse reactions: I. Alphamethyldopa and hemolytic anemia. Europ. J. Clin. Pharmacol., 3:46–50, 1970.
40. Crane, M. G., and Harris, J. J.: Effect of spironolactone in hypertensive patients. Am. J. Med. Sci., 260:311–330, 1970.
41. Dalessio, D. J.: Peripheral neuropathy associated with disulfiram (Antabus) therapy. Bull. Los Angeles Neurol. Soc., 33:136, 1968.
42. De Alarcon, R., and Carney, M. W. P.: Severe depressive mood changes following slow release intramuscular fluphenazine injection. Br. Med. J., 3:564–567, 1969.
43. De Vine, L. F., Springler, G. L., Frazier, W. E., Rhode, S. L., Pierce, W. E., Johnson, D. P., and Peckinpaugh, R. O.: Selective minocycline and rifampin treatment of group C meningococcal carriers in a new Navy recruit camp. Am. J. Med. Sci., 263:79–93, 1972.
44. De Wied, D.: Chlorpromazine and endocrine function. Pharmacol. Rev., 19:251, 1967.
45. Dodson, W. H., and Bennett, J. C.: Possible usefulness of azathioprine (Imuran) in severe rheumatoid arthritis. J. Clin. Pharmacol., 9:251–258, 1969.
46. Doll, R., and Fraser, P.: An epidemic of asthma deaths and its relationship to drug therapy. In Baker, S. B. de C., ed., Proceedings of the European Society for the Study of Drug Toxicity, ICS 220, Amsterdam, Excerpta Medica Foundation, 1971, p. 133.
47. Dollery, C. T.: Methyldopa in the treatment of hypertension. Progr. Cardiovasc. Dis., 8:278–289, 1965.
48. Doster, B., Murray, F. J., Newman, R., and Woolpert, S. F.: Ethambutol in the initial treatment of pulmonary tuberculosis therapy. U.S. Public Health Service, tuberculosis therapy trials. Am. Rev. Resp. Dis., 107:177–190, 1973.
49. Douglas, G., and Thompson, M.: A controlled trial of 'Mandrax' v. amylobarbitone sodium. Br. J. Clin. Pract., 22:19–20, 1968.
50. Douglas, W. W.: Histamine and antihistamines; 5-hydroxytryptamine, and antagonist. In Goodman, L. S., and Gilman, A., eds., The Pharmacological Basis of Therapeutics, 4th ed., New York, The Macmillan Company, 1971, p. 621.
51. Editorial: L-dopa for Parkinsonism. Drug Ther. Bull., 7:59, 1969.
52. Drug Surveillance Program: Acute adverse reactions to prednisone in relation to dosage. Clin. Pharmacol. Ther., 13:694–698, 1972.
53. Drury, M. I., and Timoney, F. J.: Experience with phenformin as an oral antidiabetic agent. J. Ir. Med. Assoc., 63:13–17, 1970.
54. Drutz, D. J., Fan, J. H., and Tai, T. Y.: Hypokalemic rhabdomyolysis and myoglobinuria following amphotericin B therapy. J.A.M.A., 211:824–826, 1970.
55. Eber, O.: Long-term therapy of hyperthyroidism with antithyroid substances in combination with synthetic thyroid hormones. Med. Clin., 66:1482–1485, 1971.

56. Ellison, R. R.: Intermittent therapy with 6-mercaptopurine (NSC-740) given intravenously to adults with acute leukopenia. Cancer Chemother. Rep., 56, Pt. 1:535–542, 1972.
57. Eshleman, J. L., Horwitz, M. R., De Courcy, S. J., Mudd, S., and Blakemore, W. S.: Atabrine as an adjuvant in chemotherapy of urinary tract infections. J. Urol., 104:902–907, 1970.
58. Fakhro, A. M., Ritchie, R. F., and Lown, B.: Lupus-like syndrome induced by procainamide. Am. J. Cardiol., 20:367–373, 1967.
59. Falco, F. G.: Review of bacteriology and practical studies and clinical pharmacology of gentamycin sulfate. Ther. Umsch. Suppl., 1:8–16, 1969.
60. Farbman, K., Wheeler, M. F., and Glich, S. M.: Arthritis induced by antithyroid medication. New York J. Med., 69:826–831, 1969.
61. Fitzgerald, J. D.: Inderal bei angina pectoris. Wien. Klin. Wochenschr., 79:332–336, 1967.
62. Forrest, W. H., Jr., Shroff, F., and Mahler, D. L.: Analgesic and other effects of nalmexone in man. Clin. Pharmacol. Ther., 13:520–525, 1972.
63. Foss, G. L., and Simpson, S. C.: Oral methyltestosterone and jaundice. Br. Med. J., 1:259–263, 1959.
64. Fracchia, A. A., Knapper, W. H., Carey, J. T., and Farrow, J. H.: Intrapleural chemotherapy for effusion from metastatic breast carcinoma. Cancer, 26:626–629, 1970.
65. Frank, L., Lichtman, H., Bird, L., and Petrou, P.: Experiences with methotrexate in psoriasis. Dermatologica, 137:87–97, 1968.
66. Fusenig, N. E., Obrecht, P., Stecher, G., and Gerhartz, H.: Ergebnisse der Therapie mit Vinca-Leukoblastin, Int. 2. Klin. Pharmakol. Ther. Toxikol., 1:40, 1967.
67. Geddes, A. M., Bridgwater, F. A. J., Williams, D. N., Oon, J., and Grimshaw, G. J.: Clinical and bacteriological studies with clindamycin. Br. Med. J., 2:703–704, 1970.
68. Gerbeaux, J., and Hanoteau, J.: Medications récentes dans le traitement de la tuberculose primaire. Ann. Pediat., 17:638–643, 1970.
69. German, J., Ehlers, K. H., Kowal, A., De George, F. V., Engle, M. A., and Passarge, E.: Possible teratogenicity of trimethodione and paramethodione. Lancet, 2:261–262, 1970.
70. Gibson, I. I. J. M.: Barbiturate delirium. Practitioner, 197:345–347, 1966.
71. Girard, J. P., Hildebrandt, F., and Faure, H.: Hypersensitivity to aspirin and clinical and immunological studies. Helv. Med. Acta, 35:86–95, 1969.
72. Giuffrida, J. C., Bizzarri, D. V., Masi, R., and Bondoc, R.: Continuous procaine spinal anesthesia for cesarean section. Anesth. Analg., 51:117–124, 1972.
73. Goldberg, H. L., and Nathan, L.: A double-blind study of Tofranil pamoate vs. Tofranil hydrochloride. Psychosomatics, 13:131–141, 1972.
74. Goldenberg, I. S., McMahan, C. A., Escher, G. C., Volk, H., Ansfield, F. J., and Olson, K. B.: Secondary chemotherapy of advanced breast cancer. Cancer, 31:660–663, 1973.
75. Goldner, M. G., Zarowitz, H., and Akgun, S.: Hyperglycemia and glycosuria due to thiazide derivatives administered in diabetes mellitus. N. Engl. J. Med., 262:403–405, 1960.
76. Gooch, W. M., Stowe, F. R., and Mogabgab, W. J.: Cephalexin in beta-hemolytic streptococcal pharyngitis. Clin. Med., 79:11–13, 1972.
77. Graham, J. R.: Cardiac and pulmonary fibrosis during methysergide therapy for headache. Am. J. Med. Sci., 254:1–12, 1967.
78. Granerus, A. K., Steg, G., and Svanborg, A.: Clinical analysis of factors influencing L-dopa treatment of Parkinson's syndrome. Acta Med. Scand. 192:1–11, 1972.
79. Greer, M. A., and McDonald, M. W.: Antithyroid drugs. DM, Oct., 20–26, 1967.
80. Gregory, D. H., Zaki, G. F., Sarcosi, G. A., and Carey, J. B.: Chronic cholestasis following prolonged tolbutamide administration. Arch. Pathol., 84:194–201, 1967.
81. Grounds, D., Davies, B., and Mowbray, R.: The contraceptive pill, side effects and personality. Br. J. Psychiatry, 116:169–172, 1970.
82. Guey, J., Charles, C., Coquery, C., Roger, J., and Soulayrol, R.: Study of psychological effects of ethosuximide (Zarontin) on 25 children suffering from petit mal epilepsy. Epilepsia, 8:129–141, 1967.
83. Gunther, R. E., and Bellville, J. W.: Obstetrical caudal anesthesia II. A randomized study comparing 1 percent mepivacaine with 1 percent mepivacaine plus epinephrine. Anesthesiology, 37:288–298, 1972.

84. Guttler, R. B., and Beauty, H. N.: Minocycline in the chemopropylaxia of meningococcal disease. Antimicrob. Agents Chemother., 1:397–402, 1972.
85. Gyory, A. N., Block, M., Burry, H. C., and Grahame, R.: Orudis in management of rheumatoid arthritis and osteoarthritis of the hip: Comparison with indomethacin. Br. Med. J., 4:398–400, 1972.
86. Hall, A. P.: Quinine infusion for recrudescences of falciparum malaria in Vietnam: A controlled study. Am. J. Trop. Med. Hyg., 21:851–856, 1972.
87. Halsreiter, E.: Long-term therapy with an inhalable dexamethasone ester. Med. Mschr., 25:34–37, 1971.
88. Hansen, H. W., and Wagener, H. H.: Diphenylhydantoin in the therapy of heart failure. Dtsch. Med. Wochenschr., 96:1866–1873, 1971.
89. Hardin, T. F.: Management of cutaneous migraines in pediatric practice: Report on 200 cases. J. Amer. Osteopath. Assoc., 68:970–972, 1969.
90. Harris, R. E.: Water intoxication secondary to oxytocin. Va. Med. Mon., 97:357–359, 1970.
91. Herman, E., and Raod, J.: Fatal hyperkalemic paralysis associated with spironolactone. Arch. Neurol., 15:74–77, 1966.
92. Herxheimer, A.: Atropine-like drugs. In Meyler, L., and Herxheimer, A., eds., Side Effects of Drugs, vol. 7, Amsterdam, Excerpta Medica Foundation, 1972, p. 243.
93. Heymann, W.: Nephrotic syndrome after use of trimethadione and paramethadione in petit mal. J.A.M.A., 202:893–894, 1967.
94. Hoffbrand, B. I., and Steward, J. D. M.: Carbenicillin and hypokalemia. Br. Med. J., 4:746, 1970.
95. Hollister, L. E.: Complications from psychotherapeutic drugs. Clin. Pharmacol. Ther., 5:322–333, 1964.
96. Horwitz, L. D., Herman, M. V., and Forlin, R.: Clinical response to nitroglycerin as a diagnostic test for coronary artery disease. Am. J. Cardiol., 29:149–153, 1972.
97. Hothersall, T. E., Mowat, A. G., Duthie, J. J. R., and Alexander, W. R. M.: Drug-induced lupus syndrome: A case report implicating isoniazid. Scott. Med. J., 13:245–247, 1967.
98. Howard, J. P.: Response of acute leukemia in children to repeated courses of vincristine (67574). Cancer Chemother. Abstr., 51:465–469, 1967.
99. Hurst, J. W., and Logue, R. B.: Treatment of heart failure. In Hurst, J. W., and Logue, R. B., The Heart Arteries and Veins, 2nd ed., New York, McGraw-Hill Book Co., 1970, p. 464.
100. Iuel, J., and Mune, O.: Peripheral arterial insufficiency in ergotism: Review of the literature and foot plethysmographic studies in ergotamine poisoning. Vasc. Dis., 4:159–166, 1967.
101. Jarzobski, J., Ferry, J., Wombolt, D., Fitch, D. M., and Eagan, J. D.: Vasculitis with allopurinol therapy. Am. Heart J., 79:116–121, 1970.
102. Jelinek, J. E.: Cutaneous side effects of oral contraceptives. Arch. Dermatol., 101:181–186, 1970.
103. Johnson, A. W.: Chlorpromazine ocular toxicity. N.C. Med. J., 28:474–476, 1967.
104. Johnson, H. K., and Waterhouse, C. H. R.: Lactic acidosis and phenformin. Arch. Intern. Med., 122:367–370, 1968.
105. Jorgensen, A. W., and Sorensen, O. H.: Digitalis intoxication. A comparative study on the incidence of digitalis intoxication during the periods 1950–1952 and 1964–1966. Acta Med. Scand., 188:179–183, 1970.
106. Kallos, P., and Kallos-Deffner, L.: Clinical and experimental evaluation of a new ergot-derivative (ergostine) in the treatment of migraine. Headache, 11:68–73, 1971.
107. Kallos, T., and Smith, T. C.: Continuous spinal anesthesia with hypobaric tetracaine for hip surgery in lateral decubitus. Anesth. Analg., 51:766–771, 1972.
108. Klempa, I., and Basler, D.: The effectiveness of pentazocine suppositories in postoperative pain. Ther. Ggw., 112:88–96, 1973.
109. Klinefelter, H. F.: Primary fibrositis and its treatment with pyrazoline derivatives, Butazolidin and Tandearil. Johns Hopkins Med. J., 130:300–307, 1972.
110. Krasno, L. R., and Kidera, G. J.: Clofibrate in coronary heart diseases. Effect on morbidity and mortality. J.A.M.A., 219:845–851, 1972.
111. Knott, D. H., and Beard, J. D.: A study of drugs in the management of chronic alcoholism. G. P., 36:118–123, 1967.

112. Kuchera, L. K.: Postcoital contraception with diethylstilbestrol. J.A.M.A., *218*: 562–563, 1971.
113. Lake, B.: Ampicillin in acute infections of general practice. A controlled trial. Med. J. Aust., *1*:636–640, 1971.
114. Lance, J. W., Anthony, M., and Somerville, B.: Thermographic, hormonal and clinical studies in migraine. Headache, *10*:90–104, 1970.
115. Langer, T., and Levy, R. I.: Acute muscular syndrome associated with the administration of clofibrate. N. Engl. J. Med., *279*:856–858, 1968.
116. Ledingham, J. G. G., and Bayliss, R. I. S.: Ethacrynic acid: Two years experience with a new diuretic. Br. Med. J., *2*:732–735, 1965.
117. Lee, J. C., Dushkin, M., Eyring, E. J., Engleman, E. P., and Hopper, J., Jr.: Renal lesions associated with gold therapy. Light and electron microscopic studies. Arthritis Rheum., *8*:1–13, 1965.
118. Leibold, J. E.: The ocular toxicity of ethambutal and its relation to dose. Ann. N.Y. Acad. Sci., *135*:904–909, 1966.
119. Levine, B., and Redmond, A.: Immunochemical mechanisms of penicillin-induced Coombs' positivity and hemolytic anemia in man. Int. Arch. Allerg., *31*:594–606, 1967.
120. Loogen, F., Risler, T., and Seipel, L.: Prevention of embolism in mitral valve lesion with anticoagulants. Long-term observations in patients with and without anticoagulant treatment. Dtsch. Med. Wochensch., *97*:1845–1849, 1972.
121. Luckey, W. T., and Schiele, B. C.: A comparison of haloperidol and trifluoperazine (a double-blind controlled study on chronic schizophrenic outpatients). Dis. Nerv. Syst., *28*:181–186, 1967.
122. Mainguet, P., Bleiberg, H., and Tijs, O.: Les ulceres de la reserpine. Acta Gastroenterol. Belg., *29*:503–514, 1966.
123. Malitz, S., and Kanzler, M.: Are antidepressants better than placebo? Am. J. Psychiatry, *127*:1605–1611, 1971.
124. Malm, U.: Intramuscular long-acting fluphenazine in the treatment of schizophrenia. Acta Psychiat. Scand., *46*:225–227, 1970.
125. Mambourg, A., Girotti, M., and Hauser, G. A.: Significance and therapy of anemia during pregnancy. Ther. Umsch., *28*:452–459, 1971.
126. Manten, A.: Antibiotic drugs. *In* Meyler, L., and Herxheimer, A., eds., Side Effects of Drugs, vol. 7, Amsterdam, Excerpta Medica Foundation, 1972, p. 389.
127. Marx, F. W., and Barker, W. F.: Surgical results in patients with ulcerative colitis treated with and without corticosteroids. Am. J. Surg., *113*:157–164, 1967.
128. Max, M., and Menguy, R.: Influence of adrenocorticotropin, cortisone, aspirin and phenylbutazone on the rate of exfoliation and the rate of renewal of gastric mucosal cells. Gastroenterology, 58:329–336, 1970.
129. McClure, P. D., Casserly, J. G., Charney, M., and Crozier, D.: Carbenicillin induced bleeding disorder. Lancet, 2:1307–1308, 1970.
130. McGuinness, B. W., and Parkin, J. B.: New long-acting formulation of chlorpheniramine maleate in hay fever. Br. J. Clin. Pract., *25*:139–141, 1971.
131. McKensie, I. F. C., Fairley, K. F., and Baird, C. W.: A clinical trial of furosemide. Med. J. Aust., *53*:879:886, 1966.
132. McKie, B. D.: Postoperative vomiting: The effects of premedication, anesthetic and oxytocic drugs. Med. J. Aust., *56*:1236–1238, 1969.
133. Choice of antihistamines. Med. Letter, *13*:102–104, 1971.
134. Middleman, E. L., Watanabe, A., Kaizer, H., and Bodey, G. P.: Antibiotic combinations for infections in neutropenic patients. Evaluation of carbenicillin plus either cephalothin or kanamycin. Cancer, *30*:573–579, 1972.
135. Miller, W. E., Gifford, R. W., Jr., Humphrey, D. C., and Vidt, D. C.: Management of severe hypertension with intravenous injections of diazoxide. Am. J. Cardiol., *24*:870–875, 1969.
136. Millichap, J. G.: Electroencephalographic evaluation of triclofos sodium sedation in children. Am. J. Dis. Child., *124*:526–527, 1972.
137. Mitchell, J. C.: Drugs for superficial fungous infections of the skin. Can. Med. Assoc. J., *93*:411–412, 1965.
138. Moldawer, M.: Anabolic agents: Clinical efficiency versus side effects. J. Amer. Med. Wom. Assoc., *23*:352–369, 1968.
139. Moore, G. E., Bross, I. D. J., Ausman, R., Nadler, S., Jones, R., Slack, N., and

Rimm, A. A.: Effects of 6 mercaptopurine (NSC-755) in 290 patients with advanced cancer. Cancer Chemother. Abstr., 52:655–660, 1968.
140. Moore, G. E., Bross, I. D. J., Ausman, R., Nadler, S., Jones, R., Slack, N., and Rimm, A. A.: Effects of 5 fluorouracil (NSC-19893) in 389 patients with cancer. Cancer Chemother. Abstr., 52:641–653, 1968.
141. Moore, G. E., Bross, I. D. J., Ausman, R., Nadler, S., Jones, R., Slack, N., and Rimm, A. A.: Effects of chlorambucil (NSC-3088) in 374 patients with advanced cancer. Cancer Chemother. Abstr., 52:661–666, 1968.
142. Mork, J. N., Thalhuber, W. H., and Swain, W. R.: Hematologic toxicity of chloramphenicol. Minn. Med., 52:1619–1624, 1969.
143. Morrison, J., and Killip, T.: Hypoxemia and digitalis toxicity in patients with chronic lung disease. Circulation, 44, Suppl. 2:41, 1971.
144. Moss, H. V.: Acne vulgaris: Treatment with three newer antibiotics. Cutis, 10: 375–376, 1972.
145. Mowat, A. P., and Arias, I. M.: Liver function and oral contraceptives. J. Reprod. Med., 3:45, 1969.
146. Muenter, M. D., Perry, H. O., and Ludwig, J.: Chronic vitamin A intoxication in adults. Hepatic, neurologic and dermatologic complications. Am. J. Med., 50:129–136, 1971.
147. Nelemans, F. A.: Report on a double-blind investigation into the influence of beta-pyridyl-carbinol on the cholesterol level of the blood. Arzneim. Forsch., 22:1410–1413, 1972.
148. New, C., Di Mascio, A., and De Mirgian, E.: Antiparkinson medication in the treatment of extrapyramidal side effects: Single or multiple daily dose? Curr. Ther. Res., 14:246–251, 1972.
149. Ng, P. S., Conley, C. E., and Ing, T. S.: Deafness after ethacrynic acid. Lancet, 1:673–674, 1969.
150. Noble, R. E.: Anorexigenic activity of intermittent dextroamphetamine with and without meprobamate. Curr. Ther. Res., 14:162–167, 1972.
151. Official Literature on New Drugs: Cytarabine (Cytosar). Clin. Pharmacol. Ther., 11:155–160, 1970.
152. Okihiro, M. M.: Neurological complications of antibiotic therapy. Clin. Proc., 34:18, 1968.
153. Olbing, H., Reishauer, H. C., and Kovacs, I.: Prospective comparison of nitrofurantoin and sulfamethoxydiazine in the longterm treatment of children with severe chronic recurrent pyelonephritis. Dtsch. Med. Wochenschr., 95:2469–2473, 1970.
154. Pannekoek, J. H.: Insulins, glucagon, and oral hypoglycaemic drugs. In Meyler, L., and Herxheimer, A., eds., Side Effects of Drugs, vol. 7, Amsterdam, Excerpta Medica Foundation, 1972, p. 577.
155. Perrot, H., and Thivolet, J.: Protoporphyrines erythropoiétiques et griséofulvin. Experientia, 26:256–257, 1970.
156. Pirila, V., Forstrom, L., and Rouhunkoski, S.: Twelve years of sensitization of neomycin in Finland. Report of 1760 cases of sensitivity to neomycin and/or bacitracin. Acta Derm. Venereol., 47:419–425, 1967.
157. Poth, J. L., Johnson, P. K., George, R. P., and Schrier, S. L.: Therapy of acute myelocytic leukemia. Daunomycin contrasted with a combination of cytosine arabinoside and 6-thioguanine. Calif. Med., 117:1–11, 1972.
158. Potts, D. M., and Swyer, G. I. M.: Effectiveness and risks of birth control. Br. Med. Bull., 26:26–32, 1970.
159. Radnot, M., and Varga, M.: Structure histologique de la cataracte causée par le piperazine. Ann. Ocul., 4:325, 1969.
160. Raskin, A.: High dosage chlorpromazine alone and in combination with an antiparkinsonian agent (procyclidine) in the treatment of hospitalized depressions. J. Nerv. Ment. Dis., 147:184–195, 1968.
161. Raskin, H. N., and Fishman, R. A.: Pyridoxine-deficiency neuropathy due to hydralazine. N. Engl. J. Med., 273:1182–1185, 1965.
162. Remenchik, A. P., Miller, C., Talso, P. J., and Wulloughby, E. O.: Depletion of body potassium by diuretics. Circulation, 33:796–801, 1966.
163. Rickels, K., Gingrich, R. L., Jr., McLaughlin, F. W., Morris, R. J., Sablosky, L., Silverman, H., and Wentz, H. S.: Methylphenidate in mildly depressed outpatients. Clin. Pharmacol. Ther., 13:595–601, 1972.

164. Rickels, K., Gratch, M. I., Gray, B. M., Laquer, K. G., Parish, L. C., Rosenfield, H., and Whalen, E. M.: Benzoctamine and chlordiazepoxide in anxious outpatients: A collaborative study. Dis. Nerv. Syst., 33:512–522, 1972.
165. Ricordan, J. F., and Walkers, G.: Effects of phenoxybenzamine in shock due to myocardial infarction. Br. Med. J., 1:155–158, 1969.
166. Rider, J. A.: Treatment of acute and chronic constipation with bisoxatin acetate and bisacodyl: Double-blind crossover study. Curr. Ther. Res., 13:386–392, 1971.
167. Riggs, M.: Ampicillin-probenecid treatment of gonorrhea. J.A.M.A., 220:420–427, 1972.
168. Rix, A., and Fisher, R. G.: Comparison of trihexyphenidyl and dihydromorphanthridine derivative in control of tremor in parkinsonism. South. Med. J., 65:1385–1390, 1972.
169. Robinson, B. B.: Pleuropulmonary reaction to nitrofurantoin. J.A.M.A., 189:239–240, 1964.
170. Rollo, I. M.: Drugs used in the chemotherapy of helminthiasis. In Goodman, L. S., and Gilman, A., eds., The Pharmacological Basis of Therapeutics, 4th ed., New York, The Macmillan Co., 1971, p. 1067.
171. Romanski, B., and Walczynski, Z.: Allergy in children with struma juvenile treated with thyroid hormones. Bull. Pol. Med. Sci. Hist., 9:92–94, 1966.
172. Rossman, M., Moskowitz, M., Fleishman, P., Sheppard, C., and Merlis, S.: The anti-anxiety effects of haloperidol and trifluoperazine in an outpatient population. Dis. Nerv. Syst., 31:130–133, 1970.
173. Rothstein, E., and Clancy, D. D.: Toxicity of disulfiram combined with metronidazole. N. Engl. J. Med., 280:1006–1007, 1969.
174. Rubens, R., Verhaegen, H., Brugmans, J., and Schuermans, V.: Difenoxine (R 15403) the active metabolite of diphenoxylate (R 1132) 5. Clinical comparison of difenoxine and diphenoxylate in volunteers and in patients with chronic diarrhea. Double-blind crossover assessments. Arzneim. Forsch., 22:526–529, 1972.
175. Russell-Taylor, W. J., Llewellyn-Thomas, E., and Sellers, E. A.: A comparative evaluation of intravascular atropine, dicyclomine, and glycopyrrolate using healthy medical students as volunteer subjects. Int. Z. Klin. Pharmakol. Ther. Toxikol., 4:358–364, 1970.
176. Sacks, O. W., Messeloff, C., and Schwarz, W. F.: Long-term effects of levodopa in the severely disabled patient. J.A.M.A., 213:2270, 1970.
177. Sagullo, C., Ansari, I., and Wallace, G.: Anesthetic use of pentazocine. Int. Surg., 57:889–892, 1972.
178. Samuels, M. L., Leary, W. V., and Howe, C. D.: Procarbazine (NSC-77213) in the treatment of advanced bronchogenic carcinoma. Cancer Chemother. Abstr., 53:135–145, 1969.
179. Shaftel, N., and Halpern, A.: The quinidine problem. Angiology, 9:34–46, 1958.
180. Shapiro, S., Slone, D., Siskind, V., Lewis, G. P., and Jick, H.: Drug rash with ampicillin and other penicillins. Lancet, 2:969–972, 1969.
181. Scharer, L., and Smith, J. P.: Serum transaminase and other hepatic abnormalities in patients receiving isoniazid. Ann. Intern. Med., 71:1113–1120, 1969.
182. Scheiner, J. J.: Evaluation of a combined muscle relaxant-analgesic as an effective therapy for painful skeletal muscle spasm. Curr. Ther. Res., 14:168–177, 1972.
183. Schultz, E., Cissee, H., and Hausemann, K.: Long-term therapy of advanced, vinblastine-resistant lymphogranulomatosis. Klin. Wochenschr., 48:1291–1299, 1970.
184. Seedat, Y. K., and Pillay, V. K. G.: Further experience with guanethidine—a clinical assessment of 103 patients. S. Afr. Med. J., 40:140–142, 1966.
185. Seigel, D. G., and Markush, R. E.: Oral contraceptives and relative risk of death from venous and pulmonary thromboembolism in the United States. Am. J. Epidemiol., 90:11–16, 1969.
186. Selwyn, J. G.: Hypersensitivity reactions to phenylbutazone. Br. Med. J., 4:487–488, 1967.
187. Serre, H., Simon, L., and Claustre, J.: Uric acid inhibitors in the therapy of gout. Sem. Hop. Paris, 50:3295–3301, 1970.
188. Siegel, R. R., Hellebusch, A., and Saliba, N.: Amphotericin B nephrotoxicity. Clin. Res., 18:447, 1970.

189. Simpson, G. M., Amin, M., Angus, J. W. S., Edwards, J. G., Go, S. H., and Lee, J. H.: Role of antidepressants and neuroleptics in the treatment of depression. Arch. Gen. Psychiatry, 27:337–345, 1972.
190. Sinanian, R., Ruoff, G., Panzer, J., and Atkinson, W.: Streptococcal pharyngitis: A comparison of the eradication of the organism by 5- and 10-day antibiotic therapy. Curr. Ther. Res., 14:716–720, 1972.
191. Sperling, I. L.: Adverse reactions with long-term use of phenylbutazone and oxyphenbutazone. Lancet, 2:535–537, 1969.
192. Stephen, S. A.: Unwanted effects of propranolol. Am. J. Cardiol., 18:463–468, 1966.
193. Sterlin, C., Ban, T. A., and Jarrold, L.: The place of Doxepin among anxiolytic sedative drugs. Curr. Ther. Res. 14:195, 1972.
194. Stewart, R. B.: Bromide intoxication from a nonprescription medication. Am. J. Hosp. Pharm., 30:85–85, 1973.
195. Stewart, R. B., and Cluff, L. E.: Gastrointestinal manifestations of adverse drug reactions. Am. J. Dig. Dis., 19:1–7, 1974.
196. Swineford, O., and Bray, E.: Aspirin and the F.D.A. A critical review of the aspirin problem. Va. Med. Mon., 98:128–132, 1971.
197. Szeplaki, S., Szmandra, J., and Szeplaki, Z.: Lidocaine treatment in coronary ischemia and angina pectoris. Munch. Med. Wochensch., 114:1997–2002, 1972.
198. Tauerner, D., Cohen, S. B., and Hutchinson, B. C.: Comparison of corticotrophin and prednisolone in treatment of idiopathic facial paralysis (Bell's palsy). Br. Med. J., 4:20–22, 1971.
199. Tompsett, R.: Pseudoanaphylactic reactions to procaine penicillin G. Arch. Intern. Med., 120:565–567, 1967.
200. Trethowan, W. H.: Haloperidol – its effective use in clinical practice. Bull. Postgrad. Comm. Med. Univ. Sydney, 25, Suppl. 1:28, 1969.
201. Tsai, S. H.: Experiences in the therapy of amebic liver abscesses on Taiwan. Am. J. Trop. Med. Hyg., 22:24–29, 1973.
202. Vandevelde, A. G., Mauceri, A. A., and Johnson, J. E.: 5-Fluorocytosine in the treatment of mycotic infections. Ann. Intern. Med., 77:43–51, 1972.
203. Van Eden, E. B., Falkson, H. C., and Falkson, G.: 1, 3-bis (2-chloroethyl)-1-nitrosourea (BCNU, NSC 409962) given concomitantly with cytosine arabinoside (NSC-63878) in the treatment of cancer. Cancer Chemother. Rep., 54, Pt. 1:347–359, 1970.
204. Van Metre, T. E., Jr., and Thomas, E.: Adverse effects of inhalation of excessive amounts of nebulized isoproterenol in status asthmaticus. J. Allergy, 43:101–113, 1969.
205. Von Pambor, R.: Klinische Untersuchung er über Augensanderungen unter der chlorochin langzeittherapie. Dtsch. Gesundheitsw., 23:2370, 1968.
206. Utz, J. P.: Chemotherapeutic agents for the systemic mycoses. N. Engl. J. Med., 268:938–940, 1963.
207. Waggoner, R. W.: The use of psychotropic drugs in general practice. J. Arkansas Med. Soc., 64:149–154, 1967.
208. Walker, J. G.: Fatal agranulocytosis complicating treatment with ethacrynic acid. Ann. Intern. Med., 64:1303–1305, 1967.
209. Wang, R. I. H., and Schuller, G.: Agranulocytosis following procainamide administration. Am. Heart J., 78:282–284, 1969.
210. Weinstein, A. W., and Allen, R. J.: Ethosuximide treatment of petit mal seizures. Am. J. Dis. Child., 111:63–67, 1966.
211. Wertheimer, L., Tinnerty, F. A., Jr., Bercu, B. A., and Hall, R. H.: Furosemide in essential hypertension. A statistical analysis of three double-blind studies. Arch. Intern. Med., 127:934–938, 1971.
212. Wenger, J., and Gross, P. R.: Acute pancreatitis related to hydrochlorothiazide therapy. Gastroenterology, 46:768, 1964.
213. White, J. M., Brown, D. L., Hepner, G. W., and Worlledge, S. M.: Penicillin-induced haemolytic anemia. Br. Med. J., 3:26–29, 1968.
214. Wiersum, J., Pugliese, W., Mesches, D., and Henriquez, C.: A comparison of erythromycin and methacycline in the treatment of common bacterial infections. Curr. Ther. Res., 11:156–164, 1969.
215. Wilkey, J. L., Barson, L. J., and Rowe, F. H.: Pentazocine for the relief of pain following urological procedures. J. Urol., 97:550–552, 1967.

216. Witton, K.: On the use of parenteral methylphenidate: A followup report. Am. J. Psychiatry, *121*:267–268, 1964.
217. Wolfromm, R., and Herman, D.: L'allergie médicamenteuse à l'ACTH: Ses manifestations cliniques, ses moyens de prévention. Sem. Hop. Paris, *43*:1252–1257, 1967.
218. Wolpert, A., Sheppard, C., and Merlis, S.: Thiothixene, thioridazine, and placebo in male chronic schizophrenic patients. Clin. Pharmacol. Ther., *9*:456–464, 1968.
219. Wombolt, D. G., Carretta, R., Egan, J. D., Atkins, L. L., and Milani, F. A.: Chronic ambulatory management of cardiac edema with ethacrynic acid. Clin. Med., *78*:24–28, 1971.
220. Woods, J. E., Anderson, C. F., De Weerd, J., Johnson, W. J., Donadio, J. V., Jr., Leary, F. J., and Frohnert, P. P.: High-dosage intravenously administered methylprednisolone in renal transplantation. A preliminary report. J.A.M.A., *223*:896–899, 1973.
221. Zacest, R., Gilmore, E., and Koch-Weser, J.: Treatment of essential hypertension with combined vasodilation and beta-adrenergic blockade. N. Engl. J. Med., *286*:617–622, 1972.
222. Zinn, W. J.: Side reactions of heparin in clinical practice. Am. J. Cardiol., *14*:36–38, 1964.

CHAPTER 6

DRUG INTERACTIONS

The purpose of this table is to provide a quick guide to clinically significant drug interactions. This listing is not a comprehensive review of the more than 6000 reported drug interactions which have appeared in the literature. Interactions that have been found to occur in animals, or those that have only been theorized, have not been included. Only those interactions reported to affect humans or those documented in experiments with humans have been included. In general, no attempt is made to list drug interactions resulting from obvious therapeutic duplication or antagonism (i.e., the CNS depressant effect of phenobarbital with chloral hydrate, or the antagonism between an antihypertensive agent used with a catecholamine which raises blood pressure). Some common trade names have also been included.

TABLE 6-1. *Drug Interactions*

Drug	Agent Interacting With	Effect	References
ANTIHISTAMINES			
	Central nervous system depressants	Antihistamines produce varying degrees of depressant effects on the central nervous system, and when combined with other depressants may result in oversedation.	12
ANTIBIOTICS			
Aminoglycosides:	Ethacrynic acid (Edecrin)	Ethacrynic acid in combination with aminoglycosides may result in transient or permanent hearing loss.	24, 36, 40
Kanamycin (Kantrex) Gentamicin (Garamycin) Streptomycin (Neomycin)	Muscle relaxants: Tubocurarine Succinylcholine Gallamine triethiodide	Synergism of neuromuscular blockade may occur when aminoglycoside antibiotics are administered concurrently with skeletal muscle relaxants. This same effect is seen with polymyxin antibiotics, including polymyxin B and colistimethate.	
Lincomycin (Lincocin)	Kaolin-pectin	Kaolin-pectin mixtures given concomitantly with lincomycin result in significant decreases in gastrointestinal absorption (90%) of this antibiotic.	57
Penicillins: Ampicillin Penicillin G Penicillin V	Probenecid	Probenecid can increase and prolong blood levels of penicillin.	25
Tetracyclines: Tetracycline hydrochloride Demeclocycline	Antacids containing aluminum, magnesium and calcium ions.	Divalent and trivalent cations inhibit the absorption of tetracyclines from the GI tract.	1, 34, 44

DRUG INTERACTIONS   263

	Ferrous sulfate	Orally administered ferrous sulfate decreases the absorption of tetracycline, oxytetracycline, methacycline and doxycycline.	
	Methoxyflurane (Penthrane)	The combination of these two drugs may result in nephrotoxicity.	
ANTINEOPLASTICS			
Azathioprine (Imuran)	Allopurinol (Zyloprim)	Allopurinol inhibits xanthine oxidase, an enzyme responsible for metabolism of azathioprine into an inactive metabolite, thereby increasing the toxicity of this antineoplastic.	21, 56
Cyclophosphamide (Cytoxan)	Allopurinol (Zyloprim)	Combination of these two drugs results in an increase in bone-marrow depression of cyclophosphamide.	2
Mercaptopurine (Purinethol)	Allopurinol (Zyloprim)	Allopurinol inhibits xanthine oxidase, an enzyme responsible for metabolism of mercaptopurine into an inactive metabolite, thereby increasing the toxicity of this antineoplastic.	21, 56
Methotrexate	Leucovorin	Administration of leucovorin immediately (2 hours) following methotrexate infusions will decrease the toxicity effect associated with methotrexate therapy. Simultaneous administration of these two agents will reduce the efficacy of methotrexate.	10, 38
ANTICOAGULANTS			
Bishydroxycoumarin (Dicumarol)	Anabolic steroids: Methandrostenolone (Dianabol)	Patients receiving anticoagulants orally in combination with anabolic steroids are exposed to an increased risk of hemorrhage.	27, 43

TABLE 6–1 continued on following page.

TABLE 6-1. (*Continued*)

Drug	Agent Interacting With	Effect	References
Warfarin sodium (Coumadin)	Norethandrolone (Nilevar) Oxymetholone (Anadrol)		
	Drugs bound to plasma proteins: Chloral hydrate Clofibrate (Atromid-S) Diazoxide (Hyperstat) Diphenylhydantoin (Dilantin) Indomethacin (Indocin) Phenylbutazone (Butazolidin) Oxyphenbutazone (Tandearil) Salicylates Ethacrynic acid (Edecrin)	These agents displace the anticoagulant from the protein binding site, resulting in increased prothrombin times and risk of hemorrhage.	20, 45
	Chloramphenicol (Chloromycetin)	Chloramphenicol increases the hypoprothrombinemic activity of oral anticoagulants. It inhibits the metabolism of bishydroxycoumarin, and may decrease production of vitamin K by intestinal flora.	6, 26

DRUG INTERACTIONS 265

Bishydroxycoumarin (Dicumarol)	Aspirin	Aspirin in large doses can inhibit the synthesis of prothrombin, cause gastric erosion, and decrease adhesiveness of platelets, resulting in increased anticoagulant effects.	
Warfarin sodium (Coumadin)	Cholestyramine (Cuemid) (Questran)	Cholestyramine binds warfarin in the gastrointestinal tract, impairing its absorption and leading to a decreased anticoagulant response.	50
	Dextrothyroxine (Choloxin)	An increased response to oral anticoagulants occurs when these agents are used concurrently.	53
	Drugs which decrease vitamin K production in the gastrointestinal tract: Kanamycin Neomycin	These drugs may decrease the amount of vitamin K available to the liver, thereby potentiating the anticoagulant effect.	26, 45
	Quinidine Quinine	These alkaloids can depress vitamin K-dependent clotting factors and patients may develop excessive hypoprothrombinemia.	29
	Glucagon	Glucagon enhances the anticoagulant effect.	28
	Inducers of hepatic microsomal enzymes: Barbiturates Carbamazepine (Tegretol) Glutethimide (Doriden)	These drugs can increase the synthesis of liver microsomal enzymes and thereby speed metabolism of anticoagulants, resulting in a decreased anticoagulant response.	7, 19, 49

TABLE 6–1 continued on following page.

TABLE 6-1. (Continued)

Drug	Agent Interacting With	Effect	References
CARDIOVASCULAR DRUGS			
Cardiac Drugs:			
Digitalis glycosides: Digoxin Digitoxin	Diuretics: Thiazides Chlorthalidone Furosemide Ethacrynic acid	Diuretic therapy which results in hypokalemia accentuates the cardiac toxicity of the digitalis glycosides.	9, 51
Digoxin	Propantheline (Pro-Banthine)	Anticholinergics may slow the passage of digoxin through the gastrointestinal tract, allowing for more complete absorption of this drug.	20
	Propranolol (Inderal)	The combined effect of these two drugs may result in increased bradycardia.	58
Quinidine	Sodium bicarbonate Acetazolamide (Diamox)	Agents which alkalinize the urine increase tubular reabsorption of quinidine and thereby lead to an increase in blood levels of this drug.	17
HYPOTENSIVES			
Guanethidine sulfate (Ismelin)	Amphetamines	Amphetamines antagonize the adrenergic neuron blockage produced by guanethidine.	16, 18
	Tricyclic antidepressants: Amitriptyline (Elavil) Desipramine (Norpramin) Imipramine (Tofranil)	The hypotensive effect of guanethidine is antagonized by concurrent administration of tricyclic antidepressants.	39, 42

CENTRAL NERVOUS SYSTEM DRUGS

Analgesics and Antipyretics: Salicylates	Sulfinpyrazone (Anturane) Probenecid	Aspirin antagonizes the ability of sulfinpyrazone and probenecid to increase the renal excretion of uric acid.	46, 59
	Indomethacin (Indocin)	Aspirin impairs the gastrointestinal absorption of indomethacin, causing a decrease in the serum levels of indomethacin.	22
Anticonvulsants: Diphenylhydantoin (Dilantin)	Chloramphenicol	Chloramphenicol inhibits the metabolism of diphenylhydantoin, resulting in an increase in the blood levels of diphenylhydantoin.	6
	Isoniazid (INH)	Isoniazid inhibits the metabolism of diphenylhydantoin in the liver. Patients who are genetically slow inactivators of INH may experience diphenylhydantoin toxicity.	35
Antidepressants: Monamine oxidase inhibitors: Pargyline (Eutonyl) Tranylcypromine (Parnate)	Amphetamines Ephedrine	Monamine oxidase inhibitors increase the amount of norepinephrine present in storage sites of the adrenergic neuron, and amphetamines result in the release of catecholamine. A number of patients have died and many others have developed severe toxic reactions from this combination.	31, 52
	Meperidine	Concomitant administration of these agents may produce severe reactions including hypertension, sweating, or hypotension.	4, 55
	Phenylephrine	Phenylephrine resembles ephedrine in pharmacologic action, and may produce hypertension, headache or vomiting when given with MAO inhibitors.	8, 37, 52

TABLE 6-1 continued on following page.

TABLE 6-1. (Continued)

DRUG	AGENT INTERACTING WITH	EFFECT	REFERENCES
HORMONES			
Corticosteroids: Prednisone Dexamethasone	Phenobarbital	Phenobarbital enhances the metabolism of corticosteroids, probably owing to enzyme induction. Patients may require increased doses of corticosteroids when receiving barbiturates.	3, 14
Chlorpropamide (Diabinese) Tolbutamide (Orinase)	Chloramphenicol (Chloromycetin)	Chloramphenicol can prolong the half-life of these oral hypoglycemic agents and may cause a hypoglycemic reaction.	6, 47
	Bishydroxycoumarin (Dicumarol)	Bishydroxycoumarin appears to inhibit the metabolism of tolbutamide and chlorpropamide, resulting in an increase in serum levels of these oral hypoglycemic agents. Patients may experience hypoglycemic reactions.	32, 33, 54
Acetohexamide (Dymelor) Tolbutamide (Orinase)	Phenylbutazone (Butazolidin)	Phenylbutazone administration increases serum levels of these oral hypoglycemic agents and may result in hypoglycemia.	5, 15
Hypoglycemic agents	Diuretics: Chlorthalidone (Hygroton) Ethacrynic acid (Edecrin) Furosemide (Lasix)	These diuretics may elevate levels of blood glucose in diabetics and may antagonize the hypoglycemic effect of antidiabetic drugs.	11
UNCLASSIFIED AGENTS			
Levodopa (Larodopa)	Pyridoxine	Vitamin B_6, in doses of 5 mg or more per day, may reduce or abolish the beneficial effects of levodopa.	13

REFERENCES

1. Barr, W. H., Adir, J., and Garrettson, L.: Decrease of tetracycline absorption in man by sodium bicarbonate. Clin. Pharmacol. Ther., 12:779–784, 1971.
2. Boston Collaborative Drug Surveillance Program: Allopurinol and cytotoxic drugs. J.A.M.A., 227:1036–1040, 1974.
3. Brooks, S. M., Werk, E. E., and Ackerman, S. J.: Adverse effects of phenobarbital on corticosteroid metabolism in patients with bronchial asthma. N. Engl. J. Med., 286:1125–1128, 1972.
4. Brownlee, G., and Williams, G. W.: Potentiation of amphetamine and pethidine by monoamine oxidase inhibitors. Lancet, 1:669, 1963.
5. Christensen, L. K., Hansen, J. M., and Kristensen, M.: Sulfaphenazole-induced hypoglycemic attacks in tolbutamide-treated diabetics. Lancet, 2:1298–1301, 1963.
6. Christensen, L. K., and Skovsted, L.: Inhibition of drug metabolism by chloramphenicol. Lancet, 2:1397–1399, 1969.
7. Corn, M.: Effect of phenobarbital and glutethimide on biological half-life of warfarin. Thromb. Diath. Haemorrh., 16:606, 1966.
8. Cuthbert, M. F., Greenberg, M. P., and Morley, S. W.: Cough and cold remedies: Potential danger to patients on monoamine oxidase inhibitors. Br. Med. J., 1:404–406, 1969.
9. Dall, J. L.: Digitalis intoxication. Am. Heart J., 70:572–574, 1965.
10. Djerassi, I., Abir, E., Royer, G. L., Jr., and Treat, C. L.: Long term remissions in childhood acute leukemia: Use of infrequent infusions of methotrexate: Supportive roles of platelet transfusions and citrovorum factor. Clin. Pediatr., 5:502–509, 1966.
11. Dollery, C. T.: Changes in carbohydrate metabolism after the use of diuretics. In Meyler, L., and Peck, H. M., eds., Drug-Induced Diseases, vol. 3, Amsterdam, Excerpta Medica Foundation, 1968, p. 95.
12. Douglas, W. W.: Histamine and antihistamines; 5-hydroxytryptamine and antagonism. In Goodman, L. S., and Gilman, A., eds., The Pharmacological Basis of Therapeutics, 4th ed., New York, The Macmillan Company, 1971, p. 639.
13. Duvoisin, R. C., Yahr, M. D., and Cote, L. D.: Pyridoxine reversal of L-dopa effects in Parkinsonism. Trans. Am. Neurol. Assoc., 94:81–84, 1969.
14. Falliers, C. J.: Corticosteroids and phenobarbital in asthma. (Letter), N. Engl. J. Med., 287:201, 1972.
15. Field, J. B., Ohta, M., Boyle, C., and Remer, A.: Potentiation of acetohexamide hypoglycemia by phenylbutazone. N. Engl. J. Med., 227:889–894, 1967.
16. Flegin, O. T., Morgan, D. H., and Oates, J. A.: The mechanism of the reversal of the effect of guanethidine by amphetamines in cat and man. Br. J. Pharmacol., 39:253P–254P, 1970.
17. Gerhardt, R. E., Knouss, R. F., Thyrum, P. T., Luchi, R. J., and Morris, J. J.: Quinidine excretion in aciduria and alkaluria. Ann. Intern. Med., 71:927–933, 1969.
18. Gulati, O. D., Dave, B. T., and Gokhale, S. D.: Antagonism of adrenergic neurone blockade in hypertensive subjects. Clin. Pharmacol. Ther., 7:510–514, 1966.
19. Hansen, J. M., Siersboek-Nielsen, K., and Skovsted, L.: Carbamazepine-induced acceleration of diphenylhydantoin and warfarin metabolism in man. Clin. Pharmacol. Ther., 12:539–543, 1971.
20. Hansten, P. D.: Drug Interactions. 2nd ed., Philadelphia, Lea & Febiger, 1973.
21. Hitchings, G. H.: Summary of informal discussion on the role of purine antagonists. Cancer Res., 23:1218–1225, 1963.
22. Jeremy, R., and Towson, J.: Interaction between aspirin and indomethacin in the treatment of rheumatoid arthritis. Med. J. Aust., 2:127–129, 1970.
23. Johanson, W. G., and Sanford, J. P.: Problems of infection and antimicrobials relating to anesthesia and inhalation therapy. Clin. Anesth., 3:300–320, 1968.
24. Johnson, A. H., and Hamilton, C. H.: Kanamycin ototoxicity – possible potentiation by other drugs. South. Med. J., 63:511–513, 1970.
25. Johnson, D. W., Kvale, P. A., and Afable, V. L.: Single-dose antibiotic treatment of asymptomatic gonorrhea in hospitalized women. N. Engl. J. Med., 283:1–6, 1970.
26. Klippel, A. P., and Pitsinger, B.: Hypoprothrombinemia secondary to antibiotic therapy and manifested by massive gastrointestinal hemorrhage. Arch. Surg., 96:266–268, 1968.
27. Koch-Weser, J., and Sellers, E. M.: Drug interactions with coumarin anticoagulants. N. Engl. J. Med., 285:547–558, 1971.

28. Koch-Weser, J.: Potentiation by glucagon of the hypoprothrombinemic action of warfarin. Ann. Intern. Med., 72:331-335, 1970.
29. Koch-Weser, J.: Quinidine-induced hypoprothrombinemic hemorrhage in patients on chronic warfarin therapy. Ann. Intern. Med., 68:511-517, 1968.
30. Koch-Weser, J., Sidel, V. W., and Federman, E. B.: Adverse effects of sodium colistimethate. Manifestation and specific reaction rates during 317 courses of therapy. Ann. Intern. Med., 72:857-868, 1970.
31. Krisko, I., Lewis, E., and Johnson, J. E.: Severe hyperpyrexia due to tranylcypromine-amphetamine toxicity. Ann. Intern. Med., 70:559-564, 1969.
32. Kristensen, M., and Hansen, J. M.: Accumulation of chlorpropamide caused by dicumarol. Acta Med. Scand., 183:83-86, 1968.
33. Kristensen, M., and Hansen, J. M.: Potentiation of the tolbutamide effect by dicumarol. Diabetes, 16:211-214, 1967.
34. Kunin, C. M., Jr., and Finland, M.: Clinical pharmacology of the tetracycline antibiotics. Clin. Pharmacol. Ther., 2:51-69, 1961.
35. Kutt, H., Brennan, R., and Dehejia, H.: Diphenylhydantoin intoxication. A complication of isoniazid therapy. Am. Rev. Resp. Dis., 101:377-384, 1970.
36. Kuzucu, E. Y.: Methoxyflurane, tetracycline, and renal failure. J.A.M.A., 211:1162-1164, 1970.
37. Lader, M. H., Sakalis, G., and Tansella, M.: Interactions between sympathomimetic amines and a new monoamine oxidase inhibitor. Psychopharmacologia, 18:118, 1970.
38. Lefkowitz, E., Papac, R. J., and Bertino, J. P.: Head and neck cancer III. Toxicity of 24 hour infusions of methotrexate (NSC-740) and protection by leucovorin (NSC-3590) in patients with epidermoid carcinomas. Cancer Chemother. Rep., 51:305-311, 1967.
39. Leishman, A. W. D., Matthews, H. L., and Smith, A. J.: Antagonism of guanethidine by imipramine. Lancet, 1:112, 1963.
40. Mathog, R. H., and Klein, W. J., Jr.: Ototoxicity of ethacrynic acid and aminoglycoside antibiotics in uremia. N. Engl. J. Med., 280:1223-1224, 1969.
41. Mielke, C. H., and Britten, A. F. H.: Use of aspirin or acetaminophen in hemophilia. N. Engl. J. Med., 282:1270, 1970.
42. Mitchell, J. R., Arias, L., and Oates, J. A.: Antagonism of the antihypertensive action of guanethidine sulfate by desipramine hydrochloride. J.A.M.A., 202:973-975, 1967.
43. Murakami, M., Odake, K., and Marsuda, T.: Effects of anabolic steroids on anticoagulant requirements. Jap. Circ. J., 29:243-250, 1965.
44. Neuvonen, P. J., Gothoni, G., Hackman, R., and Bjorksten, K.: Interference of iron with the absorption of tetracycline in man. Br. Med. J., 4:532-534, 1970.
45. O'Reilly, R. A., and Aggeler, P. M.: Determinants of the response to oral anticoagulant drugs in man. Pharmacol. Rev., 22:35-96, 1970.
46. Oyer, J. H., Wagner, S. L., and Schmid, F. R.: Suppression of salicylate-induced uricosuria by phenylbutazone. Am. J. Med. Sci., 251:1-7, 1966.
47. Petitpierre, B., and Fabre, J.: Chlorpropamide and chloramphenicol. (Letter), Lancet, 1:789, 1970.
48. Pittinger, C. B., Ergasa, Y., and Adamson, R.: Antibiotic-induced paralysis. Anesth. Analg., 49:487-501, 1970.
49. Robinson, D. S., and MacDonald, M. G.: The effect of phenobarbital administration on the control of coagulation achieved during warfarin therapy in man. J. Pharmacol. Exp. Ther., 153:250, 1966.
50. Robinson, D. S., Benjamin, D. M., and McCormack, J. J.: Interaction of warfarin and non-systemic gastrointestinal drugs. Clin. Pharmacol. Ther., 12:491-495, 1971.
51. Shapiro, S., Slone, D., Jick, H., and Lewis, G. P.: The epidemiology of digoxin. J. Chronic Dis., 22:361-371, 1969.
52. Sjoqvist, F.: Psychotropic drugs (2). Interaction between monoamine oxidase (MAO) inhibitors and other substances. Proc. R. Soc. Med., 58:967-978, 1965.
53. Solomon, H. M., and Schrogie, J. J.: Change in receptor site affinity: A proposed explanation for the potentiating effect of D-thyroxine on the anticoagulant response to warfarin. Clin. Pharmacol. Ther., 8:797-799, 1967.
54. Solomon, H. M., and Schrogie, J. J.: Effect of phenyramidol and bishydroxycoumarin on the metabolism of tolbutamide in human subjects. Metabolism, 16:1029-1033, 1967.

55. Vigran, I. M.: Dangerous potentiation of meperidine hydrochloride by pargyline hydrochloride. J.A.M.A., *187*:953-954, 1964.
56. Vogler, W. R., Bain, J. A., and Huguley, C. M., Jr.: Metabolic and therapeutic effects of allopurinol in patients with leukemia and gout. Am. J. Med., *40*:548-559, 1966.
57. Wagner, J. G.: Design and data analysis of biopharmaceutical studies in man. Canad. J. Pharm. Sci., *1*:55-68, 1966.
58. Watt, D. A. L.: Sensitivity to propanolol after digoxin intoxication. Br. Med. J., 3:413-414, 1968.
59. Yu, T. F., Dayton, P. G., and Gutman, A. B.: Mutual suppression of the uricosuric effects of sulfinpyrazone and salicylate: A study on interactions between drugs. J. Clin. Invest., *42*:1330-1339, 1963.

CHAPTER 7

CONTROL AND PREVENTION

At present it is possible to advance only broad general principles to assist the medical practitioner and the pharmacist in avoiding drug-induced diseases. Factors that affect the ways in which patients view and use their medicines, and the ways in which physicians become knowledgeable about drugs, as well as factors which may help physicians to become better prescribers, will be discussed. The potential value of the pharmacist as a drug expert and the method by which he can prepare for this new role also will be outlined.

The development and expansion of the field of drugs have outpaced our understanding of pharmacology to such an extent that only in a few instances is it possible to provide definitive guidelines for the safe administration of drugs. Factors known to predispose to drug reactions will be reviewed. Examples involving specific drugs will be given only for illustrative purposes. We will not consider as a separate topic periodic blood tests which may be given to detect early drug-induced changes (e.g., white blood cell counts or liver function studies), but this should not minimize their importance in given circumstances. The general principles outlined in this section hopefully will assist in reducing clinical problems with drugs.

A COMPENDIUM OF FACTORS INFLUENCING DRUG CONTROL AND USE

THE ROLE OF THE PATIENT

A patient's attitude toward medicines often may determine what drugs he will take, how often he will take them, and in what amounts. Many people believe that taking a drug is the way to relieve mental anguish, fear, fatigue, wakefulness, anorexia, obesity, and other miseries and discomforts. In people who hold such attitudes, excessive drug exposure, drug interactions, or overdose can lead to adverse effects. Conversely, other people are fearful of drugs or have a stoic self-image that prevents them from taking appropriately prescribed medicines, or leads them to reduce their prescribed dose so that the drug's therapeutic effect is limited or nullified.

Although age, sex, cultural, socio-economic, educational, and other factors may influence patient compliance in taking recommended drugs, many patients receive inadequate instructions and information from their physicians, or do not follow the directions stipulated on the package containing the drugs they take. Physicians certainly should increase their efforts to provide explicit instructions to patients about the drugs they recommend or prescribe. Patients also should read the instructions on the drug package carefully. In addition, the dispensing pharmacist should play a larger role in informing, instructing, and counseling patients about drugs.

Irrational drug use today is too often attributable to the public's being badly informed or misinformed. Much drug advertising aimed at the lay public is clearly geared to inculcate and reinforce the idea that medicine should be taken for any and every conceivable purpose. A lack of knowledge may not always be overcome by providing rational information, but there is no justification for condoning tactics that coerce the public to act unwisely or irrationally. Although drug advertising has improved, other means must be developed to provide the public with the information they need to use drugs judiciously.

The public must be informed that every drug is capable of causing untoward effects. A "healthy fear" of drugs brings with it the caution and care that are required to use medicines rationally. Defensive drug utilization is as important as defensive driving.

The Role of the Physician

Despite the massive expansion of the therapeutics of drugs in the past few years, there has been a decrease in many medical schools in educational programs in pharmacology and therapeutics for medical students. This has, in part, been the result of an increasing involvement of pharmacologists in molecular biology and biochemistry, with a consequent reduction in instructional efforts in the principles of pharmacology as they must be learned to use drugs effectively in the treatment of patients.

The discipline of clinical pharmacology has evolved from the basic and clinical science aspects of pharmacology. The clinical pharmacologist often assumes the role of providing instruction in the fundamentals of pharmacology and their clinical application in prescribing drugs rationally.

Continuing the education of physicians in pharmacology and therapeutics is essential. Many physicians depend too heavily on drug company detail men and advertising to obtain information about new drugs and new drug products. The manufacturer makes every effort to sell his product, and bias is a built-in feature of his promotion. Detail men should be better prepared to provide drug information than many are at present. The pharmacist can be trained to serve as an impartial drug expert, providing information needed by physicians. Medical schools have an obligation to increase their efforts in providing education for physicians in pharmacology and therapeutics. Such educational and informational programs, however, may not have a major effect upon drug utilization. Compendia of drug information that are useful and valuable as reference sources have been developed and widely distributed to physicians, but they also are not likely to alter patterns of drug use by patients significantly.

In institutional settings, drug formularies have markedly influenced drug utilization, especially if drugs not listed in the formulary are not stocked by the pharmacy and can be obtained only through restrictive procedures. The acceptability of such a restrictive formulary is predicated upon the cooperation of physicians and pharmacists who have the responsibility and authority to identify and stock only those drugs with demonstrated efficacy and safety which are required to meet the needs of patients. Community or noninstitutionalized settings present greater problems in the development and use of a restrictive formulary, but such formularies could influence prescribing practices beneficially, and would reduce the need to maintain inventories of an excessive number of different drugs and drug products. The process involved in developing, revising, and updating a formulary, requiring physicians and pharmacists to examine the evidence of a drug's value, limitations, safety, and use, can provide an important means for continuing the education of physicians in pharmacology and therapeutics. It also would force physicians to assess critically their use of particular drugs to justify addition to or retention of these drugs in the formulary. Those physicians specifically involved in establishing a formulary might become sufficiently well-informed to serve as drug experts, and possibly to develop programs for continuing the education of others.

The Role of the Pharmacist

The pharmacist's role as a drug expert has not been fully developed. Pharmacists could, and some can and do, serve as drug experts by providing professional services to meet the needs of physicians and of the public for drug information and guidance.

Training for a new and enlarged professional role should be instituted. In order for the pharmacist to realize the full potential of this new role, however, better relationships should be developed between pharmacists and physicians. Moreover, patients must recognize the pharmacist as a possible expert on drugs. Many pharmacists will have to be better informed than they are at present, and facilities for counseling patients in pharmacies will have to be developed, since such counseling cannot be provided adequately at a cash register. Hospital and clinical pharmacists also should develop the means to assist physicians and nurses in advising patients about drugs prescribed for them when they are discharged from hospitals. Those pharmacists who are prepared to provide professional services as drug experts should be certified by some professional organization, to avoid the problem of unqualified pharmacists assuming this function.

Dispensing pharmacists should develop and maintain "drug profiles" on patients to help the physician, the pharmacist, and the patient to avoid inadvertent drug interactions and drug misuse. Such files could be used by pharmacists in counseling patients about nonprescription drugs which may adversely interact with other drugs they are taking.

The Factor of Drug Dosage

Most adverse drug reactions are caused by the pharmacologic effects of the drug, which are dependent upon the concentration of the drug at its site of action. Although drug dosage in children is usually determined by age, weight, or body surface area, while drug dosage for adults is usually standardized, there is not a lower incidence of drug reactions in children than in adults. This suggests that methods now used to determine drug dosage are inadequate to prevent the occurrence of adverse pharmacologic effects in some individuals.

Effector site concentration of a drug depends on dose, bioavailability, absorption, metabolism, and excretion. Excessive blood levels of a drug can result from changes in any of these mechanisms. For example, many adverse pharmacologic effects of drugs are directly related to increased blood concentrations caused by differences in bioavailability in persons given a standardized dose or a dose determined by age, body weight, or body surface area. Avoidance of many deleterious pharmacologic effects of drugs, therefore, will depend upon prescribing individualized doses which can be determined by measurement of blood concentration or bioavailability of drugs administered to each patient. This is especially important for drugs with a steep dose response curve which also have a narrow therapeutic index or therapeutic-to-toxic ratio, such as cardiovascular and anticoagulant drugs. Techniques for determining blood concentration of some drugs have long been in use (e.g., blood salicylate levels), and new methods have recently been introduced to include a wider range of drugs (e.g., blood levels of digitalis compounds).

The Individual Drug

Adverse drug effects occur more frequently with certain drugs than with others. The incidence of adverse reactions from antineoplastic compounds is many times greater than that for most other drugs. These and other drugs that often lead to adverse effects, such as digitalis compounds, anticoagulants, hypoglycemic agents, antihypertensive agents, and others, should be used with care and in appropriately progressive doses. Other drugs, such as chloramphenicol, may be the cause of a rare but often fatal effect, in this instance aplastic anemia, and therefore should be used only for appropriate indications and not in a lax fashion.

The Number of Drugs Taken

The more drugs taken by an individual at a given time, the greater the likelihood of an adverse drug reaction. This relationship is not simply additive, but appears to be logarithmic. Individuals receiving 5 or less drugs have about a 4 per cent incidence of adverse effects, while individuals receiving three times as many drugs (11 to 15 drugs) have a 24 per cent, or six times greater, incidence of adverse effects. This is probably a result of drug interactions, synergistic effects, or cumulative effects. Also, as a rule, sicker patients receive more drugs, and there is a direct relationship between severity of illness—at least as reflected by impaired renal and hepatic function, duration of illness, and potential lethality—and the chance of a patient experiencing an adverse drug reaction. In all patients, but especially in very ill patients, therefore, it is important to restrict the number of drugs administered to those that are absolutely essential to the patient's management.

Drug Interactions

With the greater numbers and types of drugs presently available, drug interactions have become increasingly important as causes of harmful reactions, and an increasing number of adversely interacting drugs have been identified. Interactions can occur between prescription and nonprescription drugs, between nonprescription and other nonprescription drugs, and between one prescription drug and another. As patients are cared for by increasing numbers of different physicians, and as the public consumes increasing numbers of nonprescription drugs, the possibility of adverse drug interactions rises correspondingly. In order to avoid unfavorable drug interactions, a physician must be aware of which combinations of drugs produce adverse interactions and which drugs, both prescription and nonprescription, a patient is already taking.

Previous Adverse Reactions

Patients who experience or have experienced a known adverse reaction to a drug are predisposed to additional drug-induced illness, even with drugs that are unrelated to the one responsible for the initial reaction. Such patients should be told to use nonprescription drugs with caution and sparingly, and physicians also should restrict drug prescribing for such patients. The reasons for the predisposition of patients expcricncing one adverse drug reaction to additional reactions are usually not clear. In instances when allergic reactions have occurred, the causative drug and its congeners should not be readministered.

The Factor of Age

The very young and aged persons experience more adverse drug reactions than others. In infants, this is largely a result of immature hepatic enzyme systems that are unable to metabolize many drugs sufficiently. The elderly are exposed to more drugs because of a greater incidence of chronic and multiple illnesses among them. Also, there is a gradual diminution in body size and creatinine clearance in the aged which can lead to a buildup of excessive blood levels of a drug administered in a normal adult dose. Care must be exercised both in deciding upon the drug and the dosage when prescribing for patients at these opposite ends of the age spectrum.

Genetic Factors

In some individuals, sensitivity to certain drugs is caused by genetically determined disorders. Oxidant drugs produce hemolysis in individuals with erythrocyte enzymatic defects, the most common one being glucose-6-phosphate dehydrogenase (G-6-PD) deficiency. Pseudocholinesterase deficiency leads to prolonged apnea when succinylcholine is used during surgery. Individuals who are slow acetylators of isoniazid have more reactions to this drug. Most patients with these genetic traits are identified only after they have experienced a harmful effect of a drug, and thus preventing adverse drug effects in such individuals is often impossible. In patients known to have such disorders, however, troublesome drugs can be avoided.

Predisposing Diseases

Persons with certain diseases may have their illness precipitated or aggravated by certain drugs. For example, diabetes mellitus can be worsened by certain diuretics and corticosteroids; gout can be precipitated by thiazide diuretics, low doses of aspirin, and pyrazinamide; attacks of acute intermittent porphyria may be brought on by barbiturates, griseofulvin, and many other drugs. Intravenously administered tetracyclines are particularly prone to cause marked hepatic and renal damage in the fetus when given during the third trimester of pregnancy. Further, women experiencing pruritus and jaundice during the third trimester of pregnancy are prone to develop cholestatic jaundice with the later administration of oral contraceptives. Administration of drugs during pregnancy may have deleterious effects on the fetus but no adverse manifestations in the mother. No drug should be administered to a pregnant woman unless it has been satisfactorily demonstrated to be free of risk, or unless it is given for life-saving purposes.

Patients with compromised renal function are prone to adverse pharmacologic drug effects from drugs requiring renal excretion for their removal from the body. Many tables are available as guides for reducing the dosage of drugs that are dependent on the degree of the patient's renal function. Hepatic dysfunction can lead to altered metabolism and excretion of drugs. Patients with liver disease experience an incidence of adverse effects from sedatives and tranquilizers which is five times greater than that in patients with normal liver function.

Patients with gastrointestinal disease have more allergic drug reactions for unknown reasons, while individuals with atopic disease (asthma, hay fever, atopic dermatitis) are more predisposed to anaphylactic drug reactions. The presence of infection leads to an overall increase in adverse drug reactions to both antibiotics and other drugs. More allergic reactions also occur in such patients, but these are not attributable to antibiotics. However, patients with infections generally receive more drugs than patients with many other types of illnesses, and this may be an important factor in the increased incidence of adverse effects. In addition, patients with cerebral dysfunction or myocardial irritability and some forms of metabolic disorders may be predisposed to the pharmacologic effects of and experience adverse reactions to certain drugs. When the aforementioned conditions are present in a patient, potentially hazardous drugs must be avoided. It must be remembered that evidence of drug safety and action in normal subjects is not necessarily an adequate guide to safe and effective use of drugs in patients who are ill.

The complexities involved in administering many different drugs to patients with many different diseases, and who have variable degrees of predisposition to the pharmacologic and immunologic effects of drugs, clearly illustrate the need for professionally trained drug experts to assist physicians and patients in the judicious and rational use of drugs.

INDEX

Note: *Italicized* page numbers indicate figures; (t) indicates table.

Abnormalities, biochemical, as drug effects, 24–25
  fetal, drug-induced, 6, 24, 28–30
Absorption and distribution of drugs, 32–35. See also *Metabolism of drugs*.
  and active transport, 36, 37
  and drug/drug binding, 45
  changes in, related to clinical response, 44–47
  mechanism of, 32–35
  rate of, and intoxication, 45–46
  un-ionized, 33, 44
Acetaminophen (Tylenol), adverse reactions caused by, 243
Acetanilid, as cause of sulfhemoglobinemia, 106
Acetazolamide (Diamox), adverse reactions caused by, 247
  as cause of metabolic acidosis, 175
  as cause of renal calculi, 163
  as cause of renal impairment, 161
Acetohexamide (Dymelor), adverse effects caused by interactions with other drugs, 268
  as cause of liver damage, 138
Acetophenetidin (Phenacetin), adverse reactions caused by, 243
Acid-base changes, drug-induced, types of, 174–175
Acidosis, lactic, drugs causing, 175
  metabolic, as related to drug-induced disease syndromes, 175, 175(t)
    drugs causing, 175, 175(t)
  renal tubular, drug-induced, as related to hypokalemia, 173
    drugs causing, 162, 175
Acneiform drug eruptions, course of, 86
  drugs causing, 86, 86(t)
ACTH, adverse reactions caused by, 250
  acne, 86(t)
  diabetogenic effect of, 151
  diffuse hyperpigmentation, 93
  hirsutism, 96

ACTH *(Continued)*
  adverse reactions caused by,
    intravascular thrombosis, 125
    nonthrombocytopenic purpura, 111
    peptic ulceration, 128
    thrombophlebitis, 125
  exogenous, as cause of Cushing's disease, 155
Active transport, and drug absorption, 36, 37
Addiction, drug, in neonates, caused by barbiturates, 169
  caused by narcotics, 169
Adenocarcinoma, vaginal, as caused by diethylstilbestrol, 165, 170
Adenomas, hepatic, drugs causing, 141
Administration of drug, route of, and incidence of side effects, 39
  as factor in immunologic response, 63
Adrenal gland disorders, drug-induced, 155
Adrenal insufficiency, drug-induced, 155
  as related to hyponatremia, 172
  drugs causing, 155
Adrenals, adverse reactions caused by, 249
Age, as factor in predisposition to adverse drug reactions, 277
  digitalis intoxication, 118
  pharmacologic actions of drugs, 25, 26
Agonist, drug, types of, 49
Agranulocytosis, as an allergic drug reaction, 71
  drug-induced, 5, 107
  drugs causing, 107, 108(t)
Akathisia, drugs causing, 187
Albumin, serum, drug binding to, 47–48, 48(t)
Alkaline phosphatase levels, changes in liver function tests, drugs causing, 138
Alkalosis, metabolic, as related to drug-induced disease syndromes, 174–175, 175(t)
  drugs causing, 174–175, 175(t)

279

280 INDEX

Alkylating agents, as cause of skin discoloration, 94
Allopurinol (Zyloprim), adverse reactions caused by, 248
    renal calculi, 163
Alopecia, drugs causing, 94–95, 95(t)
Alpha-adrenergic blocking agents, as cause of hypotension, 124, 125(t)
AMA Drug Evaluation, 9
Amenorrhea, as related to drug-induced disease syndromes, 164
    drug-induced, 156
    drugs causing, 156, 164
American Medical Association, regulation of drug use, 9
Amines, sympathomimetic, as cause of anxiety, 194
    as cause of glaucoma, 209
    as cause of hypertension, 122
Aminoglycosides, adverse effects caused by interactions with other drugs, 262–263
Aminopterin, as cause of multiple congenital anomalies, 166
Aminopyrine, as cause of agranulocytosis, 5, 107
    as cause of anaphylaxis, 203
Aminorex, as cause of pulmonary hypertension, 146
Aminosalicylic acid (P.A.S.), adverse reactions caused by, 233
Amitriptyline (Elavil), adverse reactions caused by, 245
    as cause of seizures, 189
Ammonium chloride, as cause of metabolic acidosis, 175
Ammonium compounds, quaternary, as cause of myasthenia gravis, 186
Amobarbital (Amytal), adverse reactions caused by, 247. See also *Phenobarbital*.
Amodiaquine (Camoquin), as cause of skin discoloration, 94
Amphetamine(s), as cause of anxiety, 194
    as cause of central nervous system excitation, 188
    as cause of depression, 195
    as cause of drug fever, 198
    as cause of euphoria, 194
    as cause of seizures, 189
Amphetamine intoxication, as cause of psychosis, 196
Amphotericin B (Fungizone), adverse reactions caused by, 230
    drug fever, 198(t)
    immune hemolysis, 104
    renal impairment, 160
    renal tubular acidosis, 162
    spinal cord lesions, 192
Ampicillin, adverse reactions caused by, 230
    in interactions with other drugs, 262

Ampicillin intoxication, as cause of psychosis, 196
Analgesics, adverse reactions caused by, 243
    decrease in kidney function, 158, 159(t)
    in interactions with other drugs, 267
    megaloblastic anemia, 105
Anaphylactic drug reactions, as related to atopic disease, 278
Anaphylactoid purpura, as allergic drug reaction, 69
Anaphylaxis, drug-induced, as immunologic reaction, 67
    drugs causing, 202–203, 202(t)
Androgens, adverse reactions caused by, 249
    acne, 86(t)
    cholestatic jaundice, 132, 133
    hirsutism, 95
    virilizing effects, 157
Anemia(s), aplastic, drug-induced, 23, 97, 100
    drugs causing, 97, 98(t), 99, 99(t), 100
    hemolytic, drug-induced, types of, 100–102
    immunologic hemolytic, mechanisms of, 70–71
    iron deficiency, as related to drug-induced disease syndromes, 105
    drug-induced, 105
    drugs causing, 105
    megaloblastic, drug-induced, 104–105
    drugs causing, 104–105, 105(t)
Anesthetics, halogenated, as cause of hepatocellular jaundice, 135
    local, adverse reactions caused by, 250–251
Angina pectoris, drug-induced, mechanisms of, 115–116
    drugs causing, 115–116
Angiomata, spider, drugs causing, 94
Angioneurotic edema, as an allergic drug reaction, 90–91
    drugs causing, 90–91
Antagonist, drug, types of, 49
Anthelmintics, adverse reactions caused by, 229
Antiarrhythmic drugs, as cause of hypotension, 124, 125(t). See also *Cardiac drugs, Digitalis*.
Antiarthritics, as cause of hepatocellular jaundice, 137
    as cause of peptic ulcer and gastrointestinal bleeding, 128
Antibiotics. See also *Antimicrobials*.
    adverse reactions caused by, 230–233
    in interactions with other drugs, 262
    allergic reactions to, 6
    aminoglycoside, as cause of neuromuscular blockade, 146, 147, 147(t)

INDEX

Antibiotics *(Continued)*
 aminoglycoside, as cause of renal impairment, 159
  as cause of tinnitus and deafness, 213
 antifungal, adverse reactions caused by, 230
 as cause of candidiasis, 205
 as cause of drug-resistant organisms in bacterial infection, 204
 as cause of hairy tongue, 126
 as cause of myasthenia gravis, 186
 as cause of peripheral neuropathies, 184
 as cause of ulcerative proctitis, 130
 polymixin, as cause of neuromuscular blockade, 146, 147, 147(t)
  as cause of renal impairment, 159
Antibodies. See also *Immunoglobulins*.
 as cause of immunologic reactions to drugs, 66–72
 as factors in distribution of antigen in lymphoid tissue, 64
 interaction with drug, mechanisms of, 64
 role of IgG, IgE, and IgM, in drug fever, 71
 role of IgG, IgM, and IgA, in immunologic hemolytic anemia, 70
 specific, interaction with antigen, 64
Anticholinergic(s), as cause of central nervous system excitation, 188
 as cause of dry mouth, 126
 as cause of glaucoma, 209
 as cause of seizures, 190
 as cause of urinary retention, 163
 intoxication, as cause of psychoses, 196
 parenteral, role of in small bowel lesions, 129
Anticholinesterases, as cause of apnea, 147
 as cause of cataracts, 208
 as cause of myasthenia gravis, 186
Anticoagulants, adverse reactions caused by, 22, 239
 adrenal insufficiency, 155
 fetal hemorrhage, 167
 gangrenous lesions, 89
 hematuria, 163
 hemopericardium, 116
 in interactions with other drugs, 263
  in bleeding disorders, 112, 112(t)
 intracerebral hemorrhage, 191
 neonatal bleeding, 168
 pericardial damage, 116
 pulmonary hemorrhage, 146
 spinal cord lesions, 192
 subconjunctival hemorrhage, 207
 oral, as cause of hemorrhage, 111
  displacement from binding sites by drugs in coagulation defects, 111
  interaction with drugs to cause changes in prothrombin time, 111, 112(t)

Anticoagulants *(Continued)*
 oral, interaction with disease syndromes to change prothrombin time, 112, 112(t)
  role of in small bowel lesions, 129
Anticonvulsants, adverse reactions caused by, 244–245
 hepatocellular jaundice, 136(t)
 in interactions with other drugs, 267
 pseudolymphoma syndrome, 113
 hydantoin, adverse effects of, 23
Antidepressants, adverse reactions caused by, 245
 in interactions with other drugs, 267
 peripheral neuropathies, 185
 tricyclic, as cause of anxiety, 194
 as cause of central nervous system depression, 190
 as cause of cholestatic jaundice, 133, 133(t)
Antidiabetics, adverse reactions caused by, 249–250
 sulfonylurea, as cause of cholestatic jaundice, 134
Antidiuretic hormone secretion, inappropriate, drug-induced, 150
 as related to hyponatremia, 172
 drugs causing, 150
Antigen(s), distribution in lymphoid tissue, factors affecting, 63
 interaction with specific antibodies, 64
 use of drugs as, 60–66
Antigenicity of tissue, as affected by drug distribution, 62
Antihistamines, adverse reactions caused by, 229
 central nervous system depression, 190
 drug fever, 198(t)
 in interactions with other drugs, 262
 seizures, 189
Antihypertensives, adverse effects of, 22
 hypotension, 124, 125(t)
 myocardial infarction, 115–116
Anti-infective agents, adverse reactions caused by, 229
Antilipemics, adverse reactions caused by, 241
Antimalarials, adverse reactions caused by, 234
 hemolysis in glucose 6-phosphate dehydrogenase deficiency, 101(t)
 retinal disorders, 210
Antimicrobials. See also *Antibiotics*.
 as cause of azotemia, 159
 as cause of drug-resistant organisms in bacterial infection, 204
 as cause of renal impairment, 159
Antineoplastics, adverse reactions caused by, 23, 235–237
 as predisposing factor in infections, 205

Antineoplastics *(Continued)*
 adverse reactions caused by, aplastic anemia, dose-related, 99
 candidiasis, 205
 cholestatic jaundice, 135
 drug-resistant organisms, 205
 hepatocellular jaundice, 137
 in interactions with other drugs, 263
 megaloblastic anemia, 104
 multiple congenital anomalies, 166
 Pneumocystis carinii pneumonia, 206
 protozoal infections, 206
 pulmonary infections, 148
 suppression of spermatogenesis, 157
 thrombocytopenia, 111
Antipyretics, adverse reactions caused by, 243
 in interactions with other drugs, 267
Antirheumatic drugs, as cause of hepatocellular jaundice, 136(t)
Antituberculous drugs, adverse reactions caused by, 233–234
 ataxia, 192
 hepatocellular jaundice, 136(t), 137
 peripheral neuropathies, 184
 rheumatic syndrome, 183, 183(t)
Anxiety, as related to drug-induced disease syndromes, 194
 drugs causing, 194–195
Aplasia, pure red blood cell, drug-induced, 105–106
 drugs causing, 105–106
Aplastic anemia, as delayed hypersensitivity reaction, 99
 drug-induced, 23, 97, 100
 drugs causing, 97, 98(t), 99, 99(t), 100
Apnea, drug-induced, 146–147
 drugs causing, 146–147
Apronalide (Sedormid), as cause of thrombocytopenia, 109
Argyria, drug-induced, 24, 93–94
Arrhythmia(s), cardiac, caused by digitalis, 117
 types of, 118–119
 drug-induced, types of, 120–121
 sinus, digitalis-induced, 118
Arsenic(als), as cause of exfoliative dermatitis, 82(t)
 as cause of hemochromatosis, 93
 as cause of lung tumors, 148
 as cause of optic neuritis, 211
 as cause of warty lesions, 94
 organic, as cause of aplastic anemia, 98
Arthritis, septic, as caused by corticosteroids, 183
Aspirin, adverse reactions caused by, 243
 aplastic anemia, 100
 asthma attacks, 142
 gastrointestinal bleeding, 127
 hepatocellular jaundice, 137
 hyperuricemia, 178

Aspirin *(Continued)*
 adverse reactions caused by, iron deficiency anemia, 105
 myocardial damage, 116
 tinnitus, 214
 urticaria, 92(t)
Asthma, drugs causing, 142–143, 143(t)
Ataxia, drugs causing, 192–193
Atopic disease, as related to anaphylactic drug reactions, 278
Atrial contraction, premature, drugs causing, 120, 121(t)
Atrial fibrillation, and digitalis intoxication, as cause of ECG changes, 119
 drugs causing, 120, 121(t)
Atrial flutter, drugs causing, 120, 121(t)
Atrial tachycardia, as caused by digitalis intoxication, 119
 drugs causing, 120, 121(t)
Atrioventricular block, first-degree, drugs causing, 120, 121(t)
 second-degree, drugs causing, 120, 121(t)
Atrioventricular dissociation, as caused by digitalis intoxication, 119
 drugs causing, 120, 121(t)
Atropine sulfate, adverse reactions caused by, 237
Auditory damage, drug-induced, types of, 213
Autonomic nervous system drugs, adverse reactions caused by, 237–239
Azapetine phosphate (Ilidar), adverse reactions caused by, 238
 in interactions with other drugs, 263
 predisposing factor in infections in renal transplant patients, 205
Azathioprine (Imuran), adverse reactions caused by, 235
Azotemia, drugs causing, 159–160

Bacterial infections, caused by drug-resistant organisms, types of, 204–205
Barbiturates, as cause of acute intermittent porphyria, 180
 as cause of addiction in neonates, 169
 as cause of anxiety, 194
 as cause of drug fever, 198(t)
 as cause of exfoliative dermatitis, 82(t)
 as cause of fixed drug eruptions, 88(t)
 as cause of megaloblastic anemia, 105
 as cause of urticaria, 92(t)
 as cause of vesiculobullous eruptions, 91
 as cause of withdrawal syndromes, 193
Behavioral effects, drug-induced, types of, 24, 194–196
Benathine penicillin G (Bicillin), as cause of myocardial damage, 116

INDEX

Benzene, as cause of aplastic anemia, 97
Benztropine methanesulfonate (Cogentin), adverse reactions caused by, 238
Betamethasone (Celestone), adverse reactions caused by, 249. See also *Prednisone.*
Bethanechol chloride (Urecholine), adverse reactions caused by, 237
Bile excretion, inhibition of by drugs in cholestatic jaundice, 139
Bilirubin, displacement of, by drugs, 48
   in drug-induced kernicterus, 140, 169
Binding, competitive, of drugs, at receptor sites, 49
   of conjugated and unconjugated haptens, and immunologic inhibition, 64
   covalent, drug, and immunologic action, 60–61
   drug, to red-cell membrane, in immunologic hemolytic anemia, 70–71
   drug-drug, and absorption and distribution, 45, 46, 48
   drug-platelet, in immunologic thrombocytopenia, 69
   hapten to dermal protein, in contact dermatitis, 72
   noncompetitive, of drugs, at receptor sites, 49
   of bilirubin in drug-induced kernicterus, 169
   plasma protein to erythrocytes, in immunologic hemolytic anemia, 70–71
Binding, reversible, of drugs, and immunologic action, 60–61, 65
Binding sites. See *Receptor Sites.*
Bioavailability, of drugs, 39–40
Biochemical abnormalities, drug-induced, kinds of, 24–25
Bisacodyl (Dulcolax), adverse reactions caused by, 248
Bishydroxycoumarin (Dicumarol), adverse reactions caused by, 239
   in interactions with other drugs, 263, 265
Bladder. See *Renal, Urinary.*
Bleeding. See also *Hemorrhage, Coagulation, Clotting, Prothrombin time.*
   gastrointestinal, drug-induced, as related to iron deficiency anemia, 105
   drugs causing, 127, 128, 128(t)
   intracerebral, drug-induced, drugs causing, 191
   neonatal, as caused by anticoagulants, 168
   drugs causing, 168
Bleeding disorders, as caused by heparin, 111
   as related to drug interaction with oral anticoagulants, 111, 112
   drug-induced, types of, 109–112

Bleomycin (Blenoxane), as cause of pulmonary fibrosis, 144
Block, atrioventricular, first-degree, drugs causing, 120, 121(t)
   second-degree, drugs causing, 120, 121(t)
Block, heart, complete, as caused by digitalis intoxication, 119
   drugs causing, 120, 121(t)
   first-degree, caused by digitalis intoxication, 119
   sinoatrial, digitalis-induced, 118
   drugs causing, 120, 121(t)
   Wenckebach, digitalis-induced, 119, 120, 121(t)
Blood-brain barrier, and absorption of drugs, 33
Blood cell diseases, red, drug-induced, types of, 97–106
   white, drug-induced, types of, 106–109
Blood disorder, drug-induced, types of, 97–114
Blood levels, drug, determination of in prevention of adverse drug effects, 275
Bone disorders, drug-induced, types of, 182
Bone growth, retarded, drugs causing, 182
Bone marrow depression, drug-induced, 23. See also *Aplastic anemia, drug-induced.*
Bowel, large, necrosis of, drug-induced, 128
   small, lesions, drug-induced, 128
   necrosis of, drug-induced, 128
Bowel disorders, drugs causing, 130
Bradycardia, sinus, digitalis-induced, 118
   drugs causing, 120, 121(t)
Breast changes, drug-induced, 155
Breast hypertrophy, drug-induced, as cause of amenorrhea, 164
Breast milk, drugs excreted in, 30, 31(t)
Bromides, as cause of acne, 86(t)
   as cause of warty lesions, 94
Brompheniramine maleate (Dimetane), adverse reactions caused by, 229
Bronchoconstriction, drugs causing, 142–143
Budd-Chiari syndrome, as caused by oral contraceptives, 139
Busulfan (Myleran), as cause of adrenal insufficiency, 155
   as cause of diffuse hyperpigmentation, 93
   as cause of nail discoloration, 96
   as cause of pulmonary fibrosis, 144
Butacaine, as cause of keratitis, 207
Butabarbital sodium (Butisol), adverse reactions caused by, 247

Calcium, serum levels, changes in, drug-induced, 176–177

Calculi, renal, drugs causing, 163
Candida vaginitis, drugs causing, 164, 205
Candidiasis, drugs causing, 205
Carbamazepine (Tegretol), as cause of psychosis, 196
Carbenicillin (Geopen), adverse reactions caused by, 231
Carbutamide, as cause of agranulocytosis, 108(t)
  drug-induced, 23
  hepatocellular, drugs causing, 141
Carcinoma(s). See also *Tumors*, and names of specific tumors such as *Adenocarcinoma, Hepatocellular carcinoma*.
Cardiac arrhythmias, caused by digitalis intoxication, 117
  types of, 118–119
  drug-induced, types of, 120–121
Cardiac disorders, as related to effect of disease syndromes on digitalis, 118
Cardiac effects of digitalis intoxication, 117–120
  of drug interaction with digitalis, 118
Cardiovascular drugs, adverse reactions caused by, 115–125, 240–241
  in interactions with other drugs, 266
Cardioversion, electric, effect on digitalis sensitivity, 118
Carisoprodol (Soma), adverse reactions caused by, 239
Cataracts, drugs causing, 208, 209(t)
Cell membrane, interaction with drug, role of in immunologic action, 61
Cellular immunity. See *Cellular hypersensitivity, Hypersensitivity reactions*.
Cephalexin monohydrate (Keflex), adverse reactions caused by, 231
Cephaloridine (Loridine), as cause of immune hemolysis, 104
  as cause of renal impairment, 160
Cephalothin (Keflin), and response to Coombs' test, 71, 103–104
  as cause of renal impairment, 160
Cerebral dysfunction, as related to pharmacologic effect of drugs, 278
Cerebral stimulants, adverse reactions caused by, 246
Chelation, by drugs, effects of, 45, *46*
  of toxic substances, 45
Chemotherapy, as cause of hyperuricemia, 178
Chickenpox, as caused by corticosteroids, 206
Children, and pharmacologic actions of drugs, adverse effects on, 25
  delayed drug-induced effects in, 169
  dental damage in from tetracyclines, 126
  determination of drug dose for, 17
  drug-induced retarded bone growth in, 182
  female, occurrence of drug-induced vaginal adenocarcinoma in, 165, 170

Chloasma, drugs causing, 93
Chloral hydrate (Noctec), adverse reactions caused by, 247
Chlorambucil (Leukeran), adverse reactions caused by, 231, 235
  cirrhosis, 140
  multiple congenital anomalies, 166
Chloramphenicol (Chloromycetin), as cause of aplastic anemia, 99
  as cause of agranulocytosis, 108(t)
  as cause of "gray syndrome" in neonates, 169
  as cause of hypotension in newborn, 124–125, 125(t)
  as cause of optic neuritis, 211
  as cause of pure red blood cell aplasia, 105
  metabolism of, in infants, 25
Chlordiazepoxide (Librium), adverse reactions caused by, 245
  ataxia, 192
  cholestatic jaundice, 133, 138
Chlornaphazine, as cause of bladder tumors, 163
Chloroquine (Aralen), adverse reactions caused by, 234
  loss of hair color, 96
  methemoglobinemia, 106
  myopathy, 181
  peripheral neuropathies, 185
  retinal damage, 210
  skin discoloration, 94
Chlorothiazide (Diuril), adverse reactions caused by, 247
Chlorpheniramine maleate (Chlor-Trimeton, Teldrin), adverse reactions caused by, 229
Chlorpromazine (Thorazine), adverse reactions caused by, 245
  agranulocytosis, 107
  cholestatic jaundice, 132–133
  corneal damage, 208
  hirsutism, 96
  immune hemolysis, 104
  myasthenia gravis, 186
Chlorpropamide (Diabinese), adverse reactions caused by, 249
  in interactions with other drugs, 268
Chlorprothixene (Taractan), as cause of seizures, 189
Chlortetracycline (Aureomycin), as cause of anaphylaxis, 203
Chlorthalidone (Hygroton), adverse reactions caused by, 247
Chlorzoxazone (Paraflex), adverse reactions caused by, 239
Cholecystographic dyes, as cause of hepatocellular jaundice, 136(t)
Cholestatic jaundice, and allergic mechanisms of drugs, 131, 132
  caused by oral contraceptives, symptoms of, 134

INDEX

Cholestatic jaundice *(Continued)*
  chlorpromazine-induced, symptoms of, 132–133
  drug-induced, types of, 131–135
  drugs causing, 132, 133, 133(t), 134, 135
Cholesterol, malabsorption of, drug-induced, 129
  serum levels, changes in, drug-induced, 178–179
Cholinergics, adverse reactions caused by, 237
Chrysiasis, drug-induced, 93–94
Cinchona alkaloids, as cause of hemolysis in glucose 6-phosphate dehydrogenase deficiency, 101(t)
Cirrhosis, biliary, drug-induced, 139
  drug-induced, types of, 139–140
  drugs causing, 139, 139(t), 140
  postnecrotic, drug-induced, 139
Clindamycin (Cleocin), adverse reactions caused by, 231
Clioquinol (Vioform), as cause of allergic contact dermatitis, 86
Clofibrate (Atromid-S), adverse reactions caused by, 241
  myalgias, 182
Clotting, intravascular, drugs causing, 125
Clotting factors, inhibition of by oral anticoagulants, 111
Cloxacillin sodium (Tegopen), adverse reactions caused by, 231
CNS. See *Nervous system, central.*
Coagulation. See also *Bleeding, hemorrhage.*
Coagulation defects, as related to drug interaction with oral anticoagulants, 111
  drug-induced, types of, 111–112
Cocaine derivatives, as cause of drug fever, 198(t)
Codeine, adverse reactions caused by, 243
Colchicine, adverse reactions caused by, 243
  malabsorption, 129
  myopathy, 181
Colistimethate sodium (Coly-Mycin), adverse reactions caused by, 231
  ataxia, 192
Colitis, pseudomembranous, as caused by antibiotics, 205
  staphylococcal, as caused by antibiotics, 205
Colon. See also *Bowel, large.*
  vascular damage to, drugs causing, 130
Coma, as caused by drug-induced disease syndromes, 191
  drugs causing, 190–191
  hypothermic, drug-induced, in hypothyroid, 154
Competitive binding, of drugs, 49
Congenital anomalies, multiple, drugs causing, 166

Congenital heart disease, drugs causing, 167–168
Congenital ocular malformations, caused by thalidomide, 212
Congestive heart failure, as related to drug-induced disease syndromes, 117
Conjunctivitis, as related to drug-induced erythema multiforme, 207
Constipation, drugs causing, 130
Contact dermatitis, as a delayed hypersensitivity drug reaction, 72
Contractions, atrial, premature, drugs causing, 120, 121(t)
  ventricular, premature, drugs causing, 118, 120, 121(t)
Contraceptives, oral, adverse reactions caused by, 249
  bowel disorders, 130
  Candida vaginitis, 205
  cataracts, 208
  chloasma and facial melasma, 93
  cholestatic jaundice, 134
  congenital heart disease, 167–168
  deep vein thrombosis, 125
  depression, 195
  depressive and schizoaffective psychoses, 195
  fibrosis of ovaries, 164
  fluid retention and edema, 176
  hepatic adenomas, 141
  hirsutism, 95
  hypertension, 122
  hypertriglyceridemia, 178, 179
  menstrual cycle changes, 156, 164
  migraine headaches, 193
  ocular vascular lesions, 212
  optic neuritis, 211
  peliosis hepatis, 141
  pseudotumor cerebri, 192
  pulmonary embolism, 125
  small bowel lesions, 129
  stroke, 191
  systolic bruits, 122
  thromboembolic pulmonary disease, 146
  thrombophlebitis, 125
  thrombosis of the hepatic vein, 139
  as predisposing factor in cystitis, 205
  pyelonephritis, 205
  diabetogenic effect of, 151
Contrast media, oral, as cause of renal impairment, 160
Coombs' test, drug-induced reaction to, in immune hemolysis, 102–104
  in immunologic hemolytic anemia, 70, 71
  with cephalothin, 71, 103–104
  with methyldopa, 102–103
  with penicillin, 102–103
Corneal disorders, drug-induced, types of, 207–208

Corticosteroids, adverse effects caused by, in interactions with other drugs, 268
  as cause of acne, 86(t)
  as cause of adrenal atrophy, 155
  as cause of candidiasis, 205
  as cause of cataracts, 208
  as cause of chickenpox, 206
  as cause of congestive heart failure, 117
  as cause of Cushing's disease, 155
  as cause of depression, 195
  as cause of enlarged liver, 139
  as cause of euphoria, 194–195
  as cause of exophthalmos, 207
  as cause of fluid retention and edema, 176
  as cause of fungal infections, 89, 206
  as cause of glaucoma, 209
  as cause of herpes zoster, 206
  as cause of hirsutism, 96
  as cause of hypertension, 122
  as cause of hypokalemia, 173
  as cause of intravascular thrombosis, 125
  as cause of joint disorders, 182–183
  as cause of manic-depressive psychoses, 195
  as cause of myopathy, 181
  as cause of nonthrombocytopenic purpura, 111
  as cause of osteoporosis, 182
  as cause of pancreatitis, 130
  as cause of peptic ulceration, 128
  as cause of Pneumocystis carinii pneumonia, 206
  as cause of protozoal infections, 206
  as cause of pseudotumor cerebri, 192
  as cause of pulmonary infections, 148
  as cause of retarded bone growth, in children, 182
  as cause of skin discoloration, 94
  as cause of thrombophlebitis, 125
  as cause of viral infections, 206
  as predisposing factor in infections in renal transplant patients, 205
  in tuberculosis, 205
  diabetogenic effect of, 151
Corticotropin. See *ACTH.*
Coumarin, as cause of neonatal bleeding, 168
Council on Drugs, 9
Creatinine clearance, and procainamide excretion, relationship of, 28
Cushing's disease, drug-induced, 155
Cutaneous. See also *Dermatologic, Skin.*
Cutaneous drug eruptions, mechanisms of, 80
Cutaneous drug reactions, adverse, types of, 81–96
  as allergic mechanisms, 69, 81
Cyanosis, as related to drug-induced methemoglobinemia and sulfhemoglobinemia, 106

Cyclandelate (Cyclospasmol), adverse reactions caused by, 242
Cyclophosphamide (Cytoxan), adverse reactions caused by, 235
  amenorrhea, 156, 164
  hemorrhagic cystitis, 163
  in interactions with other drugs, 263
  pulmonary fibrosis, 144
  renal impairment, 161
  suppression of spermatogenesis, 157
Cystitis, hemorrhagic, drug-induced, 163
Cytarabine hydrochloride (Cytosar), adverse reactions caused by, 235
Cytotoxic drugs, as cause of alopecia, 94

Deafness, drugs causing, 213, 213(t)
  fetal, as caused by streptomycin, 213
Delayed hypersensitivity reactions, as immunologic reactions to drugs, 72–73
  role of lymphocytes in, 72–73
Demeclocycline, demethylchlortetracycline (Declomycin), adverse reactions caused by, 231
  anaphylaxis, 203
  in interactions with other drugs, 262
  nephrogenic diabetes insipidus, 163
  photodermatitis, 90
Depressant drugs, effect of on neonate, 168
Depression, central nervous system, drugs causing, 190–191
  drugs causing, 195
Dermatitis, contact, allergic, drugs causing, 86
  as a delayed hypersensitivity drug reaction, 72
  drugs causing, 86, 87(t)
  exfoliative, drug-induced, 81, *81*
  drugs causing, 82, 82(t)
Dermatologic. See also *Cutaneous, Skin.*
Dermatologic drug reactions, adverse, types of, 80–96
Dexamethasone (Decadron), adverse reactions caused by, 249. See also *Prednisone.*
  in interactions with other drugs, 268
  myopathy, 181
Dextran, as cause of anaphylaxis, 203
  as cause of renal impairment, 161
Dextran iron complex, adverse reactions caused by, 239
Dextroamphetamine sulfate (Dexedrine), adverse reactions caused by, 246
  congenital heart disease, 167
Diabetes, latent, as related to drug-induced glucose intolerance, 151
Diabetes insipidus, nephrogenic, drugs causing, 150–151, 163

INDEX

Diabetes mellitus. See also *Hyperglycemia*.
  aggravation of by drugs, 151–152
Diagnostic tests for detection of immunologic disease, types of, 73–77
Diaminodiphenylsulfone, as cause of methemoglobinemia, 106
Diarrhea, drug-induced, as related to hypovolemia, 176
  as related to hypokalemia, 173
  drugs causing, 129
Diazepam (Valium), adverse reactions caused by, 246. See also *Chlodiazepoxide*.
Diazoxide, adverse reactions caused by, 241
  hyperglycemia, 151
Dibucaine hydrochloride (Nupercaine), adverse reactions caused by, 250
Diethylstilbestrol (Stilbestrol), adverse reactions caused by, 249
  vaginal adenocarcinoma in female offspring, 165, 170
Digitalis, as cause of small bowel lesions, 128–129
  as related to disease syndromes in cardiac effects, 118
  metabolism of, as affected by hyperthyroidism, 118
  as affected by hypothyroidism, 118
  pharmacologic effects of, 117
  rate of absorption of, and interaction with other drugs, 118
  role of in causing spurious heart disease, 119
Digitalis glycosides, adverse reactions caused by, 240–241
  in interactions with other drugs, 266
Digitalis intoxication, as cause of cardiac arrhythmias, 118–119
  as cause of ECG changes, 117
  as cause of nausea and vomiting, 127
  as cause of ocular disorders, 212
  as cause of premature ventricular contractions, 118
  as cause of psychoses, 196
  as related to potassium loss, 117
  cardiac effects of, 117–120
  predisposition for in aged patients, 118
  vagal effects of, 118
Digitoxin, adverse reactions caused by, 240. See also *Digitalis glycosides*.
  in interactions with other drugs, 266
  thrombocytopenia, 110
Digoxin, adverse reactions caused by, 240. See also *Digitalis glycosides*.
  in interactions with other drugs, 266
Dioctyl sodium sulfosuccinate (Colace), adverse reactions caused by, 248
Diphenhydramine hydrochloride (Benadryl), adverse reactions caused by, 229

Diphenoxylate, adverse reactions caused by, 248
Diphenylhydantoin (Dilantin), adverse reactions caused by, 244
  ataxia, 192
  of drug fever, 198(t)
  gingival hypertrophy, 126
  in interactions with other drugs, 267
  megaloblastic anemia, 105
  multiple congenital anomalies, 166
  pure red blood cell aplasia, 106
  systemic lupus erythematosus, 199
  and protein binding, 35
Diplopia, drugs causing, 207
Dipyridamole (Persantin), adverse reactions caused by, 242
Dipyrone (Pyralgin), adverse reactions caused by, 243
  agranulocytosis, 107
Disease(s), preexisting, knowledge of in prevention of adverse drug reactions, 277–278
Displacement, of bilirubin by drugs in kernicterus, 140, 169
  of one drug by another, 48, 49
Dissociation constant, as factor in drug absorption, 33, 33(t)
Distribution of drug, and inflammatory disease, effect on immunologic response, 62
  and protein binding, 47
  and tissue antigenicity, as factors in allergic drug reaction, 62
Disulfiram (Antabuse), adverse reactions caused by, 251
  psychosis, 196
Diuretics, adverse reactions caused by, 247–248
  hypokalemia, 173
  hyponatremia, 171
  hypovolemia, 176
  thiazide, diabetogenic effect of, 151. See also *Thiazide diuretics*.
DNA synthesis, drug-induced, impairment of, in agranulocytosis, 107
  in megaloblastic anemia, 105
Dose and dosage, and duration of pharmacologic action of drug, 37, 38, 275
  as factor in drug effect, 35
  as related to aplastic anemia, 99
  as related to hemolysis, 102
  as related to hepatic function, 27
  as related to renal function, 26–27, 28
  as related to thrombocytopenia, 111
  as related to weight of patient, 26, 27
  determination of, in children, 17
  individualized, in prevention of adverse drug effects, 275
  of antineoplastic drugs, in agranulocytosis, 107
  in aplastic anemia, 99
  patient errors in, 13

Dose response curve, quantal, 21, 22
Down's syndrome, as related to drug-induced sinus tachycardia, 120
Doxepin (Sinequan), adverse reactions caused by, 245
Doxycycline (Vibramycin), adverse reactions cause by, 231
Drug absorption and distribution of ionized and un-ionized drugs, 33, 44
  role of liver in, 131
Drug advertising, 18-19
  improvement of, 273, 274
  use of by physicians, 274
Drug-drug binding, and absorption and distribution, 45, 46, 48
Drug effect, as a function of time, 35-36, 36(t)
Drug eruptions, acneiform and furunculoid, 86
  cutaneous, mechanisms of, 80
  fixed, characteristics of, 88, 88
    drugs causing, 88(t)
  vesiculobullous, drugs causing, 91
Drug fever, as an immunologic reaction, 71
  as related to allergic reactions, 197-198
  as related to drug-induced disease syndromes, 197
  drugs causing, 197, 198, 198(t), 199
Drug formularies, maintenance of, 274
Drug history, patient, 13-14, 15, 42
  as maintained by pharmacist, 74, 275
  in detection of adverse drug reactions, 73-74
    role of physician in assembling, 13-14, 74
Drug impurities, as cause of allergic reactions, 66
Drug-induced disease. See also under specific diseases.
  epidemiologic study of, 11-12, 16-17
  hazards of, 3, 5
  incidence of, 11
  prevention of, 13-14
Drug interaction(s). See *Table 6-1*.
  adverse, predisposing factors of, 17
    prevention of, 14, 16
  cholestatic jaundice, 133
  coma, 191
  hypertension, 122
  hyperuricemia, 178
  hypoglycemia, 153, 153(t)
  hypotension, 124
  related to number of drugs given, 16-17
  related to number of prescribers, 15
  seizures, 190
  as related to neuromuscular blockade, 147, 148(t)
  as related to rate of digitalis absorption, 118
  knowledge of in prevention of adverse reactions, 276

Drug interaction(s) *(Continued)*
  mechanisms of, 43-52, *44*
    at receptor sites, 44(t), 49-50
    in absorption and distribution, 44(t), 44-48
    in excretion, 44(t), 51-52
    in metabolism, 44(t), 50-51
    of parenteral drugs, 52
  sites of, 44, *44*
  with antibodies, mechanisms of, 64
  with anticoagulants, in bleeding disorders, 111, 112(t)
  with cell membrane, as factor in immunologic action, 61
  with digitalis, as related to cardiac effects, 118
  with erythrocyte membranes, in autoimmune hemolytic anemia, 71
  with lymphoid tissue, and immunologic response, 63
  with monamine oxidase inhibitors, as cause of central nervous system excitation, 188-189
    as cause of hypertensive crisis, 123, 123(t)
    as cause of intracerebral hemorrhage, 191
  with proteins, 34-35, 37-48
  with serum antiplatelet factors, as cause of immunologic thrombocytopenia, 69
Drug lipid/water partition coefficient, 32, 33
Drug manufacturers. See *Pharmaceutical industry*.
Drug pKa, effect on absorption, 33, 33(t)
Drug-platelet binding, in immunologic thrombocytopenia, 69
Drug prescription, by physicians, 12-15
Drug reactions, adverse. See *Table 5-1*.
  affecting central nervous system, types of, 188-193
  affecting peripheral nerves, 184-185, 185(t)
  and inherited risk, 29(t), 277
  and patient medication errors, 40, 41, 41(t)
  as related to multiple drug use, 42, 276
  behavioral, types of, 194-196
  cardiovascular, types of, 115-125
  dermatologic, types of, 80-96
  during pregnancy, 278
  ear, types of, 213-214
  endocrine, types of, 150-157
  fetal, types of, 166-170
  gastrointestinal, types of, 126-130
  gynecologic, types of, 164-165
  hematopoietic, types of, 97-114
  infections as, 204-206
  liver, types of, 131-141
  metabolic, types of, 171-180
  monitoring of, 16

Drug reactions (*Continued*)
  adverse, multisystem, types of, 197–203
    musculoskeletal, types of, 181–183
    neonatal, types of, 166–170
    neurologic, types of, 184–193
    ocular, types of, 207–212
    of myoneural junction, types of, 185–188
    photosensitive, 89–90
    predisposing factors, 16–17, 277
    prevention of, 272–278
    pulmonary, types of, 142–146
    related to hair and nails, 94–96
    renal, types of, 158–161
    respiratory, types of, 142–149
    urinary tract, types of, 158–163
  allergic. *See under specific diseases.*
    and rate of drug excretion, 62
    as caused by drug impurities, 66
    as caused by monovalent haptens, 65
    as effect of drug metabolism by microsomal enzymes, 63
    characteristics of, 75
    cutaneous, types of, 69
    fever as a sign of, 197–198
    hematologic, types of, 69
    immunoglobulins responsible for, 66–67, 67(t)
    laboratory tests for, types of, 73, 75
    to antibiotics, 6
  anaphylactic, as related to atopic disease, 278
Drug utilization control of, 272–278
  governmental, 6–10
  cost of, 2
  medical, history of, 4–6
  patient, factors influencing, 273
  patterns of, 2, 3, 12–16
  public attitudes toward, 2–3, 273
Drugs, active, concentration of in plasma, 31, 32
  bioavailability of, and adverse effect, 39–40
  high-risk, 40(t)
  ionized, absorption of, 33, 44
  nonionized, absorption of, 33, 44
  nonprescription. *See OTC drugs.*
  parenteral, interactions of, 52
  pharmaceutical standards for, 9
  risks of, comparison of, 39, 39(t)
  unbound. *See Drugs, active.*
  un-ionized, absorption of, 33, 44
Dyskinesia, tardive, drug-induced, symptoms of, 187–188
Dystonic reactions, acute, drugs causing, 187

Ear effects, drug-induced, types of, 213–214
ECG changes, as effects of digitalis intoxication, 117, 119

Edema, drugs causing, 176
  angioneurotic, drugs causing, 90–91
  pulmonary, drugs causing, 146
Electrocardiogram. *See ECG.*
Electrolyte imbalance disorders, drug-induced, types of, 171–174
Embolism, pulmonary, drugs causing, 125
Embryo, pharmacologic actions of drugs, adverse effects on, 24, 28
Emetine, as cause of myocardial damage, 116
  as cause of myopathy, 181
  as cause of pericarditis, 116
Emotional effects, drug-induced, 24
Encephalopathy, hepatic, drugs causing, 140
  as caused by drug-induced disease syndromes, 140
Endocrine effects, drug-induced, types of, 150–157
Enzyme defects, erythrocyte, as cause of drug-induced hemolysis, 100–102
Enzyme induction, and rate of drug metabolism, 50–51, 50(t)
Enzyme inhibition, by drugs, 49–50
Enzymes, microsomal, and drug metabolism, as related to allergic reactions, 63
Ephedrine sulfate, adverse reactions caused by, 238
Epidemiologic study, of drug-induced disease, 11–12, 16–17
Epsilon-aminocaproic acid, as cause of renal impairment, 161
Ergotamine tartrate, adverse reactions caused by, 238
  myocardial infarction, 115
Erythema multiforme, as allergic drug reaction, 69
  drug-induced, as related to conjunctivitis, 207
  symptoms of, 82–83, 83
  drugs causing, 82–83, 84(t)
Erythema nodosum, drugs causing, 86, 87(t)
Erythrocyte enzyme defects, as cause of drug-induced hemolysis, 100–102
Erythrocyte membrane, action of drug on in immunologic hemolytic anemia, 70–71
Erythrocytes, binding to plasma proteins in immunologic hemolytic anemia, 70–71
  use of in serologic tests for drug allergy, 76
Erythromycin, adverse reactions caused by, 231
  as cause of drug-resistant organisms in bacterial infection, 204
Erythromycin estolate (Ilosone), as cause of cholestatic jaundice, 134
Esophagitis, peptic, aggravation of by drugs, 127

Esophagus, drug reactions affecting, 127
Estrogens, adverse reactions caused by, 249
  synthetic, as cause of cholestatic jaundice, 134
Ethacrynic acid (Edecrin), adverse reactions caused by, 247
  deafness, 214
Ethambutol hydrochloride (Myambutol), adverse reactions caused by, 233
  optic neuritis, 211
Ethchlorvynol (Placidyl), adverse reactions caused by, 247
Ethionamide, as cause of peripheral neuropathies, 184
  as cause of rheumatic syndrome, 183
Ethosuximide (Zarontin), adverse reactions caused by, 245
Euphoria, drug-induced, drugs producing, 194–195
Evaluations of Drug Interactions, 44
Exanthematic rashes, drugs causing, 87
Excretion of drug, rate of, 36
  and immunologic response, 62
  renal, 51–52
Exfoliative dermatitis, drug-induced, 81, 81, 82
  drugs causing, 82, 82(t)
Exophthalmos, drugs causing, 207
Extrapyramidal syndromes, drug-induced, types of, 186–188
  drugs causing, 187

Fat, malabsorption of, drug-induced, 129
FDA, role in drug regulation and monitoring, 6–7, 8, 9
Federal Trade Commission, 7
Ferrous sulfate, adverse reactions caused by, 239
Fetal abnormalities, drug-induced, 28, 29, 30, 30(t)
  drugs causing, 167–168
Fetal deafness, as caused by streptomycin, 213
Fetal effects, drug-induced, types of, 166–170
Fetal hemorrhage, as caused by anticoagulants, 167
Fetal intoxication, as caused by mepivacaine, 168, 190
Fetus, adverse drug reactions in, prevention of, 278
  and pharmacologic action of drugs, adverse effects on, 28, 29, 30
  dental damage in, as caused by tetracyclines, 126
  effect of smoking by pregnant mothers on, 168
  female, masculinization of, drugs causing, 168

Fetus *(Continued)*
  retarded bone growth in, drug-induced, 182
Fever, drug, as related to allergic reactions, 71, 197–198
  as related to drug-induced disease syndromes, 197
  drugs causing, 197, 198, 198(t), 199
  louse-borne relapsing, association with hypotension during treatment with tetracyclines, 124, 125(t)
Fibrillation, atrial, and digitalis intoxication, as cause of ECG changes, 119
  drugs causing, 120, 121(t)
  ventricular, digitalis-induced, 118, 119
  drugs causing, 121(t)
Fibroplasia, retrolental, drug-induced, 209
Fibrosis, hepatic, drugs causing, 139. See also *Cirrhosis.*
  of ovaries, drugs causing, 164
  pulmonary, acute, nitrofurantoin-induced, 143
    chronic, nitrofurantoin-induced, 144
    drugs causing, 143–144, 144(t)
  retroperitoneal, drugs causing, 162–163
First-order kinetics, principle of, and drug absorption, 36, 37
Flucytosine (Ancobon), adverse reactions caused by, 230
Fluid balance disorders, drug-induced, types of, 176
Fluid retention, drugs causing, 176
Fluorouracil (5-FU), adverse reactions caused by, 236
Fluoxymesterone (Halotestin), adverse reactions caused by, 249. See also *Methyltestosterone.*
Fluphenazine (Prolixin), adverse reactions caused by, 246
Flurazepam hydrochloride (Dalmane), adverse reactions caused by, 247. See also *Diazepam.*
Flutter, atrial, drugs causing, 120, 121(t)
Folate malabsorption, drug-induced, as cause of megaloblastic anemia, 105, 129
Folic acid, as cause of anaphylaxis, 203
Folic acid antagonists, as cause of megaloblastic anemia, 104
Food and Drug Administration, role in drug regulation and monitoring, 6–7, 9, 10
Freons, as cause of myocardial damage, 116
Fungal infections, drugs causing, 89, 205–206
Furazolidone (Furoxone), as cause of deafness, 214
Furosemide (Lasix), adverse reactions caused by, 248
  tinnitus, 214
Furunculoid drug eruptions, 86

INDEX

Galactorrhea, drug-induced, as cause of amenorrhea, 164
  drugs causing, 156, 156(t)
Ganglionic blocking agents, as caused by pulmonary fibrosis, 145
Gastric pH, effect on drug absorption, 33, 33(t)
Gastrointestinal bleeding, drug-induced, as related to iron deficiency anemia, 105
  drugs causing, 127, 128, 128(t)
Gastrointestinal disease, as related to immunologic effect of drug, 278
Gastrointestinal drugs, adverse reactions caused by, 248
Gastrointestinal effects, drug, types of, 126–130
Genetic factors, as cause of drug-induced hemolysis, 100–102
  knowledge of in prevention of adverse drug reactions, 27, 29(t), 277
Gentamicin (Garamycin), adverse reactions caused by, 232
  in interactions with other drugs, 262
Germicides, urinary, adverse reactions caused by, 235
Gestation. See *Pregnancy.*
Gingival hypertrophy, drugs causing, 126
Gland disorders, adrenal, drug-induced, 155
  thyroid, drug-induced, 154–155
Glands, salivary, drug reactions affecting, 126–127
Glaucoma, drugs causing, 209, 209(t)
Glomerulonephritis, as a feature of immunologic serum sickness, 69
Glucose, as cause of hypokalemia, 173
  intolerance, drug-induced, 151
Glucose 6-phosphate dehydrogenase (G-6-PD) deficiency, as cause of drug-induced hemolysis, 100–102
  among American Negroes, 100, 102
  among Mediterraneans, 100, 102
  among northern Europeans, 100
Glutathione-peroxidase deficiency, as cause of drug-induced hemolysis, 102
Glutathione-reductase deficiency, as cause of drug-induced hemolysis, 102
Glutethimide, absorption and distribution of, 32
Glyceryl trinitrate (Nitroglycerin), adverse reactions caused by, 242
Glycopyrrolate (Robinul), adverse reactions caused by, 238
Goiter, neonatal, drug-induced, drugs causing, 167
Gold compounds, as cause of aplastic anemias, 98
Gold salts, as cause of chrysiasis, 93
Gold sodium thiomalate (Myochrysine), adverse reactions caused by, 248

Gonadal changes, drug-induced, 156
Gout, drugs causing, 177, 178
  drugs used in treatment of, adverse reactions caused by, 248
Granulomas, of the liver, drugs causing, 140
  pulmonary, drug-induced, 146
"Gray syndrome," in neonates, as effect of chloramphenicol, 124–125, 169
Griseofulvin (Fulvicin), adverse reactions caused by, 230
  fungal infections, 89
  photodermatitis, 90(t)
  regional hyperpigmentation, 93
Guanethidine sulfate (Ismelin), adverse reactions caused by, 241
  in interactions with other drugs, 266
Gynecologic effects, drug-induced, types of, 164–165
Gynecomastia, drugs causing, 155, 156, 156(t)

Hair, effect of drugs on, 94–96
  loss of color, drugs causing, 96
Half-life, biologic, of drugs, 36, 37, 38
Haloperidol (Haldol), adverse reactions caused by, 246
  extrapyramidal syndromes, 187
  loss of hair color, 96
Halothane hepatitis, 136
Hapten(s), drugs as, 60
  interaction with immunologic mechanisms, 60, 61, 63–66
  role of in allergic reactions, 65
Hapten type, of drug-induced immune hemolysis, 102–103
Headaches, migraine, as caused by oral contraceptives, 193
Hearing loss, fetal, drugs causing, 167
Heart block, complete, digitalis-induced, 119
  drugs causing, 120, 121(t)
  first-degree, digitalis-induced, 119
Heart disease, congenital, drugs causing, 167–168
  spurious, caused by digitalis in combination with other drugs, 119
Heart failure, congestive, as related to drug-induced disease syndromes, 117
  drugs causing, 117
Heart valves, drug reactions affecting, 115
Hematologic reactions to drugs, types of, 69–71
Hematopoietic drug reactions, adverse, types of, 97–114
Hemachromatosis, drug-induced, 93, 179
Hematuria, drugs causing, 163
Hemoglobinopathies, as cause of drug-induced hemolysis, 102

Hemolysis, drugs causing, in glucose
6-phosphate dehydrogenase
deficiency, 100, 101(t), 102
in glutathione-peroxidase deficiency,
102
in glutathione reductase deficiency,
102
in 6-phosphogluconic dehydrogenase
deficiency, 102
immune, drug-induced, types of,
102–104
drugs causing, 102, 103, 103(t)
Hemolytic anemia, drug-induced,
autoimmune, 71
immunologic, 70–71
types of, 100–102
Hemopericardium, drugs causing, 116
Hemorrhage, as caused by oral anticoagulants, 111. See also Bleeding.
fetal, as caused by anticoagulants, 167
gastrointestinal, drug-induced, 127–128
pulmonary, drug-induced, 146
subconjunctival, as caused by
anticoagulants, 207
Henoch-Schönlein purpura, drugs
causing, 201
Heparin sodium, adverse reactions caused
by, 239
alopecia, 94
bleeding disorders, 111
osteoporosis, 182
Hepatic. See also Liver.
Hepatic adenomas, drugs causing, 144
Hepatic encephalopathy, as related to
drug-induced disease syndromes, 140
drugs causing, 140
Hepatic function, as factor in drug dosage,
27
as related to pharmacologic effect of
drug, 278
Hepatitis. See also Cholestatic jaundice,
Hepatocellular jaundice.
halothane, 136
Hepatocellular jaundice, drug-induced, as
related to viral hepatitis, 135
drugs causing, 135, 136, 136(t), 137, 138
Hepatotoxins, as compared to drugs
causing liver damage, 131
Herpes zoster, drug-induced, 206
Herxheimer reaction, characteristics of,
91–92
Hexamethonium, as cause of paralytic
ileus in neonates, 168
Hirsutism, drugs causing, 95, 95(t), 96
Histamine, release of in immunologic
anaphylaxis, 67, 68
Hormone(s), adverse reactions caused by,
249
in interactions with other drugs, 268
antidiuretic, inappropriate secretion of,
drugs causing, 150

Hydantoins, as cause of exfoliative
dermatitis, 82(t)
as cause of regional hyperpigmentation,
93
as cause of toxic epidermal necrolysis,
85(t)
Hydralazine hydrochloride (Apresoline),
adverse reactions caused by, 241
myocardial infarction, 116
peripheral neuropathies, 184
systemic lupus erythematosus, 199
Hydrazine derivatives, as cause of hepatocellular jaundice, 137
Hydrochlorothiazide (Hydrodiuril,
Esidrix), adverse reactions caused by,
248. See also Chlorothiazide.
Hydromorphone hydrochloride
(Dilaudid), adverse reactions caused by,
243. See also Codeine.
Hydroxychloroquine, as cause of retinal
damage, 210
Hydroxyzine (Atarax, Vistaril), adverse
reactions caused by, 246
Hyperaldosteronism, drug-induced, 155
Hypercalcemia, as related to drug-
induced disease syndromes, 176,
176(t), 177
drug-induced, drugs causing, 176,
176(t), 177
Hypercholesterolemia, as related to drug-
induced disease syndromes, 179
Hyperglycemia, drugs causing, 151, 152,
152(t)
Hyperkalemia, as related to drug-induced
disease syndromes, 172, 173, 173(t)
drugs causing, 172, 173, 173(t)
Hyperlipemia, drugs causing, 178–179
Hypernatremia, drugs causing, 171, 171(t)
Hyperpigmentation, diffuse, drugs
causing, 92–93
regional, drugs causing, 93–94
Hyperplasia, gingival, drug-induced,
23–24
Hypertension, drugs causing, 122, 123,
122(t)
pulmonary, drugs causing, 146
Hypertensive crisis, caused by drug
interaction with monamine oxidase
inhibitors, 123, 123(t)
Hyperthyroidism, drugs causing, 154
Hypertriglyceridemia, drugs causing, 179
Hypertrophy, gingival, drugs causing, 126
Hyperuricemia, as related to drug-
induced syndromes, 178, 178(t)
drugs causing, 177, 178, 178(t)
Hypervitaminosis A, drug-induced, 93
Hypnotics, adverse reactions caused by,
247
as cause of coma, 191
Hypocalcemia, as related to drug-induced
disease syndromes, 177

Hypocalcemia *(Continued)*
  drugs causing, 177
Hypoglycemia, drugs causing, 152, 153, 153(t), 154
  neonatal, as caused by insulin, 169
Hypoglycemic agents, adverse effects caused by interactions with other drugs, 268
  oral, as cause of symptomatic hypoglycemia, 153
Hypokalemia, as related to drug-induced disease syndromes, 173, 174, 174(t)
  drug-induced, as related to hepatic encephalopathy, 140
  drugs causing, 173, 174, 174(t)
Hyponatremia, as related to drug-induced disease syndromes, 171, 172, 172(t)
  drugs causing, 171, 172(t)
Hypoplasia, enamel, as effect of tetracyclines, 126, 169
Hypotension, drugs and drug interactions causing, 123, 124, 125(t)
Hypoparathyroidism, drug-induced, 154
Hypotensives, adverse reactions caused by, 241–242
  in interactions with other drugs, 266
Hypothermia, drugs causing, 199
Hypothermic myxedema coma, drug-induced, in hypothyroidism, 154
Hypothyroidism, drugs causing, 155
Hypoventilation, drugs causing, 146–147
Hypovolemia, as related to drug-induced disease syndromes, 176

^{131}I therapy, as cause of hypothyroidism, 154
Idoxuridine (Stoxil), as cause of corneal damage, 208
IgE antibody, role of in allergic drug reactions, 66–69
IgG antibody, role of in allergic drug reactions, 66–69
IgM antibody, role of in allergic drug reactions, 66–69
Ileus, adynamic, drugs causing, 129
  paralytic, as caused by hexamethonium, 168
  drugs causing, 129
Imipramine hydrochloride (Tofranil), adverse reactions caused by, 245
  as cause of seizures, 189
Immune complexes, role of in immunologic serum sickness, 68
Immune hemolysis, drugs causing, 102, 103, 103(t)
  types of, as related to drug-induced positive reaction to Coombs' test, 102–104
Immunity, cellular. See *Cellular hypersensitivity.*

Immunoglobulin, classes of, in allergic drug reactions, 66–67, 67(t)
Immunologic action, of drugs. See also *Drug reactions, allergic.*
  affecting the myocardium, 116
  and binding and receptor sites, 62–66
  and rate of drug excretion, 62
  and route of administration, 63
  and tissue affinity, 62
  as haptens, factors affecting, 60–66
  in agranulocytosis, 107
  in cholestatic jaundice, 131, 132
  in thrombocytopenia, 109–111
  of halogenated anesthetic agents, in causing hepatocellular jaundice, 135, 137
Immunologic diagnostics, methods of, 73–77
Immunologic hemolytic anemia, mechanisms of, 70–71
Immunologic inhibition, as result of competitive hapten binding, 64
Immunologic mechanisms. See *Immunologic action.*
Immunologic reactions, to drugs, cutaneous, types of, 69
  delayed hypersensitivity reactions as, 72–73
  types of, 66–73
Immunologic vs. pharmacologic drug reactions, comparison of, 75
Immunosuppressives as cause of candidiasis, 205
  as cause of fungal infections, 206
  as cause of Pneumocystis carinii pneumonia, 206
  as cause of pulmonary infections, 148
  as cause of viral infections, 206
  as predisposing factor in infections in renal transplant patients, 205
Indomethacin (Indocin), adverse reactions caused by, 243
  aplastic anemia, 100
Infants, and pharmacologic action of drugs, adverse effects on, 25, 30
  metabolism of chloramphenicol in, 25, 124–125
  occurrence of drug-induced kernicterus in, 140
  predisposition to adverse drug reactions, 277
Infection(s), as related to allergic drug reactions, 278
  bacterial, caused by drug-resistant organisms, 204–205
  fungal, drugs causing, 89
  monilial, drugs causing, 89
  mycobacterial, drugs as predisposing factors in, 205
  protozoal, drugs causing, 206
  pulmonary, drugs causing, 148
  viral, drugs causing, 206

294 INDEX

"Innocent bystander type," of drug-induced immune hemolysis, 103
Inpatient medication errors, and adverse drug reactions, 40, 42
Insulin, as cause of hypoglycemia, 152
  in neonate, 169
  as cause of hypokalemia, 173
  as cause of Somogyi effect, 151–152
Insulin injection (regular insulin), adverse reactions caused by, 250
Insulins and antidiabetics, adverse reactions caused by, 249–250
Intoxication. See also *Toxicity.*
  amphetamine, as cause of psychosis, 196
  ampicillin, as cause of psychosis, 196
  anticholinergic, as cause of psychoses, 196
  digitalis. See *Digitalis intoxication.*
Intracranial pressure, increased, drugs causing, 191–192, 192(t)
Iodide, as cause of hyperthyroidism, 154
  as cause of hypothyroidism, 155
Iodinated contrast media, as cause of anaphylaxis, 203
Iodine, drugs containing, as cause of neonatal abnormalities, 167
Ionization of drugs, degree of, as factor in drug absorption, 33
Iron, adverse reactions caused by, 239
  hemochromatosis, 93
  malabsorption of, caused by drugs, 129
Iron deficiency anemia, as related to drug-induced disease syndromes, 105
  drugs causing, 105
Isoniazid (INH), adverse reactions caused by, 233
  fetal abnormalities, 167
  hepatocellular jaundice, 137
  joint pain, 183
  optic neuritis, 211
  peripheral neuropathies, 184
  psychosis, 196
  rheumatic syndrome, 183
  systemic lupus erythematosus, 199
  withdrawal syndromes in infants, 193
Isopentaquine, as cause of hemolysis in glutathione reductase deficiency, 102
Isopropamide iodide (Darbid), adverse reactions caused by, 238
Isoproterenol hydrochloride (Isuprel), adverse reactions caused by, 238
Isosorbide dinitrate (Isordil), adverse reactions caused by, 242
Isoxuprine hydrochloride (Vasodilan), adverse reactions caused by, 242

Jaundice, cholestatic, drug-induced, types of, 131–135
  drugs causing, 132, 133, 133(t), 134, 135

Jaundice *(Continued)*
  drug-induced, types of, 5, 131–138
  drugs causing, 138(t)
  hepatocellular, drug-induced, 135–138
  drugs causing, 135, 136, 136(t), 137, 138
Joint disorders, as related to drug-induced disease syndromes, 183
  drugs causing, 182–183

Kanamycin (Kantrex), adverse reactions caused by, 232
  deafness, 213–214
  in interactions with other drugs, 262
Keratitis, drugs causing, 207–208
Kernicterus, in neonates, drugs causing, 140, 169
Kidney function, decrease in, drugs causing, 158–161. See also *Renal.*
Kinetics, principle of first-order reaction, and drug absorption, 36, 37
Kinin, causative role in allergic anaphylaxis, 68

Lens disorders, of anterior chamber, drug-induced, 208
Lesion, bull's-eye, retinal, drugs causing, 210
  gangrenous, drugs causing, 89
  ocular, vascular, drugs causing, 212
  small bowel, drugs causing, 128
  spinal cord, as related to drug-induced disease syndromes, 192
  drugs causing, 192
  warty, drugs causing, 94
Leukemia, acute lymphoblastic, drugs causing, 113
  acute myeloblastic, drugs causing, 113
Leukocytosis, drugs causing, 107, 108(t)
Levarterenol bitartrate (Levophed), adverse reactions caused by, 238
Levodopa (Larodopa), adverse reactions caused by, 251
  dyskinesia, 188
  immune hemolysis, 103
  in interactions with other drugs, 268
  nausea and vomiting, 127
Levothyroxine sodium (Synthroid), adverse reactions caused by, 250. See also *Thyroid.*
Lidocaine hydrochloride (Xylocaine), adverse reactions caused by, 240
  seizures, 190
Lincomycin (Lincocin), adverse reactions caused by, 232
  in interactions with other drugs, 262
Liothyronine sodium (Cytomel), adverse reactions caused by, 250. See also *Thyroid.*

INDEX

Lipid, serum levels, changes in, drugs causing, 178–179
Lipid/water partition coefficient, as factor in drug absorption, 32, 33
Lithium carbonate, as cause of exophthalmos, 207
  as cause of nephrogenic diabetes insipidus, 163
Liver, role of in drug absorption and distribution, 131
  tumors, drugs causing, 141
Liver effects, types of, drugs causing, 131–141
Liver function, as factor in drug dosage, 27
  tests, drugs affecting, 138–139
Lung, calcification of, drugs causing, 146
  tumors, drugs causing, 148
Lupus erythematosus, systemic, drug-induced, 84
  as associated with pericarditis, 116
  drugs causing, 199, 199(t), 200
Lyell's syndrome. See also *Toxic epidermal necrolysis.*
  drug-induced, symptoms of, 83, 85
  drugs causing, 84, 85(t)
Lymph disorders, drugs causing, 113–114, 113(t)
Lymph nodes, localization of drug in, and immunologic action, 64
Lymphangiography, as cause of respiratory insufficiency, 145
Lymphocytes, role of in delayed hypersensitivity reactions, 72
  sensitized, and drug interaction with specific antibody, 64
Lymphomas, histiocytic, drug-related, 114
Lysergide (LSD), as cause of psychosis, 196

Malabsorption, drugs causing, 129–130
Malignancies, drug-related, in renal transplant patients, 114
Mannitol, hypertonic, as cause of hyponatremia, 172
  intravenous, as cause of congestive heart failure, 117
  as cause of hypernatremia, 171
MAO. See *Monamine oxidase.*
Masculinization, of female fetus, drugs causing, 168
Mask of pregnancy. See *Cholasma, facial melasma.*
Mechlorethamine hydrochloride (Nitrogen mustard), adverse reactions caused by, 236
Mediastinal involvement, drugs causing, 149
Medication errors, patient, and adverse drug reactions, 40, 41, 41(t)

Mefenamic acid (Ponstel), as cause of immune hemolysis, 103
Megacolon, toxic, drugs causing, 130
Megaloblastic anemia, as caused by drug-induced folate malabsorption, 129
  drugs causing, 104–105, 104(t)
Melasma, facial, drugs causing, 93
Melphalan (Alkeran), as cause of immune hemolysis, 104
Menstrual cycle, changes in, drugs causing, 156, 164
Mepazine, as cause of agranulocytosis, 108(t)
Meperidine hydrochloride (Demerol), adverse reactions caused by, 243
Mephenesin, as cause of loss of hair color, 96
Mephenytoin (Mesantoin), as cause of aplastic anemia, 98
Mepivacaine hydrochloride (Carbocaine), adverse reactions caused by, 251
  fetal intoxication, 168, 190
Meprobamate, as cause of anaphylaxis, 203
6-Mercaptopurine (Purinethol), adverse reactions caused by, 236
  diffuse hyperpigmentation, 93
  in interactions with other drugs, 263
Mercury, as cause of nail discoloration, 96
Mescaline, as cause of psychosis, 196
Metabolic alkalosis, drugs causing, 174–175, 175(t)
Metabolic disorders, as related to pharmacologic effect of drugs, 23, 278
Metabolic effects, drug-induced, types of, 171–180
Metabolism, drug. See also *Absorption and distribution of drug, Excretion of drug.*
  as related to pharmacologic action, 31–40
  products of, immunogenicity of, 63
  rate of, and enzyme induction, 50–51, 50(t)
  of digitalis, as affected by other drugs, 118
Metahexamide (Euglycin), as cause of liver damage, 138
Metals, heavy, as cause of decrease in kidney function, 158, 159(t)
  as cause of peripheral neuropathies, 184
Metaraminol, as cause of gangrenous lesions, 89
Methadone hydrochloride (Dolophine), adverse reactions caused by, 243
Methamphetamine hydrochloride (Desoxyn), adverse reactions caused by, 246. See also *Dextroamphetamine.*
Methandrostenolone (Dianabol), adverse reactions caused by, 249. See also *Methyltestosterone.*

INDEX

Methaqualone (Quaalude), adverse reactions caused by, 247
Methemoglobinemia, drugs causing, 106, 106(t)
Methicillin sodium (Staphcillin), adverse reactions caused by, 232
  as cause of drug-resistant organisms in bacterial infection, 204
Methimazole (Tapazole), adverse reactions caused by, 250
  myocardial damage, 116
  neonatal goiter, 167
Methocarbamol (Robaxin), adverse reactions caused by, 239
Methotrexate, adverse reactions caused by, 236
  in interactions with other drugs, 263
  megaloblastic anemia, 104
  as cause of pulmonary fibrosis, 144
Methoxyflurane (Penthrane), as cause of impaired renal function, 161
Methsuximide (Celontin), adverse reactions caused by, 245
Methylcholine, as cause of asthma, 143
Methyldopa (Aldomet), adverse reactions caused by, 242
  central nervous system depression, 190
  immune hemolysis, 102, 103–104
Methylphenidate hydrochloride (Ritalin), adverse reactions caused by, 246
Methylprednisolone (Medrol), adverse reactions caused by, 249. See also *Prednisone*.
Methyltestosterone (Metandren), adverse reactions caused by, 249
Methyprylon (Noludar), adverse reactions caused by, 247
Methysergide maleate (Sansert), adverse reactions caused by, 238
  myalgias, 182
  myocardial infarction, 115
  pulmonary fibrosis, 144–145
  retroperitoneal fibrosis, 162–163
Metronidazole (Flagyl), adverse reactions caused by, 234
Microsomal enzyme-inducing drugs, interaction with oral anticoagulants, as related to bleeding disorders, 112, 112(t)
Migraine headaches, as caused by oral contraceptives, 193
Milk-alkali syndrome, drug-induced, as related to hypercalcemia, 176–177
Minocycline (Minocin), adverse reactions caused by, 232
Mithramycin (Mithracin), as cause of hypocalcemia, 177
  as cause of renal impairment, 161
Monamine oxidase, inhibition of by drugs, 49–50

Monamine oxidase inhibitors, adverse effects caused by interactions with other drugs, 267
  central nervous system excitation, 188–189
  hypertensive crisis, 123, 123(t)
  intracerebral hemorrhage, 191
  as cause of hepatocellular jaundice, 136(t)
Monilial infections, drugs causing, 89
Morbilliform rashes, as allergic drug reaction, 69
Morphine sulfate, adverse reactions caused by, 243
  urticaria, 92(t)
Mouth, dry, drugs causing, 126
Multisystem effects, drug-induced, types of, 197–203
Muscle disorders, extraocular, drugs causing, 207
Muscle relaxants, skeletal, adverse reactions caused by, 239
Musculoskeletal effects, drugs causing, 181–183
Myalgias, drugs causing, 182, 182(t)
Myasthenia gravis, drugs causing, 185–186, 186(t)
Myocardial infarction, as related to drug-induced disease syndromes, 116
  drugs causing, 115–116
Myoneural junction, drug reactions affecting, 185–188
Myopathy, as related to drug-induced disease syndromes, 181
  drugs causing, 181, 181(t)

Nafcillin (Unipen), as cause of drug-resistant organisms in bacterial infection, 204
Nails, effect of drugs on, 94–96
Nalidixic acid (NegGram), adverse reactions caused by, 235
Nalorphine hydrochloride (Nalline), adverse reactions caused by, 244
Naloxone hydrochloride (Narcan), adverse reactions caused by, 244
Narcotics, as cause of addiction of neonate, 169
  as cause of coma, 191
  as cause of hypotension, 124, 125(t)
  as cause of pulmonary edema, 146
National Formulary, 9
Nausea, drugs causing, 127
Necrolysis, toxic epidermal, drug-induced, symptoms of, 83, 85
  drugs causing, 84, 85(t)
Necrosis, aseptic, drugs causing, 182
  of small and large bowel, drug-induced, 128

Neomycin, as cause of deafness, 213–214
  as cause of malabsorption, 129
Neonate. See also *Infant.*
  drug-induced effects in, drugs causing, 166–170
  goiter in, drugs causing, 167
  risk of adverse reactions to drugs in, 30
  thyroid disorders in, drugs causing, 67
Neostigmine bromide (Prostigmin), adverse reactions caused by, 237
Nephritis, interstitial, drugs causing, 160
Nephrogenic diabetes insipidus, drugs causing, 150–151, 163
Nephropathy, drugs causing, 158–161, 159(t)
Nephrotic syndrome, drugs causing, 161, 162, 162(t)
Nerve, optic, disorders of, drug-induced, 210–212
Nervous system, central, depression, drugs causing, 190–191
  drug reactions affecting, 188–193
  excitation, drugs causing, 188–189
Neurologic effects, drug-induced, types of, 184–193
Neuromuscular blockade, as related to drug interactions, 147, 148, 148(t)
  drugs causing, 146–147, 147(t)
Neuropathies, peripheral, drug reactions affecting, 184–185, 185(t)
Newborn. See *Neonate.*
NF. See *National Formulary.*
Nicotinyl alcohol (Roniacol), adverse reactions caused by, 242
Nitrofurans, as cause of hemolysis in glucose 6-phosphate dehydrogenase deficiency, 101(t)
  as cause of peripheral neuropathies, 184
Nitrofurantoin (Furadantin), adverse reactions caused by, 235
  acute pulmonary infiltrates, 143
  anaphylaxis, 203
  chronic pulmonary fibrosis, 143–144
  hemolysis in glutathione-peroxidase deficiency, 102
Nodal premature beats, digitalis-induced, 119
Nodal rhythm, drugs causing, 119, 120, 121(t)
Nodal tachycardia, digitalis-induced, 119
Noncompetitive binding, of drugs, 49
Norepinephrine (Levophed), as cause of gangrenous lesions, 89
Norethandrolone (Nilevar), as cause of hypoglycemia, 153
Nortriptyline hydrochloride (Aventyl), adverse reactions caused by, 245. See also *Amitriptyline.*
Novobiocin, as cause of drug fever, 198(t)
  as cause of kernicterus, 140, 169
Nystatin (Mycostatin), adverse reactions caused by, 230

Ocular effects, drug-induced, types of, 207–212
Ocular malformations, congenital, as caused by thalidomide, 212
Oculogyric crisis, drugs causing, 207
Oils, aspiration of, as cause of lipoid pneumonia, 145
Ophthalmoplegia, drugs causing, 207
Opiates, as cause of withdrawal syndromes, 193
Optic nerve, disorders of, drug-induced, 210–212
Optic neuritis, drugs causing, 211, 211(t)
Osteoporosis, drugs causing, 182
OTC drugs, harmful effects of, 5
  importance of in patient drug history, 73
  promotion of, 18, 19
  public use of, 1–2, 12, 19
Outpatient medication errors, and adverse drug reactions, 41
Ovaries, fibrosis of, drugs causing, 164
Over-the-counter drugs. See *OTC drugs.*
Oxygen therapy, as cause of pulmonary insufficiency, 145
  as cause of retrolental fibroplasia, 209
Oxyphenbutazone (Tandearil), as cause of acute leukemia, 113
  as cause of aplastic anemia, 100
  as cause of parotitis, 126
Oxytocin (Pitocin), adverse reactions caused by, 251
  inappropriate antidiuretic hormone secretion syndrome, 150
  myocardial infarction, 115

Pancreatitis, as related to drug-induced disease syndromes, 130
  drugs causing, 130, 130(t)
Pancytopenia. See *Aplastic anemia.*
Papilledema. See also *Pseudotumor cerebri.*
  drugs causing, 211–212
Para-aminosalicylic acid, as cause of drug fever, 198(t)
  as cause of immune hemolysis, 104
  as cause of malabsorption, 129
  as cause of myocardial damage, 116
  as cause of thrombocytopenia, 110
Paraldehyde, as cause of metabolic acidosis, 175
Paramethadione (Paradione), as cause of nephrotic syndrome, 162
Parasympatholytics, adverse reactions caused by, 237–238
Parasympathomimetics, adverse reactions caused by, 237
Parenteral drugs, interactions of, 52
Pargyline (Eutonyl), adverse reactions caused by, 242
  in interactions with other drugs, 267

Parkinsonism, drugs causing, 187
Parotitis, drugs causing, 126–127
P.A.S. See *Para-aminosalicylic acid*.
Patient(s), aged, predisposition to adverse drug reaction, 277
  predisposition to digitalis intoxication, 118
  role of in drug use, 13–15, 272–273
Patient drug history, 13–14, 15, 42
  as aid in detecting adverse drug reactions, 73–74
  pharmacist's role in, 74, 275
  physician's role in, 74
Patient medication errors, and adverse reactions, 40, 41, 41(t)
Patch test, used in detecting drug allergy, 75
PBI levels, drugs causing changes in, 154
6-PDG deficiency. See *6-Phosphogluconic dehydrogenase deficiency*.
Pelger-Huët anomaly, pseudo, drug-induced, 109
Peliosis hepatis, drugs causing, 141
Penicillamine, as cause of optic neuritis, 211
Penicillin, allergic reaction to, case history, 74
  as cause of anaphylaxis, 203
  as cause of drug fever, 198
  as cause of drug-resistant organisms in bacterial infection, 204
  as cause of exfoliative dermatitis, 82(t)
  as cause of fixed drug eruptions, 88(t)
  as cause of hapten type of immune hemolysis, 102–103
  as cause of hepatocellular jaundice, 137
  as cause of Herxheimer reaction, 91
  as cause of seizures, 189
  as cause of serum sickness, 201(t), 202
  as cause of Stevens-Johnson syndrome, 83
  as cause of urticaria, 92(t)
  as cause of vasculitis, 200
Penicillin G, adverse reactions caused by, 232
  in interactions with other drugs, 262
Penicillin G procaine, adverse reactions caused by, 233
Penicillin V, adverse effects caused by interactions with other drugs, 262
Pentamidine, as cause of impaired renal function, 160–161
  as cause of megalobastic anemia, 104
Pentazocine hydrochloride (Talwin), adverse reactions caused by, 244
  as cause of withdrawal syndromes, 193
Pentobarbital sodium (Nembutol), adverse reactions caused by, 247. See also *Phenobarbital*.
Peptic ulceration, drugs causing, 127, 128, 128(t)
Perianal moniliasis, drugs causing, 130

Pericarditis, drugs causing, 116
Pericardium, drug reactions affecting, 116
Perphenazine (Trilafon), adverse reactions caused by, 246. See also *Chlorpromazine*.
pH, gastric, as factor in drug absorption, 33, 33(t)
  urine, and renal drug excretion, 51–52
Pharmaceutical industry, legal regulation of, 7–8
Pharmacist, role in drug use, 15–16, 74, 274–275
Pharmacokinetics, 35–37
Pharmacologic action of drugs, adverse effects of, 21–25
  factors affecting, 31–40
  in aged patients, 25, 26
  in children, 25
  in fetus, 28, 29, 30
  in infants, 25, 30
  and absorption and distribution, 32–34
  as related to disease conditions, 30–31, 278
  as related to dose and dosage, 37–38, 275
  as related to renal drug excretion, 51–52
Pharmacologic properties, of drugs, 38
Pharmacologic vs. immunologic drug reactions, comparison of, 75
Pharmacology, study of by medical students, 273–274
Pharmacopeia, United States. See *USP*.
Phenacemide (Phenurone), as cause of hepatocellular jaundice, 137
Phenacetin, as cause of fixed drug eruptions, 88(t)
  as cause of nephropathy, 158
  as cause of renal tumors, 163
  as cause of sulfhemoglobinemia, 106
Phenazopyridine hydrochloride (Pyridium), adverse reactions caused by, 235
Phenformin hydrochloride (D.B.I.), adverse reactions caused by, 250
  lactic acidosis, 175
Phenindione (Danilone, Dindevan, Hedulin), as cause of agranulocytosis, 108(t)
  as cause of gangrenous lesions, 89
Phenobarbital (Luminal), adverse reactions caused by, 247
  acute intermittent porphyria, 180
Phenolphthalein, as cause of fixed drug eruptions, 88(t)
  as cause of nail discoloration, 96
  as cause of skin discoloration, 94
  as cause of Stevens-Johnson syndrome, 84(t)
Phenothiazines, as cause of akathisia, 187
  as cause of aplastic anemia, 100
  as cause of cataracts, 208
  as cause of cholestatic jaundice, 133

INDEX

Phenothiazines *(Continued)*
  as cause of diffuse hyperpigmentation, 93
  as cause of extrapyramidal syndromes, 187
  as cause of glaucoma, 209
  as cause of gynecologic disease syndromes, 164
  as cause of hypotension, 124, 125(t)
  as cause of oculogyric crisis, 207
  as cause of parkinsonism, 187
  as cause of regional hyperpigmentation, 93
  as cause of retinitis pigmentosa, 210
  as cause of seizures, 189
  as cause of tardive dyskinesia, 187–188
Phenothiazine antihistamines, adverse reactions caused by, 229
Phenoxybenzamine hydrochloride (Dibenzyline), adverse reactions caused by, 239
Phentolamine hydrochloride (Regitine), adverse reactions caused by, 242
  myocardial infarction, 116
Phenylbutazone (Butazolidin), adverse reactions caused by, 244
  acute myeloblastic and acute lymphoblastic leukemias, 113
  aplastic anemia, 98
  exfoliative dermatitis, 82(t)
  myocardial damage, 116
  parotitis, 126
  pseudolymphoma syndrome, 113
  toxic epidermal necrolysis, 85(t)
Phenylhydrazine, as cause of hemolysis in glucose 6-phosphate dehydrogenase deficiency, 101(t)
Phenylpropanolamine (Propadrine), adverse reactions caused by, 238
  hypertension, 122
Phenytoin. See *Diphenylhydantoin.*
Phosphates, as cause of hypocalcemia, 177
6-Phosphogluconic dehydrogenase (6-DPG) deficiency, as cause of drug-induced hemolysis, 102
Photodermatitis, drug-induced, 89, 89, 90
  drugs causing, 90, 90(t)
Photosensitive drug reactions, 89–90
Physicians, and patterns of drug prescription, 12–15
  role of in assembling patient drug history, 74
  role of in drug control and utilization, 273–274
Physiologic effects, drug-induced, kinds of, 24. See also *Nausea, Vomiting, Diarrhea, Constipation.*
Piperazine citrate (Antepar), adverse reactions caused by, 229
  ataxia, 192
Pituitary disorders, posterior, drugs causing, 150–151

Pituitary drugs, adverse reactions caused by, 250
Pituitary snuff, as cause of pulmonary fibrosis, 145
pKa, drug, as factor in drug absorption, 33, 33(t)
Plasma proteins, interaction with drugs, 34, 34(t), 47–48. See also *Albumin.*
Platelet-drug binding, in immunologic thrombocytopenia, 69
Platelet formation, suppression of in bone marrow, as cause of drug-induced thrombocytopenia, 111
Pleural involvement, drugs causing, 148–149
Pleurisy, as caused by drug-induced respiratory syndromes, 148
Pneumonia, lipoid, drugs causing, 145
Pneumocystis carinii, drugs causing, 206
Porphyria, acute intermittent, drugs causing, 179, 179(t), 180
Porphyria cutanea tarda symptomatica, drugs causing, 180, 179(t)
Potassium, loss of, as related to digitalis intoxication, 117
Potassium salts, as cause of hyperkalemia, 172
Prausnitz-Küstner reaction, 68
Prednisone, adverse reactions caused by, 249
  in interactions with other drugs, 268
  neonatal hypoglycemia, 169
Pregnancy, administration of drugs during, 166–170, 278
  and fetal risk of adverse drug reactions, 28
  in first trimester, 30
  tetracycline-induced liver damage during, 134
Primaquine phosphate, adverse reactions caused by, 234
  hemolysis, in glucose 6-phosphate dehydrogenase deficiency, 100–101
  in glutathione reductase deficiency, 102
  in 6-phosphogluconic dehydrogenase deficiency, 102
  methemoglobinemia, 106
Primidone (Mysoline), adverse reactions caused by, 245
  megaloblastic anemia, 105
Probenecid (Benemid), adverse reactions caused by, 248
Procainamide hydrochloride (Pronestyl), adverse reactions caused by, 240
  myasthenia gravis, 186
  systemic lupus erythematosus, 199
  vasculitis, 200–201
Procaine hydrochloride (Novocain), adverse reactions caused by, 251

Procarbazine hydrochloride (Matulane), adverse reactions caused by, 236
Prochlorperazine (Compazine), adverse reactions caused by, 246. See also *Chlorpromazine.*
  acute dystonic reactions, 187
Proctitis, ulcerative, drug-induced, 130
Progestins, synthetic, as cause of masculinization of female fetus, 168
Progestogen-estrogen combinations, adverse reactions caused by, 249
Promazine (Sparine), as cause of agranulocytosis, 108(t)
Promethazine hydrochloride (Phenergan), adverse reactions caused by, 229
Propantheline bromide (Pro-Banthine), adverse reactions caused by, 238
Proparacaine, as cause of keratitis, 207
Propoxyphene hydrochloride (Darvon), adverse reactions caused by, 244
  withdrawal syndromes, 193
Propranolol hydrochloride (Inderal), adverse reactions caused by, 241
  bronchoconstriction, 143
  congestive heart failure, 117
  hypoglycemia, 153
Propylthiouracil, adverse reactions caused by, 250
  agranulocytosis, 108(t)
  neonatal goiter, 167
  serum sickness, 201
  vasculitis, 200
Protein binding, drug, 34–35, 47–48. See also *Albumin.*
  and distribution of bilirubin, 48
Protein-bound iodide. See *PBI.*
Prothrombin time, changes in by anticoagulants, 111, 112, 112(t)
Pruritus ani, drugs causing, 130
Pseudoleukemoid reactions, drug-induced, 107, 109
Pseudolymphoma syndrome, drugs causing, 113, 113(t)
Pseudo Pelger-Huët anomaly, drug-induced, 109
Pseudotumor cerebri, drugs causing, 191–192, 192(t)
Psychogenic effects, drug-induced, 24
Psychoses, drugs causing, 195–196
  manic-depressive, drug-induced, 195
  schizoaffective, drug-induced, 195
Pulmonary, edema, drugs causing, 146
  embolism, drugs causing, 125
  fibrosis, drugs causing, 143–144, 144(t)
  hemorrhage, drugs causing, 146
  hypertension, drug-induced, 146
  infections, drugs causing, 148
  infiltrates, drugs causing, 143–144, 144(t)
  insufficiency, drugs causing, 145
Pulmonary disorders, as related to drug-induced disease syndromes, 145

Pulmonary disorders *(Continued)*
  drug-induced, types of, 142–146
Pure Food and Drug Act, 7
Purpura, anaphylactoid, as an allergic drug reaction, 69
  Henoch-Schönlein, drugs causing, 201
  nonthrombocytopenic, drugs causing, 111
  thrombotic thrombocytopenic, drugs causing, 201
Pyelogram, intravenous, as cause of renal impairment, 160
Pyrazinamide (Daraprim), as cause of hepatocellular jaundice, 137
  as cause of hyperuricemia, 178
  as cause of joint pain, 183
  as cause of megaloblastic anemia, 104
  as cause of rheumatic syndrome, 183
Pyrvinium pamoate (Povan), adverse reactions caused by, 229

Quantal dose response curve, 21, 22
Quinacrine hydrochloride (Atabrine), adverse reactions caused by, 229
  aplastic anemia, 100
  nail discoloration, 96
  skin discoloration, 94
Quinidine, adverse reactions caused by, 241
  drug fever, 198(t)
  fixed drug eruptions, 88(t)
  immune hemolysis, 103
  in interactions with other drugs, 266
  myasthenia gravis, 186
Quinine sulfate, adverse reactions caused by, 234
  hemolysis in glutathione reductase deficiency, 102
  immune hemolysis, 103
  myasthenia gravis, 186
  optic neuritis, 211
  tinnitus, 214

Radiation therapy, as cause of alopecia, 95
Radioiodine, as cause of hyperthyroidism, 154
  as cause of seizures, 189
Rashes, as allergic drug reactions, 69
  exanthematic, drugs causing, 87
Rauwolfia alkaloids, as cause of depression, 195
Receptor sites, of drugs. See also *Displacement, Binding.*
  and drug interactions, 44, *44*, 49–50
  as related to pharmacologic action, 21
  of anticoagulants, displacement of, in bleeding disorders, 111
Registry on Adverse Reactions, 9

Renal calculi, drugs causing, 163
Renal drug excretion, as factor in pharmacologic mechanisms, 51–52
Renal function, as factor in drug dosage, 26–27, 28
 as related to pharmacologic effect of drug, 278
 decrease in, drugs causing, 158–161
 as related to drug-induced disease syndromes, 161
Renal insufficiency, drug-induced as related to hyperkalemia, 172
Renal transplant patients, drug-related malignancies in, 114
Renal tubular acidosis, drug-induced, as related to hypokalemia, 173
 drugs causing, 162, 175
Renal tumors, drugs causing, 163–164
Renal vasculitis, necrotizing, drugs causing, 161
Rescinnamine (Moderil), adverse reactions caused by, 242. See also *Reserpine*.
Reserpine (Sandril, Serpasil), adverse reactions caused by, 242
 nasal blockage in neonate, 168
 peptic ulcer, 128
Respiratory effects, drug-induced, types of, 142–149
Retina, disorders of, drugs causing, 210
Retinitis pigmentosa, drugs causing, 210
Retroperitoneal fibrosis, drug-induced, drugs causing, 162–163
Rheumatic syndrome, drugs causing, 183, 183(t)
Rifampin, adverse reactions caused by, 234
Ristocetin, as cause of thrombocytopenia, 111
Rosacea, aggravation of by drugs, 94

Salicylates, adverse effects caused by, in interactions with other drugs, 267
 acute renal failure, 158
 anaphylaxis, 203
 coma, 191
 fixed drug eruptions, 88(t)
 gastroduodenal injury, 127
 kernicterus, 140
 tinnitus, 214
 vesiculobullous eruptions, 91
Salivary glands, drug reactions affecting, 126–127
Salvarsan, as cause of liver disease, 5
Scalded skin syndrome. See *Toxic epidermal necrolysis, Lyell's syndrome*.
 drug-induced, 83–84, 85
Secobarbital (Seconal), adverse reactions caused by, 247. See also *Phenobarbital*.

Sedatives, adverse reactions caused by, 247
 central nervous system depression, 190
 central nervous system excitation, 188
 coma, 191
Seizures, as related to drug-induced disease syndromes, 190
Seizures, drugs causing, 189, 189(t), 190
Serologic tests, for drug allergy, types of, 75, 76–77
Serotonin, causative role in allergic anaphylaxis, 68
Serum albumin, drug binding to, 47–48, 48(t)
 effect on drug response, 35
Serum antiplatelet factors, interaction with drug, 69
Serum calcium levels, changes in, drug-induced, 176–177
Serum cholesterol levels, changes in, drug-induced, 178–179
Serum glutamic oxaloacetic transaminase. See *SGOT*.
Serum lipid levels, changes in, drug-induced, 178–179
Serum sickness, as an immunologic reaction, 68
 drugs causing, 201, 201(t)
Serum uric acid levels, changes in, drugs causing, 177, 178
SGOT levels, changes in, drugs causing, in liver-function tests, 138–139
Silver salts, as cause of argyria, 93–94
 as cause of nail discoloration, 96
Sinoatrial block, drugs causing, 118, 120, 121(t)
Sinus arrest, digitalis-induced, 118
Sinus arrhythmia, digitalis-induced, 118
Sinus bradycardia, drugs causing, 118, 120, 121(t)
Sinus tachycardia, drugs causing, 120, 121(t)
Skeletal muscle relaxants, adverse reactions caused by, 239
Skin. See also *Cutaneous, Dermatologic*.
Skin discoloration, drugs causing, 94
Skin pigmentation. See *Hyperpigmentation*.
Skin tests, for drug allergy, types of, 75–76
SLE. See *Lupus erythematosus, systemic*.
Slow-reacting substances, role of in allergic anaphylaxis, 68
Smoking, pregnant mothers, effect on fetus, 168
Sodium, as cause of congestive heart failure, 117
Sodium bromide, adverse reactions caused by, 247
Somogyi effect, drug-induced, 151–152
Spectinomycin (Trobicin), adverse reactions caused by, 233

Spermatogenesis, suppression of, drugs causing, 157
Spinal cord lesions, as related to drug-induced disease syndromes, 192
  drugs causing, 192
Spironolactone (Aldactone), adverse reactions caused by, 248
  gynecomastia, 156
  hyperkalemia, 172
Spleen, localization of drug in, and immunologic response, 64
SRSA. See *Slow-reacting substances.*
Steatorrhea, drugs causing, 129, 130
Steroids, anabolic, as cause of acne, 86(t)
  as cause of cholestatic jaundice, 132, 133
  as cause of hepatocellular carcinoma, 141
  as cause of hirsutism, 95
  as cause of peliosis hepatis, 141
  as cause of vitilizing effects, 157
  androgenic, as cause of hepatocellular carcinoma, 141
  as cause of masculinization of female fetus, 168
Stevens-Johnson syndrome. See also *Erythema multiforme.*
  drug-induced, symptoms of, 82–83, 83
  drugs causing, 82–83, 84(t)
Stibophen (Fuadin), as cause of immune hemolysis, 103
Stimulants, cerebral, adverse reactions caused by, 246
Streptomycin (Neomycin), adverse effects caused by interactions with other drugs, 262
  as cause of fetal deafness, 213
  as cause of fetal hearing loss, 167
  as cause of optic neuritis, 211
  as cause of serum sickness, 201(t)
  as cause of vestibular damage, 213
Streptomycin sulfate, adverse reactions caused by, 233
Stroke, drugs causing, 191
Succinylcholine, as cause of apnea, 147
Sulfhemoglobinemia, drugs causing, 106
Sulfides, as cause of sulfhemoglobinemia, 106
Sulfisoxazole (Gantrisin), as cause of pseudo Pelger-Huët anomaly, 109
Sulfonamides, adverse reactions caused by, 234
  agranulocytosis, 108(t)
  cholestatic jaundice, 135
  drug-resistant organisms in bacterial infection, 204
  erythema multiforme, 83
  exfoliative dermatitis, 82(t)
  fixed drug eruptions, 88(t)
  hemolysis in glucose 6-phosphate dehydrogenase deficiency, 101(t)
    in glutathione-peroxidase deficiency, 102

Sulfonamides *(Continued)*
  adverse reactions caused by, hepatocellular jaundice, 137
  immune hemolysis, 104
  kernicterus, 140, 169
  myocardial damage, 116
  photodermatitis, 90(t)
  renal impairment, 159
  serum sickness, 201
  toxic epidermal necrolysis, 85(t)
  urticaria, 92(t)
  vasculitis, 200
  toxic effects of, 6, 7
Sulfones, as cause of hemolysis in glucose 6-phosphate dehydrogenase deficiency, 101(t)
  as cause of regional hyperpigmentation, 93
Sulfonylureas, as cause of hypoglycemia, 153
  as cause of photodermatitis, 90(t)
Sulfoxone, as cause of hemolysis in glutathione reductase deficiency, 102
Sympatholytics, adverse reactions caused by, 238–239
Sympathomimetics, adverse reactions caused by, 238
Sympathomimetic amines, as cause of hypertension, 122
Synthetic substitutes, adverse reactions caused by, 249
Systemic lupus erythematosus, drug-induced, 84
Systolic bruits, as effect of oral contraceptives, 122

Tachycardia, atrial, drugs causing, 119, 120, 121(t)
  bidirectional, as caused by digitalis intoxication, 119
  junctional, as caused by digitalis intoxication, 119
  nodal, digitalis-induced, 119
  sinus, drugs causing, 120, 121(t)
  ventricular, drugs causing, 118, 119, 121(t)
Teeth, discoloration of, in children as caused by tetracyclines, 126, 169
Teratogenic effects, drug-induced, 24, 28–30, 166–170
Test(s), liver function, drugs affecting, 138–139
  patch, for drug allergy, 75
  serologic, for drug allergy, 77
  tissue sensitization, for drug allergy, 77
Tetracaine hydrochloride (Pontocaine), adverse reactions caused by, 251
  keratitis, 207–208
Tetracyclines, adverse effects caused by interactions with other drugs, 262
  as cause of azotemia, 160

Tetracyclines *(Continued)*
    as cause of drug-resistant organisms in bacterial infection, 204
    as cause of enamel hypoplasia in children, 126, 169
    as cause of fetal abnormalities, 167
    as cause of hepatic damage, 134
    as cause of hypotension in treatment of louse-borne relapsing fever, 124, 125(t)
    as cause of nail discoloration, 96
    as cause of pseudotumor cerebri, 192
    as cause of renal tubular acidosis, 162
    as cause of retarded fetal bone growth, 182
    as cause of swollen or hairy tongue, 126
Tetracycline hydrochloride, adverse reactions caused by, 233
    in interactions with other drugs, 262
Thalidomide, adverse effects of, 6, 28
    congenital ocular malformations, 212
    multiple congenital anomalies, 166
Thallium, as cause of alopecia, 94
Thiabendazole (Mintezol), adverse reactions caused by, 229
    myalgias, 182
Thiazides, as cause of hypotension, 123, 125(t)
    as cause of photodermatitis, 90(t)
Thiazide diuretics, diabetogenic effect of, 151
    as cause of hypercalcemia, 177
    as cause of hyperuricemia, 177, 178
Thioguanine, adverse reactions caused by, 236
Thiopental (Pentothal), as cause of acute intermittent porphyria, 180
Thioridazine (Mellaril), adverse reactions caused by, 246. See also *Chlorpromazine*.
Thiothixene (Navane), adverse reactions caused by, 246
Thioxanthenes, as cause of extrapyramidal syndromes, 187
    as cause of parkinsonism, 187
Thorium dioxide (Thorotrast), as cause of cirrhosis, 140
    as cause of leukemias, 113, 114
    as cause of malignant liver tumors, 141
    as cause of renal tumors, 163
    as cause of spinal cord lesions, 192
Thrombocytopenia, as an allergic drug reaction, 69
    dose-related, drugs causing, 111
    immunologic, drugs causing, 109, 110(t), 111
Thrombophlebitis, as effect of oral contraceptives, 125
Thrombosis, deep vein, as effect of oral contraceptives, 125
Thyroid, adverse reactions caused by, 154, 250

Thyroid disorders, drugs causing, 154–155
Thyroid function studies, drugs affecting, 154
Tinnitus, drug-induced, drugs causing, 213
Tissue, antigenicity of, as affected by drug distribution, 62
    lymphoid, interaction with drug, effect on immunologic response, 63
    sensitization tests, for drug allergy, 77
Tolbutamide (Orinase), adverse reactions caused by, 250
    in interactions with other drugs, 268
Tongue, hairy or swollen, drugs causing, 126
Toxic agents, and chelation by drugs, 45
Toxic epidermal necrolysis. See also *Lyell's syndrome*.
    drug-induced, symptoms of, 83, 85
    drugs causing, 84, 85(t)
Toxicity. See also *Intoxication*.
    of chloramphenicol in newborn infants, 124–125
    of digitalis glycosides, and cardiac effects, 117–120
Toxicity level, and drug dose, 27
Tranquilizers, adverse reactions caused by, 245–246
    central nervous system depression, 190
    depression, 195
Transaminase levels, changes in, drugs causing, 138
Tranylcypromine sulfate (Parnate), adverse reactions caused by, 245
    in interactions with other drugs, 267
Triacetoxyanthracene, as cause of keratitis, 208
Triamcinolone (Aristocort, Kenalog), adverse reactions caused by, 249. See also *Prednisone*.
    myopathy, 181
Triamterene (Dyrenium), adverse reactions caused by, 248
    hyperkalemia, 172
    megaloblastic anemia, 104
Trichomonacides, adverse reactions caused by, 234
Trifluoperazine (Stelazine), adverse reactions caused by, 246. See also *Chlorpromazine*.
Trihexyphenidyl hydrochloride (Artane), adverse reactions caused by, 238
Trimeprazine tartrate (Temaril), adverse reactions caused by, 229
Trimethadione (Tridione), adverse reactions caused by, 245
    aplastic anemia, 98
    nephrotic syndrome, 162
Trimethobenzamide hydrochloride (Tigan), adverse reactions caused by, 248

Triparanol, as cause of alopecia, 95
  as cause of loss of hair color, 96
Tripelennamine citrate (Pyribenzamine), adverse reactions caused by, 229
  of anaphylaxis, 203
Triprolidine hydrochloride (Actidil), adverse reactions caused by, 229
Tuberculosis, corticosteroids as predisposing factor in, 205
d-Tubocurarine, as cause of myasthenia gravis, 186
Tumors. See also *Carcinoma*.
  liver, drugs causing, 141
  lung, drugs causing, 148
  renal, drugs causing, 163–164
Tyramine, interaction with monamine oxidase inhibitors, as cause of hypertensive crisis, 123, 123(t)

Ulcer, peptic, drugs causing, 127–128
Uric acid, serum levels, changes in, drugs causing, 177, 178
Urinary germicides, adverse reactions caused by, 235
Urinary tract effects, types of, drugs causing, 158–163
Urine pH, and drug excretion, 51–52
Urticaria, as an allergic drug reaction, 69
  drug-induced, characteristics of, *91*
  drugs causing, 90–91, 92(t)
USP (United States Pharmacopeia), 4, 8, 9

Vagal effects, of digitalis intoxication, 118
Vaginal adenocarcinoma, as caused by diethylstilbestrol, 165, 170
Vaginitis, Candida, drugs causing, 164
Vancomycin, as cause of drug-resistant organisms in bacterial infection, 204
Vasculitis, drugs causing, 200, 200(t), 201
  renal, necrotizing, drugs causing, 161
Vasodilators, adverse reactions caused by, 242
Vasopressin (Pitressin), as cause of inappropriate antidiuretic hormone secretion syndrome, 150
  as cause of myocardial infarction, 115
Vestibular damage, drugs causing, 213
Ventricular contractions, premature, drugs causing, 120, 121(t)
Ventricular fibrillation, drugs causing, 118, 119, 121(t)
Ventricular tachycardia, drugs causing, 118, 119, 121(t)
Vinblastine sulfate (Velban), adverse reactions caused by, 237
  peripheral neuropathies, 185

Vincristine sulfate (Oncovin), adverse reactions caused by, 237
  peripheral neuropathies, 185
Viomycin (Viocin), as cause of deafness, 213–214
Viral hepatitis, as related to drug-induced hepatocellular jaundice, 135
Viral infections, drugs causing, 206
Virilizing effects, drugs causing, 157, 164
Vitamin A, adverse reactions caused by, 251
  hypervitaminosis A, 93
  pseudotumor cerebri, 192
Vitamin B_{12}, malabsorption of, drug-induced, 129
Vitamin D, adverse reactions caused by, 251
  hypercalcemia, 177
Vitamin K, derivates, as cause of hemolysis in glucose 6-phosphate dehydrogenase deficiency, 101(t)
  adverse reactions caused by, 251
  hepatocellular injury, 138
  fat-soluble, malabsorption of, drug-induced, 130
  synthetic, as cause of kernicterus in neonates, 169
Vitreous disorders, drug-induced, types of, 208
Vomiting, drug-induced, as related to hypovolemia, 176
  drugs causing, 127

Warfarin sodium (Coumadin), adverse reactions caused by, 239. See also *Bishydroxycoumarin*.
  in interactions with other drugs, 264, 265
Weight, as factor in drug dosage, 26, 27
Wenckebach phenomenon, digitalis-induced, 119, 120
Withdrawal, drug, as cause of seizures, 190
Withdrawal syndromes, drugs causing, 193
  in neonates, 169
Women, tetracycline-induced liver damage in, 134
World Health Organization, drug monitoring system of, 10

Zoxazolamine (Flexin), as cause of hepatocellular damage, 137–138
  as cause of renal impairment, 161

A separate index of Proprietary Drugs begins on p. 305.

INDEX OF PROPRIETARY DRUGS

(Page numbers in **boldface** type indicate pages on which the drug is listed in Table 5–1, Individual Drugs and Their Adverse Effects, and Table 6–1, Drug Interactions. See also generic drug names listed in the general Index.)

Aarane, 142, 143
Achromycin, 134
Actidil, **229**
Aldactone, 156, 172, 173, **248**
Aldinamide, 136, 137
Aldomet, 103, 122, 123, 124, 125, 136, 138, 156, 164, 176, 190, 198, 199, **242**
Alkeran, 95, 98, 103, 104
Altafur, 184, 185, 207
Amebarsone, 133
Amicar, 136, 159, 160
Aminorex, 146
Amytal, 104, 112, **247**
Anadrol, 133, 141, **264**
Analexin, 111, 112
Anavar, 133
Ancobon, **230**
Anectin, 147
Antabuse, 111, 112, 196, **251**
Antepar, 189, 190, 193, **229**
Antivert, 167
Anturane, **267**
Apresoline, 116, 124, 125, 184, 199, 201, **241**
Aralen, 167, 181, 210, **234**
Aramine, 89, 123
Aristocort, 181, **249**
Artane, 94, **238**
Atabrine, 87, 88, 94, 95, 96, 99, 100, 101, 131, 136, 138, **229**
Atarax, **246**
Atromid-S, 48, 95, 112, 150, 182, **241**, **264**

Aureomycin, 134, 202, 203
Aventyl, 123, 133, **245**
Axotyl, 211
Azulfidine, 101, 130

Bactrim, 159
Benadryl, 90, **229**
Benemid, 101, 136, 162, 178, 189, 190, 201, 202, **248**
Bicillin, 116
Blenoxane, 144
Bonine, 167
Bromsulphalein, 87, 92, 134, 202
Butazolidin, 48, 87, 98, 104, 108, 110, 112, 113, 116, 126, 127, 128, 129, 136, 140, 153, 154, 158, 159, 161, 176, 199, 200, 201, **244**, **264**, **268**
Butisol, **247**

Camoquin, 94
Carbasone, 136
Carbocaine, 168, 190, **251**
Catron, 211
Cedilanid, 110
Celestone, **249**
Celontin, 199, **245**
Chloromycetin, 87, 99, **264**, **268**
Chlor-Trimeton, 98, **229**

305

INDEX OF PROPRIETARY DRUGS

Cholografin, 136
Choloxin, **265**
Cleocin, **231**
Cogentin, **238**
Colace, **248**
Coly-Mycin, 147, 159, 160, 184, 185, 186, 189, 193, 207, **231**
Compazine, 90, 108, 133, 187, 196, 207, 210, **246**
Coumadin, 139, **239, 264, 265**
Cuemid, **265**
Cyclospasmol, **242**
Cytomel, **250**
Cytosar, **235**
Cytoxan, 95, 98, 111, 136, 143, 150, 152, 156, 157, 159, 161, 163, 164, 166, 172, **235, 263**
Cytran, 133

Dalmane, **247**
Danilone, 89, 108, 133, 136, 159, 162
Daraprim, 99, 104
Darbid, **238**
Darvon, 92, 146, 193, **244**
DBI, 175, **250**
Decadron, 181, **249**
Decholin, 202
Declomycin, 85, 90, 96, 151, 163, 202, 203, **231**
Demerol, 110, **243**
Desoxyn, **246**
Dexedrine, **246**
Diabinese, 84, 90, 98, 105, 108, 110, 133, 134, 143, 150, 153, 154, 172, 179, 180, 201, **249, 268**
Diamox, 91, 98, 108, 110, 140, 159, 161, 163, 175, **247, 266**
Dianabol, 133, 141, **249, 263**
Diatrin, 108
Dibenzyline, 124, 125
Dicumarol, 139, **239, 263, 265, 268**
Dilantin, 48, 84, 87, 88, 95, 98, 104, 105, 108, 110, 111, 112, 113, 120, 124, 125, 126, 129, 136, 137, 140, 149, 152, 166, 179, 180, 198, 199, 200, 201, 207, **244, 264, 267**
Dilaudid, **243**
Dimetane, 85, 154, **229**
Dindevan, 89, 108, 133, 136, 154, 159, 160, 162
Diuril, 87, 90, 98, 130, 133, 200, 201, **247**
Dolophine, **243**
Dopar, 103, 123, 127, 139, 188
Doriden, 112, 189, 190, 193, **265**
Dulcolax, **248**
Dymelor, 133, 136, 139, 153, **268**
Dyrenium, 104, 172, 173, **248**

Edecrin, 108, 117, 124, 125, 128, 140, 151, 152, 171, 178, 213, 214, **247, 262, 264, 268**
Elavil, 50, 123, 124, 125, 126, 133, 156, 164, 185, 188, 189, 190, 194, **245, 266**
Entero-Vioform, 86, 136
Erythrocin, 134
Esidrix, **248**
Euglycin, 133, 136, 138, 139
Eutonyl, 123, **242, 267**

Fedrazil, 167
Flagyl, 108, 196, **234**
Flexin, 136, 137, 159, 161
Florinef, 173
Fluothane, 135, 136, 139
Fuadin, 103, 110, 136
Fulvicin, **230**
Fungizone, 98, **230**
Furacin, 87, 101, 184, 185
Furadantin, 101, 105, 133, 143, 144, 184, 185, 202, 203, **235**
Furoxone, 101, 123, 213, 214

Gantrisin, 90, 98, 101, 109
Garamycin, 147, 159, **232, 262**
Geopen, **231**

Haldol, 86, 89, 90, 96, 112, 124, 156, 164, 187, **246**
Halotestin, 133, **249**
Hedulin, 89, 108, 133, 136, 159, 160
Humatin, 159, 160
Hydrodiuril, 90, 123, 143, 144, **248**
Hydromox, 138
Hygroton, 108, 130, 151, 152, 178, **247**
Hyperstat, **264**

Ilidar, **238**
Ilosone, 133, 134
Imferon, 198, 201, 202, **239**
Imuran, 111, 114, 128, 130, 136, 138, 166, 195, 205, **235, 263**
Inderal, 117, 120, 124, 125, 142, 143, 153, 196, **241, 266**
Indocin, 48, 98, 112, 127, 128, 133, 136, 142, **243, 264, 267**
INH, **233, 267**
Intal, 142, 143
Ismelin, 118, 120, 122, 124, 125, 127, **241, 266**

INDEX OF PROPRIETARY DRUGS 307

Isordil, **242**
Isuprel, 120, 127, 142, 143, 194, **238**

Kantrex, 147, 159, 185, 186, 213, **232, 262**
Keflex, **231**
Keflin, 103, 139, 159, 160, 198, 202, 204
Kenacort, 181
Kenalog, **249**
Kynex, 84, 98

Larodopa, 103, 123, 127, 139, 188, **251, 268**
Lasix, 117, 124, 125, 140, 151, 152, 171, 178, 213, 214, **248, 268**
Leukeran, 136, 139, 140, 166, **235**
Levophed, 89, 123, **238**
Levoprome, 199
Librium, 90, 98, 108, 133, 136, 138, 156, 164, 179, 193, 195, **245**
Lincocin, 46, **232, 262**
Loridine, 103, 159, 160, 198, 202
Luminal, **247**

Marezine, 167
Marplan, 123, 136
Marsilid, 135, 136, 137, 139
Matulane, 157, **236**
Maxibolin, 133
Medicel, 84
Medrol, **249**
Mellaril, 108, 121, 133, 156, 210, **246**
Meloxine, 136
Meltrol, 175
Mesantoin, 88, 98, 113, 136, 199
Mestinon, 186
Metandren, 132, 133, 141, **249**
Milontin, 113
Minocin, **232**
Mintezol, 182, **229**
Mithracin, 136, 139, 159, 161, 177
Moderil, **242**
Mucomyst, 142, 143
Myambutol, 211, **233**
Mycostatin, **230**
Myleran, 143, 155, 156, 164, 166
Myochrysine, **248**
Mysoline, 98, 104, 105, 113, 129, 199, **245**

Nalline, 191, **244**
Naqua, 95
Narcan, 191, **244**
Nardil, 49, 123, 136

Navane, 187, **246**
NegGram, 101, 192, 212, **235**
Nembutal, 130, **247**
Neo-mercazole, 99
Neomycin, **262**
Neo-Synephrine, 209
Neutrapen, 202
Niacin, 133
Niamid, 123, 136
Nilevar, 133, 153, **264**
Nitroglycerin, **242**
Noctec, **247**
Noludar, **247**
Norpramin, 123, 133, **266**
Novocain, 202, **251**
Nupercaine, **250**

Oncovin, 95, 98, 111, 127, 130, 150, 157, 172, 185, **236**
Orabilex, 136, 159, 160
Orinase, 85, 90, 98, 105, 108, 110, 128, 133, 134, 153, 154, 162, 179, 180, **250, 268**
Ornade, 122

Pacatal, 133
Paradione, 88, 162
Paraflex, **239**
Parnate, 50, 123, 137, **245, 267**
Peganone, 113, 136
Penthrane, 135, 136, 137, 159, 160, **263**
Pentothal, 179
Percorten, 173
Permitil, 133
Persantin, **242**
Pertofrane, 108, 123
Phenacetin, **243**
Phenergan, 87, 90, 108, 133, **229**
Phenobarbital, 104
Phenurone, 136, 137
Pitocin, 115, **251**
Pitressin, 115, 122
Placidyl, 112, 189, 190, 193, **247**
Plaquenil, 108
Plasmochin, 108
Polycillin, 138
Ponstel, 103, 128, 142
Pontocaine, **251**
Potaba, 138
Povan, **229**
Preludin, 167
Presidon, 108
Pro-Banthine, 118, **238, 266**
Prolixin, 133, **246**
Pronestyl, **240**
Propadrine, **238**

INDEX OF PROPRIETARY DRUGS

Prostaphlin, 133, 138, 159, 160
Prostigmin, 186, **237**
Purinethol, **263**
Pyralgin, **243**
Pyribenzamine, 98, 108, 201, 202, 203, **229**
Pyridium, **235**

Quaalude, **247**
Questran, 112, 129, 130, 132, **265**

Regitine, 116, 122, 123, 124, 125, **242**
Rela, 88
Releasin, 202
Renografin, 60, 160
Ritalin, 120, 123, **246**
Robaxin, **239**
Robinul, **238**
Rondec, 90
Roniacol, **242**

Sandril, **242**
Sansert, 115, 144, 162, 182, **238**
Seconal, 104, 112, **247**
Sedormid, 109, 110
Septra, 159
Serpasil, **242**
Sinequan, 123, **245**
Soma, 88, **239**
Sparine, 90, 98, 108, 133, 148, 199
Spontin, 98
Staphcillin, 159, 160, 202, **232**
Stelazine, 133, 156, 164, **246**
Stilbestrol, **249**
Stoxil, 208
Sucostrin, 147
Synkayvite, 101
Synthroid, **250**

Talwin, 122, 146, 193, **244**
Tandearil, 48, 98, 100, 108, 110, 112, 126, 128, 136, 140, 153, 176, **264**
Tapazole, 99, 108, 116, 133, 136, 167, **250**

Taractan, 156, 164, 187, 189
Tegopen, **231**
Tegretol, 84, 99, 110, 133, 136, 150, 196, **265**
Teldrin, **229**
Telepaque, 136
Temaril, 90, 133, **229**
Thorazine, 87, 90, 93, 95, 96, 98, 103, 104, 107, 108, 124, 132, 133, 139, 154, 186, 191, 199, 200, 208, 210, **245**
Thorotrast, 99, 139, 140, 141, 163, 192, 205
Tibione, 108
Tigan, 136, **248**
Tofranil, 108, 123, 124, 125, 133, 143, 154, 156, 164, 185, 188, 189, 191, 198, **245, 266**
Tolinase, 153
Trecator SC, 95, 136, 137
Tridione, 84, 87, 88, 95, 98, 100, 108, 136, 162, 166, 186, 199, **245**
Trilafon, 133, 154, 199, **246**
Trobicin, **233**
Tylenol, **243**

Ultran, 156
Unipen, 139, 205
Urecholine, **237**

Valium, 148, 168, 195, 196, **246**
Vancocin, 185
Vasodilan, **242**
Velban, 95, 98, 127, 185, **237**
Vesprin, 98
Vibramycin, **231**
Viocin, 201, 213
Vioform, 86
Vistaril, **246**
Vivactl, 123

Xylocaine, 120, 148, 189, 190, **240**

Zarontin, 108, 199, **245**
Zyloprim, 136, 140, 161, 163, 178, 198, **248, 263**